Current Topics in Caesarean Section

Edited by Panagiotis Tsikouras,
Nikolaos Nikolettos, Werner Rath
and Georg Friedrich Von Tempelhoff

Published in London, United Kingdom

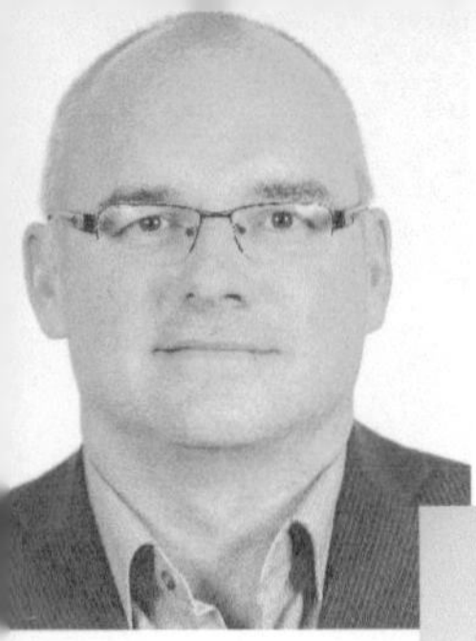
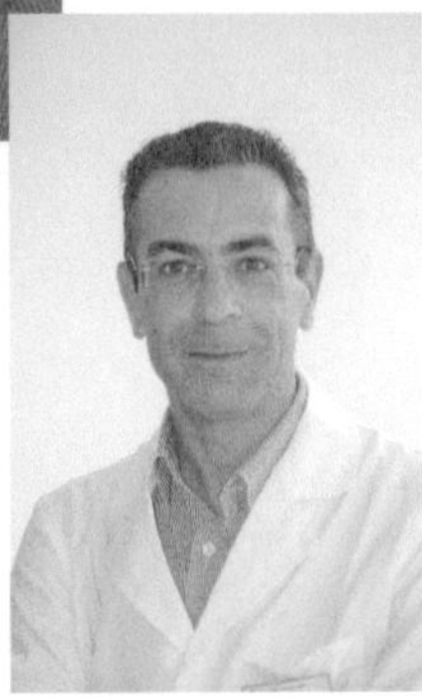
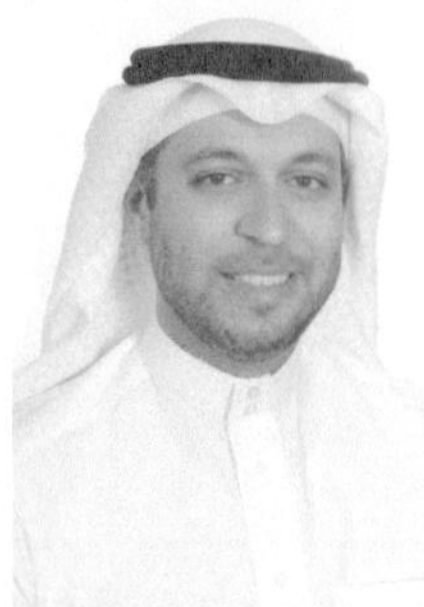
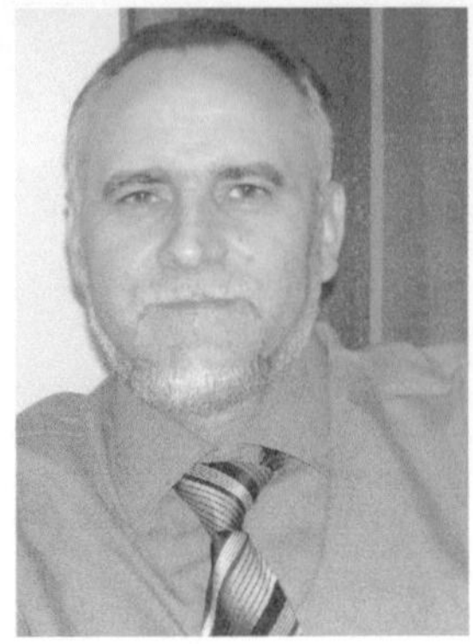
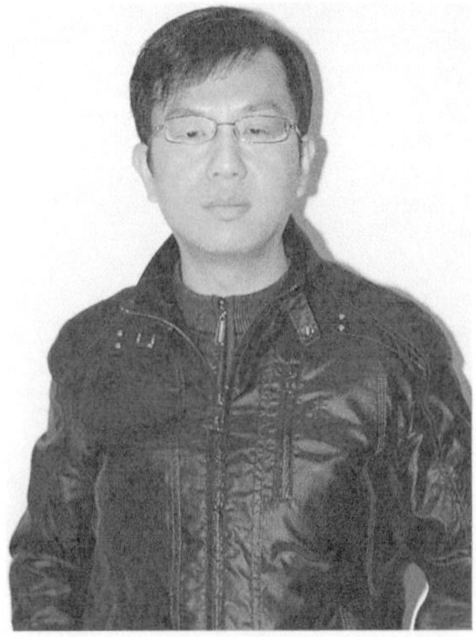
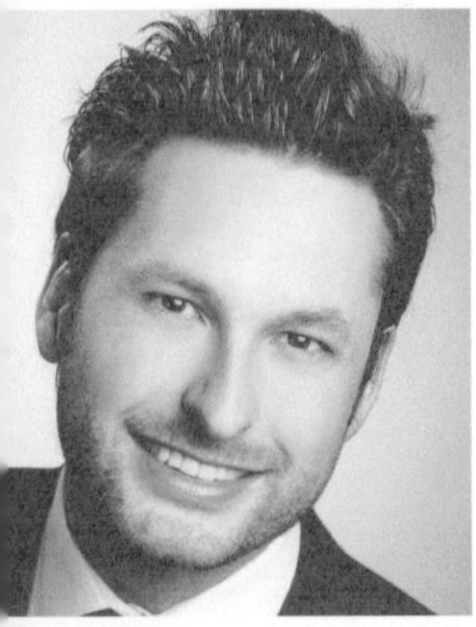
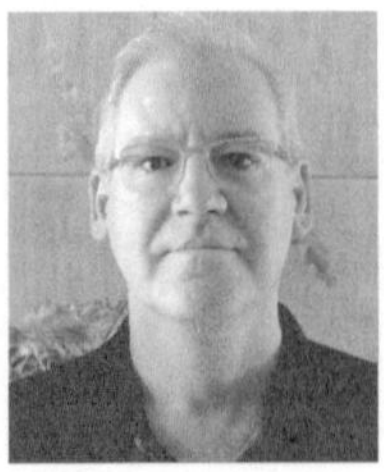

IntechOpen

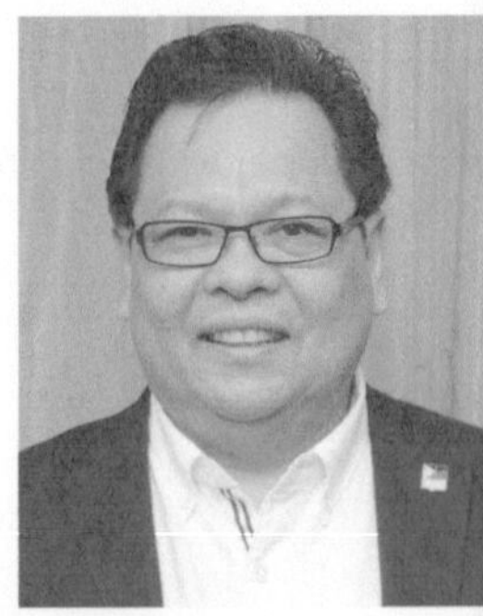
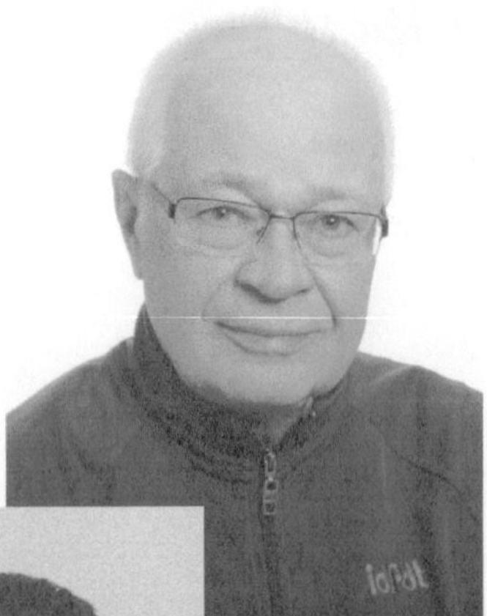
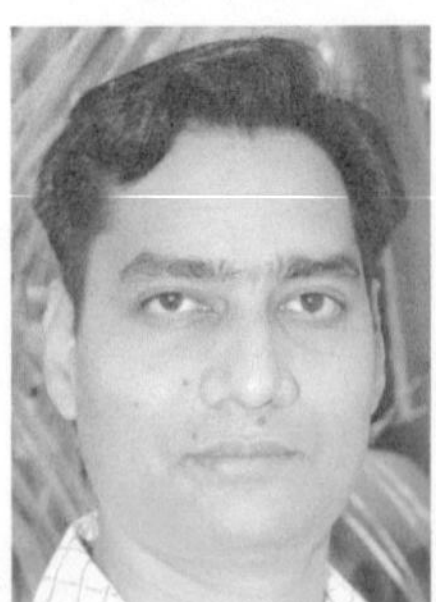
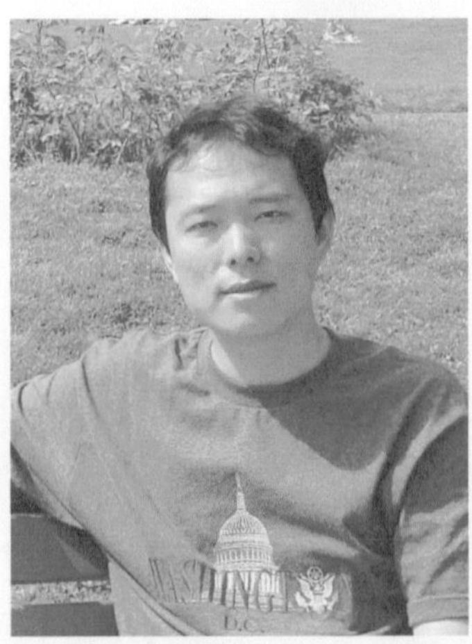
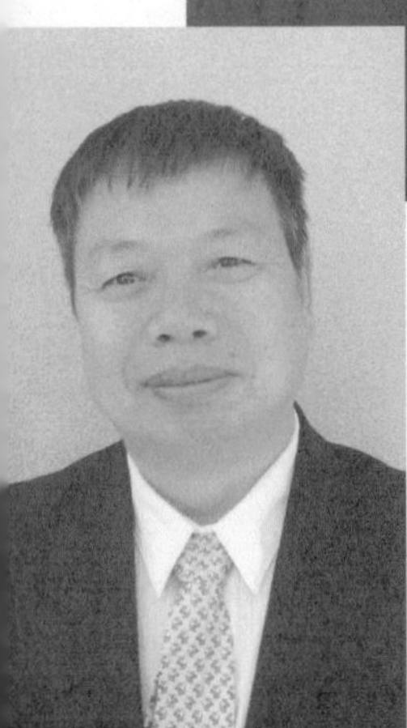
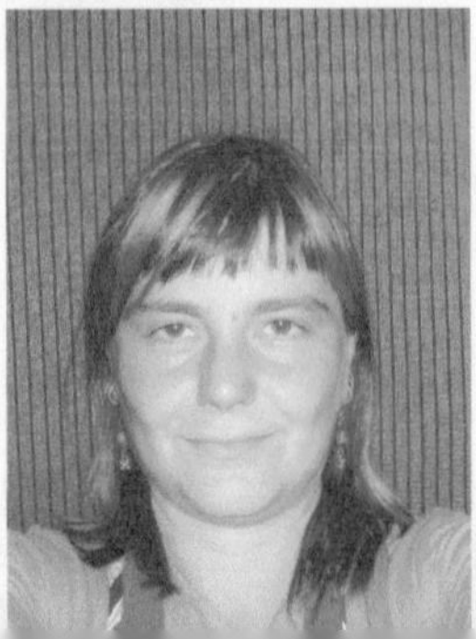

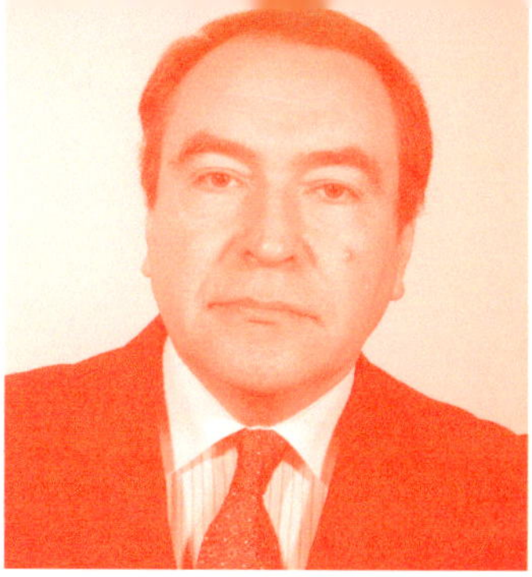
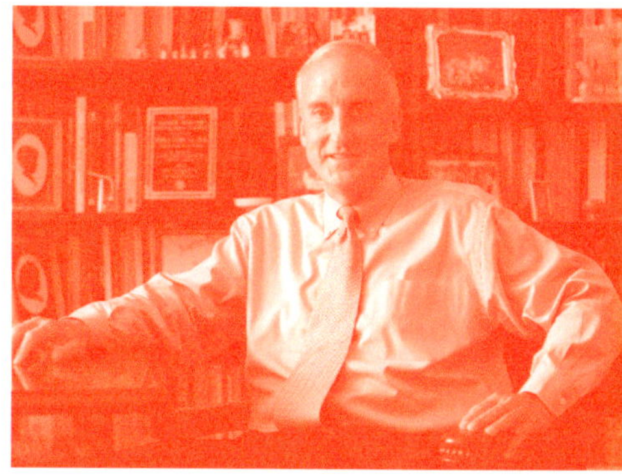
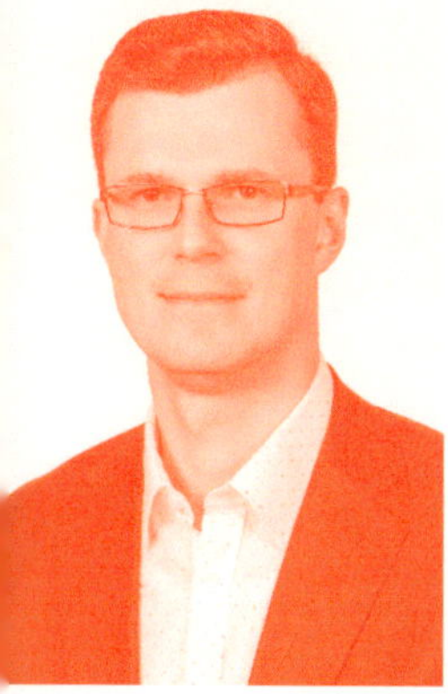
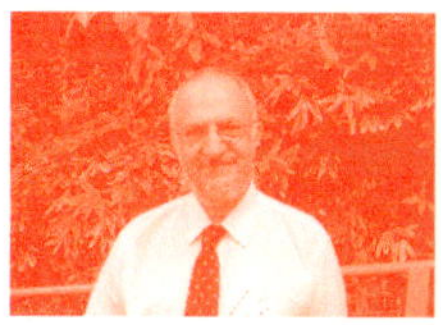
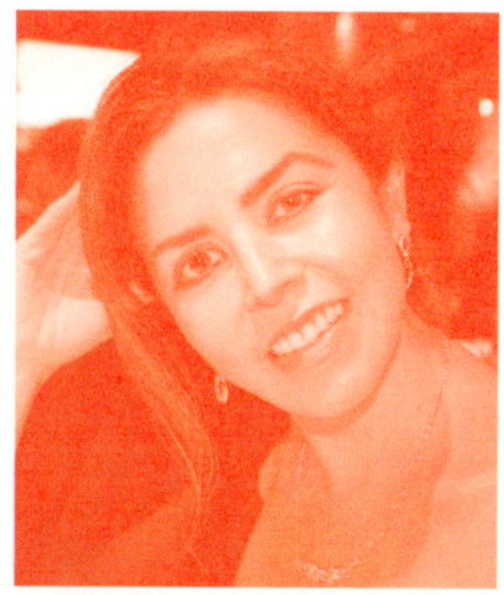

Supporting open minds since 2005

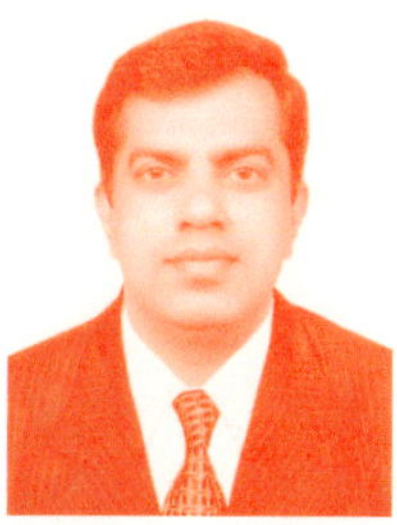
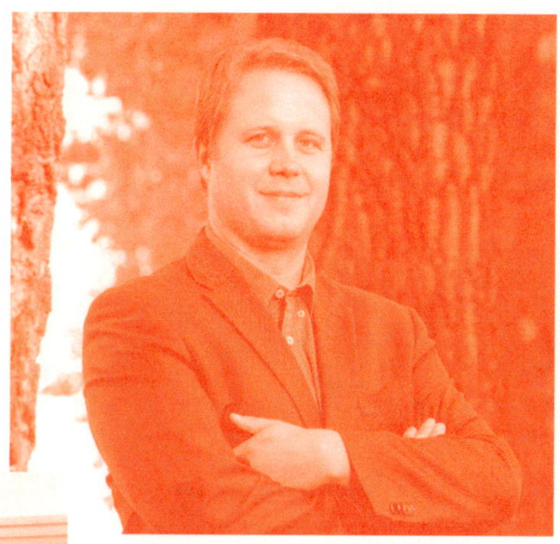
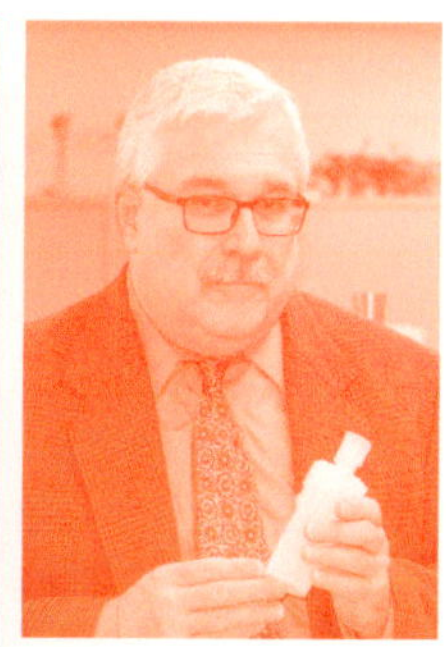
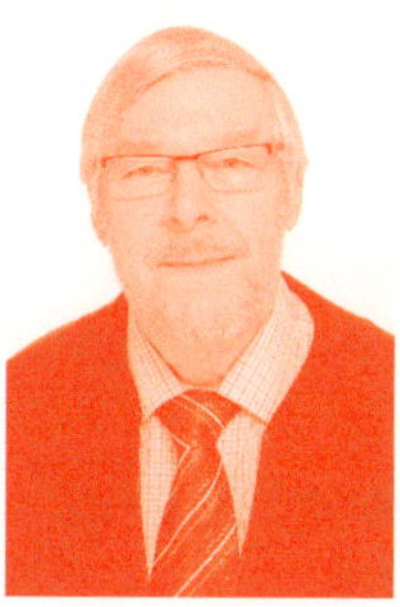
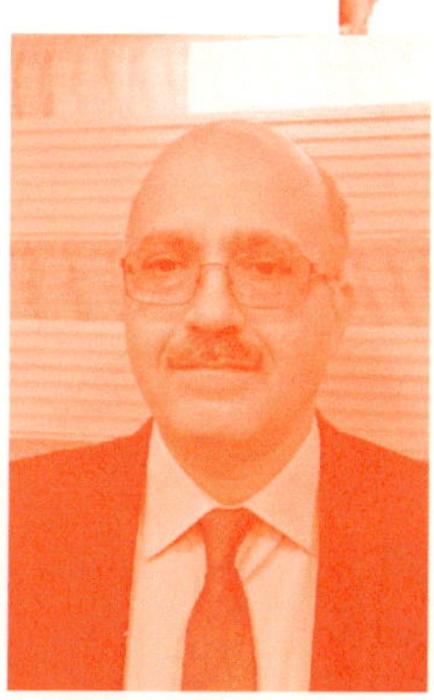
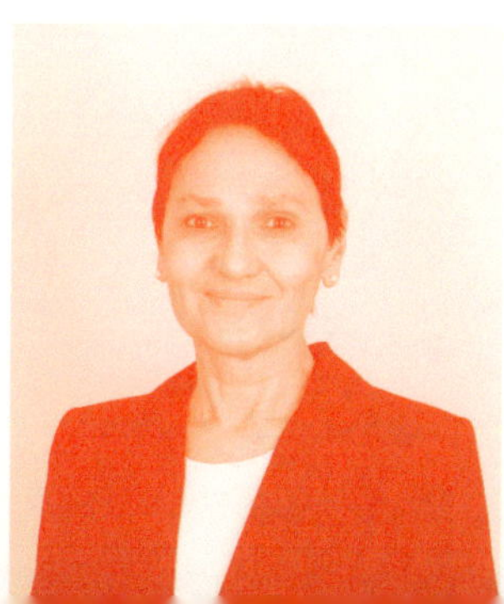
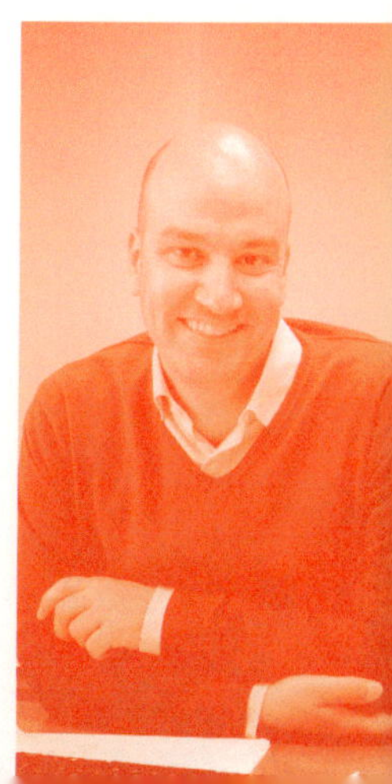

Current Topics in Caesarean Section
http://dx.doi.org/10.5772/intechopen.92475
Edited by Panagiotis Tsikouras, Nikolaos Nikolettos, Werner Rath and Georg Friedrich Von Tempelhoff

Contributors
Melinda Matyas, Mariusz Dubiel, Szymon Bednarek, Małgorzata Głogiewicz, Rafał Adamczak, Jigna Shah, Bhavya Baxi, Anet Papazovska Cherepnalkovski, Vesna Pavlov, Ivanka Furlan, Marija Bucat, Pontius Bayo, Juliet Ajok, Teodoro Durá-Travé, Isabel San Martín-García, Fidel Gallinas-Victoriano, María Malumbres-Chacón, Paula Moreno-González, María Urretavizcaya-Martinez, Panagiotis Tsikouras, Anna Chalkidou, Anastasia Bothou, Angeliki Gerede, Xanthoula Anthoulaki, Spyridon Michalopoulos, Efthimios Demmosthenous, Ioannis Tsirkas, Fotini Gaitatzi, Eirini Bampageorgaka, Apostolos Lazarou, Natalia Sachnova, Michael Koutsogiannis, Konstantinos Nikolettos, Theopi Nalbanti, Panagiotis Petsidis, Stefanos Zervoudis, Georgios Iatrakis, Werner Rath, Georgios Galazios, Nikolaos Nikolettos, Georgios Dragoutsos, Ifigenia Apostolou, Alexios Alexiou, Tshililo Mashamba, Awoke Giletew Wondie, Jayaraman Nambiar, Thiencherry Rema, Angeliki Antonakou, Dimitrios Papoutsis, Frederico José Amédeé Péret, Liv Braga De Paula, Padmasri Ramalingappa, Raksha Shivaramegowda, Shruthi Holavanahalli SrinivasaMurthy, Jaqueline Ferreira, Angela Köninger, Annegret Schnabel, Christian Litzka, Maria Emilia Solano

First published in London, United Kingdom, 2021 by IntechOpen
IntechOpen is the global imprint of INTECHOPEN LIMITED, registered in England and Wales, registration number: 11086078, 5 Princes Gate Court, London, SW7 2QJ, United Kingdom
Printed in Croatia

British Library Cataloguing-in-Publication Data
A catalogue record for this book is available from the British Library

Additional hard and PDF copies can be obtained from orders@intechopen.com

Current Topics in Caesarean Section
Edited by Panagiotis Tsikouras, Nikolaos Nikolettos, Werner Rath and Georg Friedrich Von Tempelhoff
p. cm.
Print ISBN 978-1-83969-178-2
Online ISBN 978-1-83969-179-9
eBook (PDF) ISBN 978-1-83969-180-5

For EU product safety concerns:
IN TECH d.o.o., Prolaz Marije Krucifikse Kozulić 3, 51000 Rijeka, Croatia, info@intechopen.com or visit our website at intechopen.com.

Meet the editors

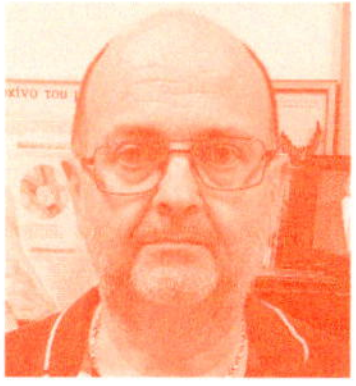

Dr. Panagiotis Tsikouras is a specialist in obstetrics-gynecology, perinatal medicine, and contraception at the School of Medicine, Democritus University of Thrace, Greece. He is also the headmaster of the Family Planning Centre and Gynecological Cytology Laboratory at the same university. Dr. Tsikouras is a fellow of the International Academy of Clinical and Applied Thrombosis/Hemostasis. His scientific activities focus on paediatric and adolescence medicine, gynecological oncology, high-risk pregnancies. He is a reviewer for several international journals and has numerous scientific publications to his credit, including papers and book chapters. He has also contributed to international and national guidelines on coagulation and thrombosis in obstetrics-gynecology.

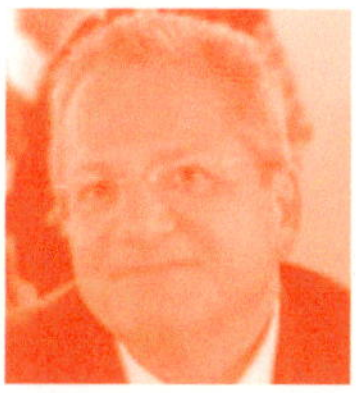

Dr. Nikos Nikolettos is a specialist in obstetrics, gynecology and assisted reproduction at the Democritus University of Thrace, Greece. He is trained in gynecological endocrinology, human reproduction, and in vitro fertilization. From 2007 to 2011, Dr. Nikos served as director of the In Vitro Fertilization Unit, University Regional General Hospital of Alexandroupolis, Greece. From 2012 to 2018, he was director of the Laboratory of Reproductive Physiology - Artificial Fertilization. In 2018 he became Professor of Assisted Reproduction at the Democritus University of Thrace, Greece. In 2019 he took over the management of the University Obstetrics-Gynecology Clinic, Medical Department, Democritus University of Thrace. His scientific work includes more than 100 publications in international journals and many lectures by invitation to international and Greek conferences.

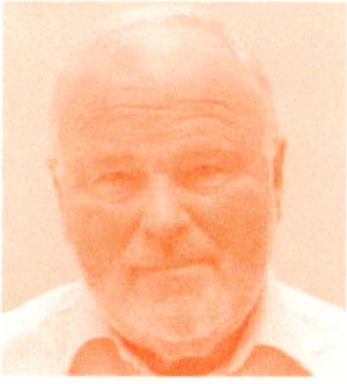

Dr. Werner Rath is a specialist in obstetrics and gynecology, gynecologic oncology, perinatal medicine, and hemostaseology. He is currently a professor in the Gynecology and Obstetrics Faculty of Medicine, University of Kiel, Germany, and honorary doctor at the Democritus University of Thrace, Alexandroupoli University Hospital He previously served as chief of the *Department of Gynecology and Obstetrics at University Hospital RWTH Aachen, Germany*. Dr. Rath is a reviewer for numerous journals and chief editor of *Geburtshilfe und Frauenheilkunde* (GebFra). He has several publications, including thirteen book chapters, to his credit.

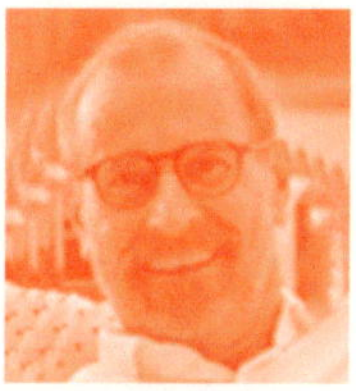

Dr. Georg Friedrich von Tempelhoff is a specialist in obstetrics and gynecology, gynecologic oncology, perinatal medicine, and hemostaseology. He is chief of the Department of Gynecology and Obstetrics, St. Vinzenz Hospital Hanau, Germany, and head of the Institute for Thrombosis and Coagulation Disorders in Gynecology and Obstetrics, Germany. He is a fellow of the International Academy of Clinical and Applied Thrombosis/Hemostasis. His scientific focus is hemostaseological and hemorheological disorders in women with miscarriages, preeclampsia, and thrombosis. Dr. von Tempelhoff is a reviewer for numerous journals and, in addition to his publications and book chapters, has also contributed to international and national guidelines on coagulation and thrombosis in gynecology.

Contents

Preface

It is estimated that 1.2 million caesarean sections are performed in the United States each year, accounting for 31.7% of all births. In most European countries, the rate of caesarean delivery also exceeds 30%. The medical effects of this phenomenon remain unclear.

Factors that contribute to the increased frequency of C-sections include improved technical performance combined with increased security, reduction of maternal mortality rates (estimated at 6–22 women per 100,000 operations), and an overall significant decline in the frequency of forceps delivery.

The increased frequency of primary caesarean incisions has led to an increased number of pregnant women with previous C-sections despite a moderate increase in the rate of vaginal delivery after caesarean delivery.

The estimated total percentage of caesarean deliveries in women older than 35 years is 35%, according to a study by the World Health Organization (WHO). The study certified an increase in the frequency of caesarean births in both primigravidae and multigravidae. Full-term pregnancies with a head presentation in women without previous C-section accounted for 60% of births, whereas pregnancies in women with previous C-section accounted for 11.4% of births. Primigravidae with a head presentation with spontaneous or induced labor accounted for 15.3% and 18.3% of births, respectively. The tendency to have a fewer number of children led to a greater percentage of primigravidae who are at increased risk for caesarean section. The widespread application of assisted reproduction methods has led to increased rates of twin (35%) and multiple (77%) pregnancies and thus an increase in the percentage of C-sections.

According to meta-analyses, the use of cardiotocographic monitoring of the fetoplacental unit led to a 20% increase in the frequency of cesarean sections. Two studies of low-risk pregnancies found that the frequency of C-sections doubled with continuous cardiotocographic monitoring. This is due to an overestimation of the records regarding the presence or absence of perinatal asphyxia.

Several blind studies have compared C-section rates after induction or waiting in prolonged pregnancies without fully documented findings and without significant differences. There are several studies that show that induction of labor is associated with a significant reduction in the frequency of C-sections compared to adherence to waiting. However, these studies focused mainly on pregnancies > 41 weeks or those that were high risk. Several researchers have investigated whether the adoption of a regular induction of labor between 37 and 38 + 6 weeks is associated with a reduction in the frequency of stillbirths, but results have been conflicting. However, there is a trend that supports the view that the induction of childbirth between 39 and 40 weeks of pregnancy helps to reduce the incidence of stillbirths.

Caesarean section is a surgical procedure that should be done only when clinically indicated, as it can lead to potential consequences such as infection, thrombosis, bleeding, emergency hysterectomy, persistent pelvic pain, infertility, and even death.

Active birth control is mainly used to reduce cesarean sections. However, epidural analgesia may increase the frequency of CS (13% vs. 8% in the United States).

The passage of the newborn through the mother's vagina, skin contact after childbirth, and breastfeeding give the newborn the opportunity to colonize with the beneficial germs of the mother. Their penetration into the digestive system of the newborn contributes to the creation of normal intestinal flora as well as the activation of the newborn's defense system with the possibility of maximum development. Microbes that a mother does not have are dangerous to the newborn. When a field of labor is sterile, such as in caesarean section, the newborn will be colonized by the first germs it comes into contact with, which are not those of the mother. From a microbiological point of view, the newborn needs to be in contact with a single person, the mother.

If a neonate is born by caesarean section, it is possible to alternate the "host" of the microbiome, which is of great importance in the transfer of beneficial bacteria from mother to neonate during birth, since the first microbiomes to be colonized are hospital germs, for which the newborn has no antibodies at all. This immune system dysfunction and changes in metabolism, scientists believe, are responsible for the development of diseases. Population studies have shown that infants born via C-section have a 20% increased risk of developing asthma, type 1 diabetes, obesity in adulthood, and a slightly lower risk of developing gastrointestinal disorders such as Crohn's disease or celiac disease (gluten intolerance). Consequently, the infant born via C-section does not develop an immune system like that of an infant delivered vaginally.

Literature confirms that vaginal delivery allows the newborn gastrointestinal tract to be colonized by maternal bacteria, whereas cesarean delivery results in the neonatal gastrointestinal tract being colonized by hospital bacteria. Given that the gastrointestinal tract is where immune cells mature, its invasion by foreign microbiomes has a decisive effect on the pancreas and the physiology and pathology of the infant's immune system.

Scheduled cesarean section is usually performed between 37 and 40 weeks, which is considered full-term, although research has shown that many newborns of this age are not yet mature and may have serious health problems. A study of 13,258 newborns from 12 hospitals (35.8% delivered at 39/40 weeks, 6.3% delivered at 37/40 weeks, and 38.4% delivered at 38/40 weeks) showed that newborns born between 37 and 38 + 6/40 weeks developed respiratory problems and hypoglycemia. They also exhibited low levels of catecholamines, on average five times less compared to newborns delivered vaginally. Most were admitted to the neonatal intensive care unit, so it is best to schedule a cesarean section for no earlier than 39 weeks when possible. It appears that C-section after completion of the 39th week of pregnancy is associated with a decrease in maternal and neonatal morbidity, at least in relation to certain parameters.

Although a caesarean section is considered safe, there are some risks, including increased maternal morbidity and mortality, blood loss, neonatal respiratory distress syndrome, neonatal injuries, joint dystocia, Joint dystocia sometimes occurs in association to C-section due to the position of the embryo and placental abnormalities. Thus, avoidance of C-section is safe, there are some risks, including increased maternal morbidity and mortality, blood loss, neonatal respiratory distress syndrome, neonatal injuries, joint dystocia, and placental abnormalities.

The role of the obstetrician-gynecologist is to responsibly and objectively inform the pregnant woman about any special conditions of the specific pregnancy and any relevant scientific guidelines. It is also important to inform the pregnant person of the possibility of caesarean section as well as associated risks and potential effects on future pregnancies and deliveries. Ultrasound plays an important role in the decision to avoid or perform a caesarean section in time for the benefit of the mother and fetus.

I would like to thank all the authors who contributed their work to this volume.

Dr. Panagiotis Tsikouras and Dr. Nikolaos Nikolettos
Democritus University of Thrace,
Komotini, Greece

Dr. Werner Rath
Kiel University,
Germany

Dr. Georg Friedrich Von Tempelhoff
St. Vinzenz Hospital Hanau,
Germany

Section 1

Caeasarean Section in General

Chapter 1

Second Stage Cesarean Section

Jayaraman Nambiar and Thiencherry Rema

Abstract

The incidence of second stage cesarean section is on the rise. Second stage cesarean section is associated more chances of maternal and fetal injury. Though various techniques are mentioned to deliver the fetal head in second stage cesarean section, the "pull" method is associated with lesser complications. It is important to train Obstetricians in second stage section as it needs extra skill to deliver a deeply engaged head. Judicious use of oxytocin and assisted vaginal deliveries may decrease the need for second stage cesarean section.

Keywords: Cesarean section, second stage, assisted delivery, vacuum, forceps, pull method

1. Introduction

Incidence of second stage cesarean section is increasing. Its technically difficult to deliver a head which is deeply impacted inside the pelvis. Its associated with maternal trauma and sometimes even fetal trauma. The purpose of this chapter is to analyze various methods that are used to deliver the head in second stage section. The chapter also deals with complications of second stage cesarean section and its management.

2. Complications associated with second stage cesarean section

Incidence of cesarean section is increasing throughout the world, so is the second stage cesarean section. There is a steady increase in the incidence of Cesarean Section. A 10-year study showed a rising incidence of Cesarean section at full dilatation, and currently, the incidence of second stage Cesarean section is around 2% [1]. Unexpected complications, like unsatisfactory progress or fetal distress, may occur in the second stage of labour. Second stage section is usually done for CPD or fetal distress. With fewer Obstetricians not using assisted vaginal deliveries, the incidence of the second stage is increasing. Management of delay in the second stage requires a lot of skill and judgment. To deliver a head which is deeply impacted in the pelvis is difficult. Opting for a vaginal delivery with assistance requires considerable skill and judgment. In general, fewer people attempt assisted vaginal deliveries now. More and more cases are taken for a section rather than difficult assisted deliveries. Within the national maternity hospital in Dublin in a center with more than 9000 deliveries per year, While the cesarean section incidence has increased from 18.3% to 23.5% from 2005 to 2014, there is a sharp decline in assisted vaginal deliveries from 14–11% [2]. In the year 2014, there were 8000-second stage cesarean section in the UK [3].

Second stage Cesarean sections are associated with more complications than first stage cesarean sections. Cesarean section done at full dilatation of cervix with head deeply engaged in the pelvis is a potential risk factor for maternal and fetal injury. Second stage cesarean section is associated with more genital trauma and perinatal morbidity. Second stage cesarean sections can be related to trauma, bleeding, peripartum Hysterectomy. Analysis of second stage complications ere studied by V M Allen et al. in a study in 2005. They looked at the difficulties associated with second stage sections over five years. A total of 549 cases of second stage sections. Incidence of intraoperative trauma was 6.4%, and two patients underwent peripartum Hysterectomy. 57(4.7%) of cases had early postpartum bleeding. 9(1.1%) subjects had postoperative febrile morbidity. The relative risk of maternal trauma is 2.6, and perinatal Asphyxia was 1.5 in the above study by V M Allen at al [4]. In a study by Murphy et al. Second stage sections were associated with more chances of bleeding. Out of 209 women who underwent section in the second stage, 20(10%) had bleeding more than 1000 mL. Almost 50 (24%) of cases had extension of the cesarean wound after the second stage section [5].

Newborn injuries are more common following assisted vaginal deliveries than sections. Incidence of newborn trauma was (22% of 184 deliveries in Cesarean section versus 9% of 209 assisted vaginal deliveries). Severe fetal injuries, like Brachial plexus trauma, was also more common following operative vaginal deliveries [4]. Operative trauma like intracranial hemorrhage is also more common following operative vaginal deliveries. The incidence of intracranial bleeding was 1 of 860 infants delivered by vacuum extraction, 1 of 664 delivered using forceps and 1 of 907 delivered by cesarean section during labour [6]. Hence avoiding a difficult assisted vaginal delivery will decrease the incidence of severe fetal trauma. However, neonatal complications like Asphyxia and intensive care admissions are more common in second stage sections. Reduced Apgar scores and lower umbilical artery pH was 11 per cent in women who underwent cesarean section at full dilatation versus 6% among women who underwent vaginal assisted delivery [4]. However, this may be due to prolonged labour and may not be directly related to delivery mode. There was no significant neurodevelopmental delay between babies delivered by assisted vaginal delivery and Cesarean section when followed up for five years. The overall incidence of neurodevelopmental delay was low [7].

Since the Cesarean section at full dilation is associated with increased maternal and neonatal morbidity every attempt should be made to reduce the second stage cesarean section. Judicious use of Oxytocin and monitoring of labour by partogram may reduce the incidence of second-stage cesarean section. A senior consultant obstetrician's presence can result in more vaginal deliveries and can reduce cesarean section at full dilatation [8]. Instrumental delivery is more likely to fail in occiput posterior position than anterior positions. Hence a careful vaginal examination and use of ultrasound should determine the position of the head before attempting an instrumental delivery [9].

3. Technique of delivering a deeply engaged head

Impaction of the fetal head occurs when the station of head is below the level of ischial spines, and then onwards the delivery of the head becomes difficult. A deeply engaged head is hard to deliver and can cause difficulty [10]. A careful vaginal examination should be done before Cesarean section to ascertain the findings.

The incision that preferred for second stage cesarean section is Joel-Cohen incision. This is an incision 3 cm above the public symphysis. It is associated with lesser operating time [11]. When performing cesarean section in the second stage, a higher incision is preferred on the Uterus. Blunt dissection of Uterus with fingers is associated with lesser blood loss than sharp dissection using scissors [12]. An incision lower in the Uterus may be associated with more chances of injury and extension of the uterine incision. Chances of bladder injury are more likely if the incision is lower. With a lower incision, sometimes inadvertent delivery through the vagina may also occur. Hence, it is always better to put an incision higher in the lower segment during the second stage sections. The fetal head is deeply impacted in the second stage of labour and delivering poses a challenge. The Uterus is a state of contraction, and Oxytocin infusion should be stopped before taking the patient for cesarean section. There is no evidence that Nitroglycerin relaxes the Uterus [13]. Moreover, the use of uterine relaxants may be associated with more chances of postpartum bleeding. There is no evidence that the use of tocolytics ease the delivery at second stage cesarean section [14]. Sometimes if constriction ring dystocia is suspected a low vertical incision may be used in the lower segment. A vertical lower segment incision has a risk of extension on to the bladder or upper uterine segment. It may be associated with higher chances of rupture in subsequent pregnancies. The only advantage of a vertical lower segment incision is that there are lesser chances of extension laterally into the broad ligament area.

Deepening the plane of aesthesia may help to disengage the fetal head. Upward pull of fetal shoulder may help to disengage the fetal head. The operating hand should be placed in a cup-shaped fashion and delivered to the fetal head. This conventional method of delivering the head as cephalic without assistance may result in the uterine wound's extension and is dangerous when the head is deeply engaged in the pelvis. Hence, it would be advisable to resort to one of the two commonly used "pull" or "push" method techniques. In the "push" method head is pushed from below. In the "pull" the baby is delivered as breech using a reverse breech extraction. A head low position may help the delivery of the deeply engaged head.

When the push method is used, the patient should be in semi lithotomy position. There is a risk of introducing infection into the uterine cavity, and all aseptic measures should be taken. Pressure should be uniform over the fetal head, and stress at any one point on the fetal head must be avoided. Flexion should be maintained while pushing the head up. Steady pressure applied by the operating surgeon abdominally on fetal shoulders may help ease fetal head delivery during the push method [15].

In the pull method baby is delivered as breech. One or both feet are caught and delivered. There is flexion of the thoracolumbar spine and head is lifted out of pelvis by a pull on the feet. This is called a "reversed breech extraction" of the baby. In the revere breech extraction by pull method, the risk of injury to surrounding structures was much less than the push method, especially in cases with cephalo pelvic disproportion [16].

Patwardhan's maneuver is a useful maneuver in the delivery of a deeply engaged head. If the back is anterior, one arm is delivered followed by other arm, and then the trunk is delivered. Finally, the legs are pulled out. If the back is posterior one arm followed by same side leg, other side leg and arm are delivered. In a study by Lal et al. in India, the Patwardhan's maneuver was associated with significantly fewer chances of injury and lesser need for blood transfusion [17].

The pull method has been shown to have better outcomes compared to the push method. In a study done in Nigeria, the pull method was associated with better results than the push method. The pull method was associated with lesser blood loss than the push method (1257 ml versus898 ml) and lesser uterine wound extension (33% versus 11%). Though the incidence of low Apgar scores was lesser in the pull method, there was no increase in neonatal morbidity or death between groups [18]. Levy et al. in a study compared both pull and push method. There were 48 cases of difficult extraction of the head. When the pull method used, the incidence of extension of uterine incision was 15% compared to 50% when pushing method as used. Also, the incidence of postpartum fever was only 5% in the pull method and was very high (46%) when the push method was used. Hence the pull method of delivering the head appears safer than the push method [19].

The fetal head can get deeply impacted in pelvis following attempted vaginal delivery, especially with vacuum application and delivery, may be extremely difficult. The use of the pull method here is associated with less trauma than the push method [20].

Many other techniques which are not validated have been described for delivering a deeply engaged head. Use of Whitmore position where the legs are abducted and hips flexed at 135 degrees has been tried in the second stage section [21]. Use of non-dominant hand to lift the presenting part and use of low patient bed are other techniques that may facilitate a deeply engaged head. However, these techniques are not validated scientifically and need more studies.

Fetal disimpacting system is a silicon device that is placed in vagina and filled with saline, elevating the fetal head. It can elevate the head by 3 cm. Initial reports are promising and may be of help in delivering a deeply impacted head [22]. In a study done in India by Subartha L Seal et al., the incision to delivery was much shorter when a fetal pillow was used (297.2 ± 27.1 seconds when fetal pillow as not used versus 176.5 ± 14.0 seconds when fetal pillow was used). Significant uterine extension occurred more frequently 39/120 when fetal pillow was not used, and it occurred only in 6/120 cases when fetal pillow was used. Fetal pillow may be a possible alternative to other methods that can be of help deliver the fetal head [23].

C-snorkel is a soft, malleable tube with holes and can be placed between the vagina and the fetal head. Aeration through the tube can help to disengage the fetal head. There are no adequate trials with this equipment [24].

There is a need for adequate training in second stage sections. Second stage sections often happen in odd hours, and help from senior faculty may not be available. There is an urgent need of training a junior faculty in training for second stage sections.

4. Managing complications associated with second stage sections

Second stage sections may be associated with many complications. Extension of uterine incision and bleeding is one of the most typical difficulties in the second stage section. The deeply engaged head, lack of amniotic fluid and the thinned out lower segment predispose uterine wound extension during delivery. It is important to make an adequate incision on the abdominal wall. The loose fold of peritoneum should be picked up incised, and upper limit of the bladder should be identified to avoid injury to the bladder. The incision on the Uterus may be placed relatively at a higher level to prevent uterine incision extension. A careful delivery of head using a "push" or "pull" technique should be used. Extension of the lower segment uterine incision is one of the most typical injuries during a section. The chances extension of the uterine incision is directly proportional to the length of the second stage of labour. The uterine wound extension as 25% if the second stage of labour was 1–3 hours and increasing to 32% if the duration of the second stage of labour was 4–5 hours. Uterine wound extension commonly occurred into the lower segment, followed by the cervix [25]. If the incision has extended the edges of the incision should be identified and sutured. If there is excess bleeding Uterine artery ligation or internal iliac artery ligation may need to be done. Uterine artery ligation is done by passing an absorbable suture material like No 1 Polygalactin suture through the myometrium medial to the Uterine artery. The suture is brought forward through an avascular area through the anterior and posterior wall of the broad ligament and sutured. Internal iliac artery ligation may be needed in cases where there is severe bleeding. When all measures have failed, sometimes Hysterectomy may be required in the extreme extension of Uterine incision. In rare instances of lateral extension of uterine incision, sometimes ureters may be injured and wise to help a Urologist repair these injuries.

Bladder injuries can sometimes occur during the second stage cesarean section due to extension. The torn bladder edges should be identified and sutured in 2 continuous layers by 3.0 or 4.0 delayed absorbable sutures. The bladder should be drained continuously for 2 to 3 weeks with continuous bladder drainage. If there is suspicion of injury to ureteric orifices, help should be taken from urologist to repair the defect.

Occasionally when the section is done in the second stage of labour, the baby may be delivered accidentally through an incision on the vagina. Hence it is essential to identify the lower segment and correct incision to deliver the baby through the lower uterine segment [26].

Patients who underwent Cesarean section in the second stage may be at increased risk of preterm labour in subsequent pregnancies [27].

5. Conclusion

Cesarean sections rates are increasing so is the increase in second stage cesarean sections. Judicious use of Oxytocin and monitoring may help to reduce the incidence of second-stage cesarean sections. Second stage cesareans sections are associated with complications like bleeding and other maternal tissue injuries. Currently, the pull method of delivering the head seems to be associated with fewer complications than the push method. Obstetricians must get trained for second stage cesarean section.

Acknowledgements

We appreciate the help provided by Abhishek Nambiar during the course of preparation of this article.

Conflict of interest

The authors declare no conflict of interest.

Author details

Jayaraman Nambiar[1*] and Thiencherry Rema[2]

1 Professor, Department of Obstetrics and Gynaecology, Kasturba Medical College, Manipal, India

2 Sonologist, Balan Nivas, Misisonary Hills, Ooty, India

*Address all correspondence to: drramnambiar@gmail.com

References

[1] Loudon JAZ, Groom KM, Hinkson L, Harrington D, Paterson-Brown S. Changing trends in operative delivery performed at full dilatation over a 10-year period. J Obstet Gynaecol 2010;30:370-375. DOI: 10.3109/01443611003628411.

[2] National Maternity Hospital, Holles St., Dublin 2. Annual Reports 2006 to 2015.

[3] Vousden N, Cargill Z, Briley A, Tydeman G, Shennan AH. Caesarean section at full dilatation: incidence, impact and current management. Obstet Gynaecol 2014;16:199-205. DOI:org/10.1111/tog.12112

[4] Allen VM, O'Connell CM, Baskett TF. Maternal and perinatal morbidity of caesarean delivery at full cervical dilatation compared with caesarean delivery in the first stage of labour. BJOG 2005;112:986-990.DOI: 10.1111/j.1471-0528.2005.00615.x.

[5] Murphy DJ, Liebling RE, Verity L, Swingler R, Patel R. Early maternal and neonatal morbidity associated with operative delivery in second stage of labour: a cohort study. Lancet 2001;358:1203-1207. DOI: 10.1016/S0140-6736(01)06341-3

[6] Towner D, Castro MA, Eby-Wilkens E, Gilbert WM. Effect of mode of delivery in nulliparous women on neonatal intracranial injury. N Engl J Med. 1999 Dec 2;341(23):1709-1714. DOI: 10.1056/NEJM199912023412301

[7] Bahl R, Patel RR, Swingler R, Ellis M, Murphy DJ. Neurodevelopmental outcome at 5 years after operative delivery in the second stage of labor: a cohort study. Am J Obstet Gynecol. 2007 Aug;197(2):147.e1-147.e6. DOI: 10.1016/j.ajog.2007.03.034

[8] Lewis EA, Barr C, Thomas K. The mode of delivery in women taken to theatre at full dilatation: does consultant presence make a difference? J Obstet Gynaecol 2011; 31 (3):229-231. DOI: 10.3109/01443615.2011.553692

[9] Ebulue V, Vadalkar J, Cely S, Dopwell F, Yoong W. Fear of failure: are we doing too many trials of instrumental delivery in theatre? Acta Obstet Gynecol Scand 2008;87(11):1234-1238. DOI: 10.1080/00016340802443848

[10] Kadhum TJ Head pushing versus reverse breech extraction for delivery of impacted head during cesarean section Kuf Med J 2009;12:200-205. DOI: 10.36740/WLek202005135

[11] Sandars J, Beattie B, Chaudry S, Chippington Derrisk D, Demilew J, James D,et al. National Institute for Health and Clinical Excellence: Caesarean Section Clinical Guidance. London: NICE; 2011[http://www.nice.org.uk/nicemedia/live/13620/57162/57162.pdf].

[12] Magann EF, Chauhan SP, Bufkin L, Field K, Roberts WE, Martin JN Jr. Intra-operative haemorrhage by blunt versus sharp expansion of the uterine incision at caesarean delivery: a randomised clinical trial. BJOG. 2002 Apr;109(4):448-452. DOI: 10.1111/j.1471-0528.2002.01296.x

[13] Morgan PJ, Kung R, Tarshis J. Nitroglycerin as a uterine relaxant: a systematic review. J Obstet Gynaecol Canada 2002;24:403-409. DOI: 10.1016/s1701-2163(16)30403-0

[14] Waterfall H, Grivell RM, Dodd JM. Techniques for assisting difficult delivery at caesarean section. Cochrane Database Syst Rev. 2016 Jan 31;(1):CD004944. DOI:10.1002/14651858.CD004944.pub3.

[15] Landesman R, Graber EA. Abdominovaginal delivery:

modification of the cesarean section operation to facilitate delivery of the impacted head. Am J Obstet Gynecol. 1984 Mar 15;148(6):707-710. DOI: 10.1016/0002-9378(84)90551-9

[16] Chopra S, Bagga R, Keepanasseril A, Jain V, Kalra J, Suri V. Disengagement of the deeply engaged fetal head during cesarean section in advanced labor: conventional method versus reverse breech extraction. Acta Obstet Gynecol Scand. 2009;88(10):1163-1166. DOI: 10.1080/00016340903214932

[17] Lal M, Goyal P, Shamim S. Evaluation of Patwardhan Technique in Second Stage Caesarean Section. Int Arch BioMed Clin Res [Internet]. 2018Mar.20 [cited 2021Jan.26];4(1): 47-9.

[18] Fasubaa OB, Ezechi OC, Orji EO, Ogunniyi SO, Akindlele ST, Loto OM, et al. delivery of the impacted head of the fetus at caesarean section after prolonged obstructed labour: a randomised comparative study of the two methods. J Obstet Gynaecol 2002;22:375-378 DOI: 10.1080/01443610 220141290

[19] Levy R, Chernomoretz T, Appelman Z, Levin D, Or Y, Hagay ZJ. Head pushing versus reverse breech extraction in cases of impacted fetal head during Cesarean section. Eur J Obstet Gynecol Reprod Biol. 2005 Jul 1;121(1):24-26. DOI: 10.1016/ j.ejogrb.2004.09.014

[20] Blickstein I. Difficult delivery of the impacted fetal head during cesarean section: intraoperative disengagement dystocia. J Perinat Med. 2004;32(6): 465-469. DOI: 10.1515/JPM.2004.152

[21] Khosia A. Cesarean section in a wedged head. Ind J Med Sci 2003;57:187-191. PMID: 14514249.

[22] Singh M, Varma R. New developments. Reducing complications associated with a deeply engaged head at caesarean section: a simple instrument. TOG 2008;10:38-41. https://doi.org/10.1576/toag.10.1.038.27376

[23] Seal SL, Dey A, Barman SC, Kamilya G, Mukherji J, Onwude JL. Randomized controlled trial of elevation of the fetal head with a fetal pillow during cesarean delivery at full cervical dilatation. Int J Gynaecol Obstet. 2016 May;133(2):178-182. DOI: 10.1016/j.ijgo.2015.09.019

[24] Clinical Innovations. Murray Utah. C-snorkel: Impacted Fetal Head ReleaseDevice by Softlift. 2012.[http://www.clinicalinnovations.com/products/c_snorkel].

[25] Sung JF, Daniels KI, Brodzinsky L et al. Cesarean deliveryoutcomes after a prolonged second stage of labor. Am J ObstetGynecol 2007; 197 (3): 306.e1-306.e5 DOI: 10.1016/j.ajog.2007.07.005

[26] Peleg D, Perlitz Y, Pansky S, Levit A, Ben-Ami M. Accidental delivery through a vaginal incision (laparoelytrotomy) during caesarean section in the second stage of labour. BJOG. 2001 Jun;108(6):659-660. DOI: 10.1111/j.1471-0528.2001.00133.x

[27] Wood SL, Tang S, Crawford S. Cesarean delivery in the second stage of labor and the risk of subsequent premature birth. Am J Obstet Gynecol. 2017;217:63.e1-63.10. DOI: 10.1016/j.ajog.2017.03.006

Chapter 2

Twin Pregnancies Labour Modus and Timing

Panagiotis Tsikouras, Anna Chalkidou, Anastasia Bothou, Angeliki Gerede, Xanthoula Anthoulaki, Spyridon Michalopoulos, Ioannis Tsirkas, Fotini Gaitatzi, Irene Babageorgaka, Apostolos Lazarou, Natalia Sachnova, Michael Koutsogiannis, Konstantinos Nikolettos, Theopi Nalbanti, Eythimios Demosthenous, Georgios Dragoutsos, Ifigenia Apostolou, Alexios Alexiou, Panagiotis Petsidis, Stefanos Zervoudis, George Iatrakis, Werner Rath, George Galazios and Nikolaos Nikolettos

Abstract

Twin pregnancies are categorized according to three factors, zygosity, chorionicity and amnionicity. Dizygotic twins are always dichorionic and diamniotic, where each twin has its own chorionic and amniotic sac. Monozygotic twins account for 1/3 of twin pregnancies and show higher morbidity and mortality. In monozygotic twins, chorionicity and amnionicity are determined by the time of zygote division. Chorionicity and amnionicity determine the risks of twin pregnancy. Morbitidies are shown notable decreasing tendency depending on improving of high risk obstetric and neonatal care, however is still discussed the optimum labour management in twin pregnancies Vaginal delivery in twin pregnancies is possible when both have cephalic presentation and in the late weeks of pregnancy during which the risks of prematurity are minimized. The aim of this review was the assessment and evaluation the impact of the labour modus and timing of termination of twin pregnancies due to rise of their occurrence based on scientific aspects of the new published literature on perinatal outcome.

Keywords: twin pregnancies, modus of terminating births, perinatal outcome

1. Introduction

The definition of multiple pregnancies describes the presence of more than one fetus in a single pregnancy. Usually the reference to multiple pregnancies refers to twins, which means that two fetuses coexist in the same pregnancy in one uterus. Twin pregnancy results from the fertilization of two ova from a corresponding sperm (dizygotic twins) or from the fertilization of an ovum after separation of the resulting zygote with the final result of the creation of two embryonic monozygotic twins. Each fetus is surrounded by two membranes, one external (well known as chorionic) and one internal (well known as amniotic). Possibly, more than two embryos will be created in multiple pregnancies, but the more there are, the less likely to survive in the future. The frequency of multiple pregnancies in the human species can be calculated based on Hellin's rule and therefore the following data emerge: for twin pregnancy 1: 85 (1.18%), for triple pregnancy 1:85^2 (0.013%) and for quadruple pregnancy 1:85^3 (0.0061%) [1–4].

The 2/3 of them are polygenic pregnancies and 1/3 are monogenic pregnancies. Regarding twin pregnancies, about 70% are dizygotic and 30% are monozygotic twins. The incidence of multiple pregnancies has generally increased in recent years from 1/100 to 1/60–1/70 births. The exact frequency of twins is very difficult to determine because in the first trimester they have a high frequency of miscarriages, much higher than single pregnancies and compared to that in the third trimester of pregnancy to be doubled. Spontaneous abortion of one twin without affecting the other is often asymptomatic. While the frequency of monogenic pregnancies does not depend on the race, heredity, age of the mother, as well as her ability to fertilize after administration of drugs to induce ovulation, the frequency of polygenesis is influenced by the above factors [1–4]. Twin pregnancies account for 1% to 3.5% of total births and have a 15% perinatal mortality rate. In Greece, the incidence of twin spontaneous pregnancies is about 1% and in women with IVF is about 25%. The percentage of perinatal mortality in the US has been declining from 12.6% in 1980 to 6.8% in 2001, a decrease of 46%. According to the literature, about 50% of twin pregnancies are associated with prematurity and low birth weight. Compared to single pregnancies, twin pregnancies have four times the risk of perinatal mortality, while in triple and upper multiple pregnancies there is up to nine times the similar risk. Especially in adolescent twin pregnancies and twin pregnancies in women over 35 years are 46.28% and 16.68% respectively [1–8].

1.1 Epidemiology

The frequency of monozygotic twins is 3.5/1000 to 4/1000 births or 0.4% of pregnancies completely stable regardless of the mother's age, race and heredity is determined by the analysis of the morphology of the placenta or genotype. The dizygotic twins affected because of follicular growth by levels of follicle stimulating hormone FSH, and luteinizing hormone LH affected by racial hereditary factors. The fluctuation rates of the twin pregnancies considered to be due in dizygotic twins, since monozygotic twins have stable effect 3.5/1000 to 4/1000 births. The frequency of dizygotic twins is associated with multiple ovulation heredity and shows high geographical variation. The incidence of spontaneous twin pregnancies varies around the world, with rates ranging from 8/1000 to 17/1000 births. In particular, it ranges from 57/1000 in Nigeria, 12/1000 in the United Kingdom, 12.4/1000 in Scotland, 4/1000 in Japan. In particular, in the USA there was an increase of 65% from 68339 in 1980 to 125134 in 2002. In particular the twins have a fivefold increased incidence in various parts of Africa as a whole of 1/50 or 16/1000 pregnancies, due to high levels of gonadotropins, about half the incidence in Asia 1/150 averaged 3/1000 pregnancies in particular in the yellow race Japanese 2.4%. The incidence of twin pregnancies is in the white race 1/90 or 8/1000 pregnancies [9–12].

Twin pregnancies are more common in older mothers. There is a positive correlation between increased maternal age and increased FSH secretion. There is an approximately 2% increase in women over 35 years old due to increased FSH levels after 37 years (twin decrease and increase in miscarriages in high interest rates) 2% increase after the fourth pregnancy, regardless of age and frequency of contact. There is an increase from adolescence to 39 years per year 0.8% per subsequent pregnancy and then a sharp decline, increased rate of uterine anomalies (1:20) [12–14]. The rate of spontaneous conception is increased due to increased FSH and LH during the summer months with a corresponding reduction in winter. Worldwide, the incidence of twin pregnancies is 1/80, which may be due to different levels of gonadotropins. Women with dizygotic twins have statistically significantly increased serum FSH levels during the early follicular phase, as well as an increased rate of FSH release during impulses. With regard to twin pregnancies, there is a direct correlation with the mother's ethnicity, while on the other hand, the father's ethnicity does not affect. In addition, the probability of giving birth to twins is affected by the heredity of the parents, at a rate of 2% on the part of the mother and 0.8% on the part of the father. The various toxic substances present in water and food are also dynamic factors that play a role in the frequency of dizygotic twins. Regarding this fact, in 1988 there was an increase of twins from 3‰ to 20‰ in areas contaminated with polychlorinated hydrocarbons. Finally, in cases of twin pregnancies after in vitro fertilization, 85% of them are dizygotic and 15% monozygotic. The incidence of twins in developed countries is higher than normal due to assisted reproduction methods (IVF, induction of ovulation)) [12–14]. The incidence of twin pregnancies after widespread use of assisted reproduction has increased significantly. From 1/80 pregnancies nearly the frequency has been tripling. Particular the percentage of twin pregnancies using the "in vitro fertilization" (IVF) or" intra cytoplasmic sperm injection" (ICSI) is 18–53%, while with the use of insemination and of controlled ovarian overstimulation (IUI - COH) with induction of ovulation is 6.8% to 11.7% [10–18]. Most twins resulting from assisted reproduction are dizygotic. Significant is the increase in the frequency of twins from 10/1000 births in 1980 to an average of 20/1000 births with the help of assisted reproduction methods. A total of 25% of pregnancy and 1/64 in the United Kingdom are the result of assisted reproduction methods) [14–18]. The incidence of assisted reproductive twins can be significantly reduced depending on the use of the embryo selection method and the selective transfer of an embryo. However, the incidence of monozygotic twin pregnancies after assisted reproduction is higher compared to spontaneous monozygotic twin pregnancies. The incidence of monozygotic twin pregnancies due to assisted reproduction is 0.9%. According to bibliographic sources, blastocyst transfer and maternal age (under 35 years) are associated with an increased risk of both either monozygotic or monochorionic twins after IVF [10–22]. According to literature reports the risk of miscarriage in the first trimester is 43% in twins after spontaneous conception, 51% after assisted reproduction while the respective risk rates of miscarriages are 19% and 21% [10–22]. Twin pregnancy is the result of fertilization of 2 eggs from 2 sperm (dizygotic twins 1.2% of pregnancies) or the division of a fertilized egg by the separation of the zygote into 2 separate entities, forming two embryos that can develop individually (monozygotic twins: 0.4% of births or 4/1000 births) [10–22]. The incidence of monochorionicity due to IVF is 3.2% [10–22]. The percentage of monozygotic twins is stable, in contrast the percentage of dizygotic twins depends on race, various genetic factors, mother's age, endogenous gonadotropins, sex fetus and the use of assisted reproduction methods [10–22].

2. Diagnosis

Imaging of the chorion from 5 to 6 weeks after LMP (Last Menstrual period).
Imaging of the fetal poles from the 7th week after LMP.
Fetal heartbeat from the 7th week after LMP.

and in transvaginal ultrasound we have:

Imaging of the chorion from the end of the 4th week after LMP.

Imaging of the amniotic sacs from the 5 'week after LMP.

Imaging of fetuses from the end of the 6th week after LMP.

Fetal heart rate from the 6th week after LMP.

Ultrasound monitoring of a twin pregnancy has two main objectives: to determine the chorionicity and zygosity of the pregnancy due to the higher risk of conceiving a chromosomally abnormal fetus compared to single pregnancies, the risk of twin-twin transfusion syndrome and intrauterine growth restriction.

In particular, the determination of chorionicity that is easier between 11 and 13 weeks (identification of placental points L and T, number of amniotic sacs) is a prerequisite for monitoring twin pregnancies, early detection FFT syndrome, screening for congenital abnormalities. It is often difficult to diagnose monoamniotic twins because it is difficult to visualize them due to the small thickness of the membrane or in cases of oligamnion. The existence of entangled umbilical cords confirms the existence of a single amniotic cavity. The estimation of the thickness of the diaphragm has 83% prognostic value for dichorionic pregnancy, in cases of thin membrane 83% prognostic value for monochorionic diamniotic pregnancy. In dichorionic pregnancies, two placentas are visualized but in monochorionic pregnancies when two layers are detected during the examination of the diaphragm, then these are monochrorionic diamniotic pregnancies, if they are four layers then these are dichorionic diamniotic pregnancies. Ultrasound examination in twins with a single placental mass in the presence of a triangular protrusion of the placental tissue, a peak sign of a twin pregnancy or a lambda or a double apex indicates the existence of two placentas therefore a dichorionic, diamniotic pregnancy. In cases of non-detection of the lambda point but certification of the T sign at the membrane entrance, it indicates monochorionic twin pregnancies. In monochorionic placentas the selective discontinuation of one twin leads to an increase in thromboplastin and poses a risk of amniotic fluid embolism for both the other fetus and the pregnant mother. Fetuses of different genders are always dichorionic and diamniotic. The initial measurements of twin fetuses based on Crown-rump length (CRL) and nuchal translucency do not differ from those of single pregnancies. Amniocentesis is the method of choice in many cases. The rate of spontaneous abortion after amniocentesis does not differ in twin pregnancies achieved by assisted reproduction methods compared to those achieved by spontaneous conception. In pregnancies achieved through assisted reproduction technology, there are high levels of β-HCG with an increased rate of premature maturation and also an increased rate of placental abnormalities, as well as a vaginal spotting. Twin pregnancies have a higher rate of aneuploidy [22–30].

2.1 Monitoring of multiple pregnancy

Chorionicity should be determined on the first ultrasound at the first visit. Possible prenatal screening problems should be highlighted, several visits are necessary for intensive monitoring of both the pregnant mother and the fetus.

2.1.1 Frequency of visits

2.1.1.1 Monochorionic/diamniotic twins

Every 2 weeks until the 16th–24th week of pregnancy in order to exclude TTTS. Especially, during 18th week of pregnancy it should be performed for a detailed examination of fetal development and during 22–24 weeks of pregnancy for a detailed fetal heart ultrasound. After 24th week, until 32nd week of pregnancy, it should also be performed every 2 weeks, and after 32nd week of pregnancy it should be performed every week until the time of delivery, in order to evaluate in time the possible pathology of the intrauterine fetal development.

2.1.1.2 Estimated fetal weight (EFW)

A difference of estimated fetal weight between 2 embryos less than 25% is considered to be normal.

2.1.1.3 Monochorionic/monoamniotic

The frequency of visits for these twins is mainly determined by the course of the pregnancy and the follow-up should be more frequent because of the fact that the possible complications occur at higher rates, including TTTS and umbilical cord compression [22–30].

2.1.1.4 Dichorionic

18 weeks detailed fetal development test.

22–24 weeks detailed fetal heart ultrasound.

Every 2 to 4 weeks from the 24th to the 32nd week and every week until the birth to assess intrauterine development pathology in a timely manner.

EFW A difference of less than 25% between the EFWs of the two fetuses is considered normal.

Regular testing for hypertension (preeclampsia) should be done to avoid intravenous medication. The early diagnosis of gestational diabetes mellitus is done with increased glucose curve (increased complications in multiple pregnancies).

During these visits, weight gain, blood pressure and changes in the cervix (ultrasound or vaginal examination) should be carefully recorded.

In addition to the amniotic fluid index (AFI), important Doppler ultrasound indicators are: Doppler flow rate tachycardia (UA), umbilical artery pulse index (UAPI), middle cerebral artery Doppler, venous duct (DV) [22–30].

2.2 Complications of twin pregnancy

2.2.1 Maternal complications

Maternal complications in multiple pregnancies occur at higher rates compared to single pregnancies.

2.2.1.1 Hyperemesis

Hyperemesis appears due to increased placental mass and increased β-HCG levels. It is increasing and is a previous complication.

2.2.1.2 Preeclampsia

Compared to a single pregnancy, when there is an increased chance of preeclampsia, it doubles and quadruples. Atypical preeclampsia without hypertension is also common, but with hepatic and renal disorders. The incidence rate is

8.1% in dichorionic embryos, 6% in monochromatic ones, while respectively it is only up to 5% in single pregnancies. If other aggravating factors coexist, such as advanced maternal age of first pregnancy and BMI ≥35 Kg/m2, then 75 mg aspirin is recommended.

2.2.1.3 HELLP syndrome

As an acute fatty liver of pregnancy reaches a 9% incidence in twin pregnancies, in contrast to a single pregnancy it is only 0.9%.

2.2.1.4 Anemia

Anemia particularly iron deficiency anemia due to increased plasma volume without being fully explained. Possible cause of hospitalization.

2.2.1.5 Gestational diabetes

The incidence is 14% in twin pregnancies and 8% in single pregnancies.

2.2.2 Bleeding during pregnancy and postpartum bleeding

Low lying placenta or placenta previa are more common in twin pregnancies. Placenta abruption is also more common is multiple pregnancy than it is in single pregnancies. Twin pregnancies cause uterus overdistention, which results in 10% of the cases in uterine atony. Umbilical umbilical cord bulging is ten times more common in twins than in singleton pregnancies. Velamentous umbilical cord insertion is ten times more common in twin pregnancies than in single pregnancies.

2.2.3 Other complications

Bleeding (10% risk of uterine atony)
Transfusion
Endometritis
Increased incidence of umbilical cord prolapse (9 times more frequent versus single and 8.5% in twin pregnancies)
Solitary umbilical artery (3 times more frequent than single pregnancy)
Velamentous cord insertion (10 times more frequent than single pregnancy)
Increased Morbidity (8 times more frequent versus single) [30–34].

2.2.4 Fetal complications

Preterm labor
Low birth weight
High rate of fetal respiratory distress
Risk of cerebral palsy 4.5 times higher than in single pregnancies
Prematurity, respiratory distress syndrome and neonatal infections are the main causes of neonatal mortality.

Selective reduction in dichorionic twin pregnancies is recommended to be performed in the 12th week of pregnancy or in the 20th week of pregnancy.

Selective reduction at 12 weeks of gestation the abortion rate is 5% and the prematurity rate less than 33 weeks is 6%.

Selective reduction at 20 weeks the abortion rate is 14% and the prematurity rate less than 33 weeks is 20% [31–38].

3. Complications in monochorionic twins

3.1 Pathology of fetal weight develpoment

In about 10% of monochorionic twins, there is an uneven distribution of placental tissue between the fetuses and therefore a pathological increase in the weight of one fetus from the second trimester of pregnancy.

3.1.1 Twin to twin transfusion syndrome (TTTS)

In the placenta of monochorionic twins there are vessels - anastomoses on the surface of the placenta. Through these vessels there is an uneven distribution of blood between the two embryos, with one embryo receiving much more blood than the other. As a result, there is a difference in amniotic fluid, with the bigger fetus having increased amniotic fluid and the smaller fetus having very little fluid. TTTS observed only in monochorionic twin pregnancies due to the existence of vascular anastomoses and therefore common fetal circulation. In this syndrome there are intraplacental arteriovenous anastomoses (and more rarely arterial–arterial anastomoses without arteriovenous anastomosis), in which the blood deviates from one twin (donor) to another (recipient). Its incidence is 4 to 35% of monochorionic pregnancies and it shows high rates of perinatal mortality>50%. The diagnosis is ultrasound, usually between 16 and 26 weeks. 1 in 10 monochorionic twins will develop TTTS syndrome [34–40]. However, vascular anastomoses occur in>95% of monochorionic pregnancies. After some time, the twin recipient fetus shows great growth for gestational age (macrosomia, organomegaly), is profuse and hydropic and shows polycythemia, hypertension, congestive heart failure and hydramnios. The donor shows anemia and hypovolemia and, ultrasound, shows growth restriction and oligohydramnios. In TTTS, detected by some of the above characteristic manifestations from the first weeks of the second trimester, the perinatal mortality of both twins is almost 100%. Along with previous ultrasound findings, the hydropic placenta was described as the first manifestation of TTTS. The intense hydramnios of the recipient could be treated with drainage amniocentesis, which may result in>50% survival for both twins. Often, a drainage amniocentesis is sufficient but a repeat amniocentesis may be required. In recent years, with the help of embryoscopy, laser anatomy of the anastomoses is performed. The procedure involves a risk of miscarriage/premature birth at a rate of 10–15% within the next 6 weeks of surgery [34–38]. However, after this operation, an increased incidence of congenital heart disease was reported in both recipient and donor twins. Rarely, there may be similar development of twins and a normal amount of amniotic fluid in both sacs. Selective termination of a pregnancy is one of the possible "therapies." Interventions (along with hydramnios drainage and photocoagulation of anastomoses) with a potentially increased risk of other pregnancies from possible embolism. It has been argued that the donor's death will stop the transfusion into the recipient while in the recipient killing there is a risk of increased resistance to the vascular network of the placenta, which will burden the already anemic donor. Dying of a fetus has the most serious risk of diffuse intravascular coagulation (usually after a few weeks). An extreme manifestation of TTTS is the presence of a normal anatomically twin donor ("twin pump" [TP]) who usually has a large heart and signs of heart failure (resulting in mortality>50%) and "transfuses" blood (with arterial–arterial placental anastomosis). In a cardiac receptor twin (1% of monochorionic twin births) that does not have a direct vascular connection to the placenta (twin reversed arterial perfusion [TRAP]). The Acardiac twin (AT) recipient usually has other, very serious, anatomical abnormalities (Acardiac monster) (may be brainless or headless) while the normal fetus (if it survives) after birth usually has, remission of signs of heart failure. Transfusion from fetal donor to embryo recipient is done through anastomoses especially through arterial artery and less venous anastomoses in the placenta. The etiology of TRAP syndrome is reported to be either non-conformation of the fetal heart or reversal of blood flow leading to heart aplasia. In a continuing pregnancy, with TRAP, 1–2 times a week ultrasound monitoring of AT is recommended to look for hydrops. With the same frequency, Doppler should be performed in the DA to look for abnormalities of the umbilical artery, umbilical vein and venous pore. Given the increased risk of preterm birth, corticosteroids should be administered between 24 and 34 weeks of gestation (WG). As a prenatal treatment, amniotic fluid (due to coexistence and hydramnios) was removed in the past, the cardiac duct was removed by "caesarean section" (uterine cross-section) or alcohol was administered into the umbilical cord of the AT. Today, among other treatments (waiting or delivery), an attempt can be made to block the umbilical cord circulation of the cardiac twin (BUCCT). In particular, between 18 and 27 WG, BUCCT can be performed using laser, bipolar diathermy or the use of "radiofrequency ablation (RFA]), which are performed under local anesthesia and administration ofconscious sedation. Usually, under ultrasound control, a 2–3 mm fetoscope is inserted into the amniotic cavity (). An alternative but less common method is embryonic umbilical cord ligation [34–40]. Finally, there is a significant risk of structural abnormality in monochorionic twins, with 4% of cases the abnormality concerns only one of the two fetuses. TTTS syndrome is a complication that affects only monochorionic twins and is the most common cause of fetal loss and disability in monochorionic twins. It is characterized by a significant difference in amniotic fluid between the two embryos, increased amniotic fluid around the recipient fetus and minimal amniotic fluid around the donor fetus. The cause of the development of the syndrome is placental vascular anastomoses between the two fetuses. TTTS syndrome occurs in the early stages of pregnancy, when delivery is not an option because the fetuses are still very premature. Therefore, there is significant mortality and morbidity without therapeutic intervention, with possible miscarriage or fetal loss of one or both fetuses [34–40].

3.2 Complications in dichorionic twins

3.2.1 Intrauterine growth restriction (IUGR)

In a 20% of dichorionic twins there is a significant difference in their development, with one of the fetuses not developing well. Probable cause is placental insufficiency in one of the two placentas. This probability is more common when the difference in the development of twins exceeds 18–20% [34–40].

3.2.2 Structural anomaly

The risk of structural abnormality does not increase in dichorionic twins. But since they are two babies, the chance of a structural abnormality in pregnancy, at least in one of the two babies, is twice as high as in a single pregnancy [34–40].

3.3 Monozygotic twins

They show a high frequency of structural anomalies that are classified into three categories.

1. **Conjoined twins** 1/33000 births monoamniotic monochorionic. It can be thoracopagus or omphalopagus. 70% are females.

2. **Congenital abnormalities** resulting from vascular exchange vascular anastomoses in monochorionic placentation.

3. **Acardiac twin** in TTTS, frequency of occurrence 1% of monochorionic twin pregnancies [34–40].

3.4 Cases of intrauterine fetal death of a twin

The risk of intrauterine fetal death is higher in twin pregnancies compared to single pregnancies.

During the ultrasound examination between the 10th and 14th week, the rate of fetal loss in single pregnancies is 2%.

4% in dichorionic pregnancies

1% in monochorionic pregnancies

Intrauterine death of both fetuses

in the first trimester 1.6% in dichorionic twins

2% in monochorionic twins

After the 14th week intrauterine death 2% in dichorionic twins

4% in monochorionic twins

Intrauterine death of both 0.2% sequentially

6% in monochorionic twins

Towards the end of pregnancy risk of endometrial death

1/3333 in the 33rd week of gestation

1/313 35 weeks of gestation

1/69 39 week of gestation

1st trimester of pregnancy vanishing twin common phenomenon no effect on the other twin.

In pregnancies over 20 weeks of gestation there is intrauterine death of a twin 5% of all twin pregnancies.

In monochorionic twins acute hypotension is observed anemia ischemia leading to morbidity or death of the other.

In pregnancies over 26 weeks of gestation risk of imminent death of a twin so there is a need to organize the delivery.

After the death of one twin, administration of corticosteroids to the other twin.

Daily checkup of PT, PTT, Platelets and Fibrinogen is needed. Weekly checkup of biophysical profile and delivery at 37 weeks of gestation is recommended.

The prognosis of the survivor depends on the chorionicity and less on the gestational age at which the uterine death occurred [40–44].

4. Method and time of termination of pregnancy

Abnormal presentations of twins A, B or both are among the common complications during delivery. For the delivery, there should be organization in the Maternity Hospital and constant vigilance of Obstetricians, Neonatologists and Anesthesiologists, continuous cardiotocographic examination and maximum readiness for the execution of a possible emergency caesarean section. The various presentations of fetuses in twin pregnancies are.

4.1 Vaginal delivery-ceasarean section

In general, both in single pregnancies and in twin pregnancies, the best way to complete delivery is vaginal delivery due to:

1. Development of the newborn's lungs due to the stress of vaginal delivery and therefore less likely to develop pulmonary distress syndrome.

2. In vaginal delivery the bacteria of the normal flora of the mother's vagina settle in the intestine of the newborn and cause activation of the immune system of the newborn. In particular, it is suggested by the American College that in head presentation, regardless of prematurity, cesarean section has no advantage over vaginal deliveries, provided that it was a low-risk pregnancy (No pregnancy pathology such as preeclampsia, intrauterine growth restriction). Regarding intracranial hemorrhage, cerebral palsy, chorioamnionitis there is no influence on the head presentation of the method of termination of pregnancy, only correlation is reported with the degree of prematurity therefore the gestational age of the newborn. In contrast to breech presentation, the rates of cerebral palsy are reported to be increased. According to the American College head presentation in both newborns there is no difference in morbidity of neonates with vaginal delivery compared to neonates born by caesarean section. The views of the American College are confirmed by several studies that concern selected low-risk pregnancies, aged >35 weeks of gestation with a head presentation of the 1st fetus that suggest the choice of vaginal delivery of the 2 fetuses [44–50].

No adverse effects of vaginal delivery were observed with regard to morbidity and mortality of the latter even when its projection is not head-on. After the birth of the first baby, the presentation of the second is often changed, as a result the second twin may have a vertical shape, an abnormal presentation and therefore a caesarean section is preferred. The second twin in case of change of presentation has an increased risk of perinatal asphyxia and therefore the organization of an emergency caesarean section is extremely necessary. Important factors for how to complete the birth of twins are:

Presentation of the first twin

Estimated birth weight

In the majority of cases 75–85% the fetus iswith head presentation and if there are no risk factors in diamniotic twins' vaginal deliveryis indicated. The big problem is in the second twin, especially when it is not in head presentation, there are contradictory data from the literature, while some authors report that there are no advantages of caesarean section over vaginal delivery, other authors emphasize the risks of vaginal delivery such as increased perinatal morbidity, mortality and fetal distress.

Disadvantages of cesarean sections are increased maternal morbidity and increased cost of health benefits. In newborns weighing less than 600 gr, or in 26 weeks of gestation, vaginal delivery is recommended due to low survival rates [48–58].

Between 600 and 2000 g weight, or in 27–8 weeks of gestation, if the first fetus is not in head presentation, then a caesarean section is recommended to avoid umbilical cord prolapse and twin interlocking.

If the first fetus is in head presentation should made an effort for vaginal delivery. If the se fetus is not in head presentation at internal cephalic version should attempt immediately and in failure organization of an emergency cesarean section. In cases where the second twin is not in head presentation but has a weight of over 2000 g external cephalic version should attempt and in case of failure internal cephalic version should attempt under local anesthesia and in repeated failure emergency cesarean section should be done. In cases of weight difference from 500 g of the weights of the two fetuses cesarean section in monoamniotic twins should be performed. Cesarean section is a routine method for termination of labor to prevent umbilical cord prolapse and twin interlocking in IUGR, conjoined twins or twins with TTTS [55–58].

4.2 Main complications of vaginal twin delivery

Inter-anchoring of twins in a longitudinal lie can occur in either cephalic presentations or in breech presentations.

Acute twin-to-twin transfusion syndrome is rare and is associated with changes in intravascular pressure along large vascular anastomoses and intrauterine pressure during labor, creating a risk of heart failure and exchange transfusion between twins.

It is recommended in low-risk twin pregnancies of dichorionic twins a birth planning for 37th week and of monochorionic twins for 36th week.

In monochorionic monoamniotic pregnancies, caesarean section is preferred to avoid overlapping (1/1000 births). According to the Bibliography the number of cesarean sections required to prevent a neonatal death is between 264 and 1451.

The above reports are disadvantageous in terms of their validity because the data on how to arrange the birth of the 2nd fetus, the interval between the 1st and 2nd births as well as the type of obstetric manipulations are missing or insufficient. Therefore, the potential benefits to the newborn of a Caesarean section should be weighed against the potential short-term and long-term risks of complications from the mother.

According to recent data on short-term and long-term maternal morbidity, scheduled Caesarean section is not recommended in all low-risk twin pregnancies. In contrast, scheduling vaginal delivery in twin pregnancies >35 weeks with a head projection of the 1st fetus is a relatively safe and acceptable method, provided that staff are experienced in arranging the 2nd fetal delivery.

The way of terminating the labor in twin pregnancies is increasingly troubling the modern obstetrician due to the large number of twin pregnancies that result from the application of assisted reproduction methods. The frequency of stillbirths and perinatal morbidity and mortality are higher in twin pregnancies.

Retrospective studies have shown that caesarean section has the advantage of reducing the morbidity of the 2nd fetus [55–58].

Many meta-analyzes of studies comparing selective Cesarean section with vaginal delivery do not find an advantage in performing cesarean section. Due to the small number of the above studies, more and larger ones need to be carried out. Future research should also look at the possible causes of increased stillbirths in twin pregnancies as well as investigating the role of chorionicity in the normal or non-development of childbirth [55–58].

Due to the dramatic increase in the frequency of Caesarean sections observed in recent years and the increase in the frequency of twin pregnancies, and despite the higher risk of perinatal asphyxia compared to single pregnancies, it is suggested by many studies near the probable date of delivery. According to most recent literature, it is recommended between 37^{+3} and 37^{+5} weeks of pregnancy [55–58].

Nowadays, there is an increase in the frequency of twin pregnancies after spontaneous conception in developed countries, which is explained by the choice to have children at an advanced age (approximately 6% compared to 2.3% 4 years ago). In addition, over the last decade there has been an increase in the incidence of twin pregnancies worldwide as a result of the increasing demand for assisted reproduction methods. Especially in Canada this increase amounted to 15% during 2007–2012.

Twin pregnancies are characterized by increased perinatal morbidity and mortality require larger amounts of surfactant after admission to the Neonatal Intensive Care Unit department especially in the early week and are accompanied by increased maternal morbidity and mortality attributed mainly to the increased risk of bleeding [44–58].

4.3 Increased mortality of full-term twins

According to bibliographic sources in twin pregnancies there is an increase in the relative risk of stillbirth and the risk of unpleasant events during childbirth is increased.

The neonatal mortality of twins compared to single pregnancies is 4.3‰ against 3.8‰ for newborns weighing 2501-3000gr, and 7.4‰ against 2.2‰ for newborns weighing 3000gr. Double mortality during childbirth is also reported.

Due to the evolution of perinatal neonatal care, there is a decrease in the risk of perinatal death of twins during the last three decades. Higher perinatal mortality was also observed in twin neonates with birth weight > 2500gr compared to corresponding weights of single pregnant neonates.

Referring to retrospective studies involving large numbers of twin births, selective caesarean section can also reduce perinatal mortality of full-term twins by 75%. Also important factors that influence the obstetrician to the choice of elective caesarean section are the often observed relatively high (> 35 years) age of the interest rates, as well as the fact that the majority are first-borns. In cases of premature births or severe retardation of intrauterine growth, most recommend caesarean section in pregnancies <32 weeks or when the weight of the fetus is <1500gr.

Regarding the method of conception, twin pregnancies after IVF, ICSI show a higher frequency of premature births, births of infants with residual weight as well as other events. The risk of stillbirth increases after the completion of the 37th week of pregnancy and is 6–9 times higher in dichorionic twins and even more in monochorionic. It is recommended to perform selective Caesarian section in the dichorionic twins in the 37th week and the 36th in the monochorionic twins [44–58].

4.4 Delivery termination time

The International Society for Twin Studies and SOGC recommend giving birth before the 38th week of pregnancy. It is considered a reasonable choice to design a selective low transverse cesarean section during the 38th week.

4.4.1 Absolute indications

Monoamniotic twins due to high risk of umbilical cord prolapse.
Siamese twins

When the presentation of the 1st is not cephalic.

When the 1st of the embryos is in breech presentation, it is recommended to perform a Caesarean section due to the insertion and impossibility of descent of the protruding parts through the pelvic tube, especially when the 2nd embryo is in cephalic presentation. Although the above development is very rare, it is accompanied by high perinatal mortality.

Even when the projection is head-shaped, vaginal delivery remains a controversial choice, due to the increased likelihood of obstetric complications, which usually occur after the birth of the first fetus (placental obstruction, umbilical cord prolapse, fetal bradycardia). Moreover, we should note that the maternal postoperative infections are more frequent, as it becomes necessary to perform an emergency cesarean section for the second fetus.

Empirically and traditionally, the attempt for vaginal delivery is made when the projection of the first fetus is head and there are no other complications, but this has not been proven by well-designed prospective studies. According to the same study, the main cause of neonatal death in relation to the projection of the birth of the second fetus is suffocation-acidosis of the fetus, while the above cause can also cause cerebral palsy.

Remarkably, in most of the younger Obstetricians there is a lack of sufficient capacity, training and experience to deal with success with the increased obstetric requirements of the second fetus, especially when the projection is not cephalic.

According to studies that openly state the choice of whether or not to perform a caesarean section when the projection of the 2nd was not cephalic, 84% of caesarean sections were confirmed with similar rates of neonatal morbidity and mortality between the 2 fetuses. The manner of termination of childbirth in twin pregnancies is increasingly problematic for the modern obstetrician due to the large number of twin pregnancies resulting from the application of assisted reproduction methods. The frequency of stillbirths and perinatal morbidity and mortality are higher in twin pregnancies.

Several studies have shown that vaginal delivery of the 2nd fetus is accompanied by increased perinatal morbidity and mortality and they consider it necessary to perform a selective Cesarean section. In all twin pregnancies, the 2nd fetus can be significantly protected.

Based on the above, it is proposed the vaginal arrangement of the birth of twins only in cases of interest rates: multipara women, aged <35 years, with cephalic presentation of both fetuses, in full-term, without pathology pregnancies, the duration of which does not exceed 38 weeks and which occurred after normal conception. In all other cases, the execution of Caesarian section is proposed [44–58].

5. Discussion

Twin pregnancies have had a steady 70% increase since 1980 and are associated with increased perinatal mortality about 4 times higher than single pregnancies. The main cause of morbidity is preterm birth with an average birth of 35 weeks, the following are: intrauterine growth restriction, intrauterine death, hydramnio (about 10% of cases), preeclampsia (triple incidence in congenital pregnancies), congenital abnormalities, iron deficiency anemia, postpartum hemorrhage, placental abruption and precursor placenta [40–50].

Multiple pregnancies are high-risk pregnancies and are associated with increased neonatal morbidity and mortality, mainly due to prematurity. To understand how a multiple pregnancy increases the rates of adverse neonatal outcomes, it is necessary to record for each incident:

a. the mode of conception (natural conception or assisted reproduction)

b. the possibility of fetal death (automatic initially or after meiosis)

c. the family history of multiple pregnancies

d. the descriptive anatomy of the placenta

The successful use of assisted reproduction techniques is a milestone in the treatment of infertility. The increase of multiple pregnancies is a very important issue, open for solution, since they are accompanied by numerous medical and social problems. Preventing multiple pregnancies with the prudent use of available techniques will contribute significantly to solving this problem [6, 16].

Premature birth before 32–33 weeks of gestation is a major cause of complications in multiple pregnancies. The average age of spontaneous delivery is about 35.5 weeks while in multiple pregnancies it is 33 weeks. Premature birth occurs in 20–50% of twin pregnancies, which means 7–10 times more often compared to single pregnancies. The increased likelihood of twins' complications is mainly due to the high incidence of low birth weight infants as a result of premature or intrauterine growth restriction.

Prematurity is directly responsible for the high neonatal morbidity and mortality of twin pregnancies, due to the high probability of respiratory distress syndrome, intra-abdominal bleeding and necrotic enterocolitis. Also, there are increased rates of residual development of one fetus, or both of them, congenital abnormalities and complications associated with the Twin to twin Transfusion Syndrome (TTTS). Twin pregnancies complicated by premature birth burden the family financially and psychologically, because it requires the transfer of the pregnant woman or the newborn to tertiary hospitals, which have special intensive care units [58–65]. The incidence of depression is increased in mothers of twins, which requires special attention from the clinical doctor.

Newborns born from twin and triplet pregnancies are accompanied by the long-term consequences of perinatal complications. Cerebral palsy is the most common complication of multiple pregnancies. The rates of cerebral palsy are five times higher among twins and ten times higher among triplets, compared with other newborns. The case described in our study with persistent paraplegia was due to fetal hypoxia, cerebral palsy due to placental abruption in the 26th week of pregnancy [58–65].

A particularly important issue is the delivery time of a twin pregnancy and the growing tendency for premature termination of multiple pregnancies, as the increased tendency for preterm delivery in multiple pregnancies and the performance of premature cesarean section have significantly contributed to the increase in neonatal in multiple pregnancies. However, it is noteworthy that the selective neonatal decreases fetal mortality. The explanation for this lies in the fact that the duration of multiple pregnancies after a period of time increases the likelihood of endometrial death. In triplets, in particular, it is reported that after 34 weeks, fetal mortality increases significantly and requires close obstetric monitoring [65–68].

On the other hand, the preventive administration of corticosteroids as a routine, now, in all centers to enhance the pulmonary maturity of the fetus and the use of the surfactant, immediately after birth in premature infants, have the effect of drastically reducing deaths from respiratory distress syndrome in neonates of multiple pregnancies. There is evidence to suggest that the estimate of fetal weight of multiple pregnancies, with the growth curves created for single pregnancies, is incorrect.

Recent data from population studies show that optimal survival of neonates from multiple pregnancies is observed at a younger gestational age and lower body weight than in neonates of single pregnancies [68–70].

The developmental curves of the embryos used in the daily obstetric practice and in our country, are the result of the analysis of data from hospital databases, in non-European populations. According to studies, the distribution of fetal weight in relation to gestational age varies significantly, depending on the population and the time period. There is a difference of up to 11% in the average birth weight of newborns of different populations, at a certain gestational age, while the differences are even greater, exceeding 45% for the third percentage growth curve of the populations of these newborns [68–74].

Residual intrauterine development of fetal twin pregnancies is traditionally diagnosed using single growth curves from single pregnancies. Twins grow at rates similar to those of single pregnancies by the 30th week, followed by slower growth rates, while the same applies to the way triplets develop in relation to twins. Therefore, the developmental curves of the newborns should be revised and adjusted according to the number of fetuses and the gestational age, in order to become more rational.

Systematic monitoring of multiple pregnancies and the correct guidance of the doctor to the pregnant woman for a conservative lifestyle, are the cornerstone for avoiding prematurity. Ultrasound plays an irreplaceable role in the monitoring of multiple pregnancies, with the timely determination of the number of fetuses, the chorionic villus sampling, the position of the placenta and the continuous assessment of the development of the fetus in terms of weight [65–74].

In addition, the use of Doppler contributes to the early diagnosis of intrauterine growth disorders and fetal distress. The use of ultrasound in combination with cardiotocography and the systemic administration of corticosteroids, in all multiple pregnancies between 27 and 33 weeks, are the modern arsenal of the Obstetrician for the diagnosis and treatment of prematurity in these pregnancies. Also, the measurement of fetal fibronectin in the cervix, the ultrasound determination of the length of the cervix or the measurement of estradiol in the saliva of the pregnant woman, are techniques that are experimentally applied for the early diagnosis of premature birth [65–74].

Regarding the method of childbirth in multiple premature pregnancies, both worldwide and in our country, there is a tendency to increase caesarean sections, which is statistically significantly associated with a reduction in intrauterine deaths, single pregnancies. This risk is only 1% in a single pregnancy, while it increases by 10% in dichorionic twins and 15% in monochorionic twins, due to the occurrence of complications from placental anastomoses [65–74]. Therefore, measuring the length of the cervix during the ultrasound examination in the first and second trimester helps to prevent and properly treat impending prematurity. Twin pregnancies are high-risk pregnancies. The average gestational age for twins is about 35 weeks. Newborns of multiple pregnancies have a low birth weight, with an average of 2,500 g for twins. About 10% of twins and 25% of triplets have a birth weight of less than 1,500 g. Low birth weight results in high perinatal mortality, especially in monochorionic pregnancies accompanied by an increased rate of prematurity [65–74].

Multiple pregnancies resulting from infertility are at increased risk of preterm birth versus twin pregnancies with normal conception. This is due to pre-existing risk factors in women with a history of infertility such as uterine abnormalities pelvic infections surgery. Assisted reproduction methods increase monozygotic twins 12 times 13% after ovulation induction 22% for triplets with monozygotic twins. It is estimated that in multiple pregnancies the increased infant mortality is accompanied by almost twice the probability of severe neonatal disability compared to single pregnancies [65–74].

According to an analysis of the International Bibliography, they were certified at a high frequency of complications from fetuses, but the assessment of the above data should be done with consideration and strict criteria according to the guidelines.

Many researchers have found that along with the increase of pregnant's women age, there is a corresponding increase in the frequency of multiple pregnancies. Other researchers have found an increased incidence of multiple pregnancies in high births compared to first-borns, although the widespread use of assisted reproduction methods now tends to reduce this increase [65–74]. The large increase in the frequency of caesarean sections (41%) is one of the most dramatic changes in the last 40 years regarding the manner of delivery. This large increase is attributed to the fear of possible legal involvement and to the increased perinatal morbidity and mortality of the second neonate, especially when the shape is not vertical. Perinatal mortality has decreased in recent years, hovering internationally at 9.6% without a statistically significant difference between newborn twins [65–74]. An important contribution to the formation of perinatal mortality has the birth of multiple newborns weighing less than 1500gr. According to many researchers, no significant difference was found in the Apgar score between 1st and 2nd twins, as well as a relationship between the score and the way the childbirth was completed. According to others in twins born with a normal birth, the Apgar score of the 1st minute of the 2nd was lower compared to that of the 1st. There has also been a recent increase in the Apgar score, especially in the second duo indicative of a better perinatal outcome.

An important role in reducing perinatal mortality and improving perinatal status was played by the early diagnosis of multiple pregnancies in the last 20 years, as well as the systematic application of ultrasound and Doppler ultrasound in their monitoring [65–74]. The above resulted in a more accurate estimate of the probable birth weight, shape and projection, as well as the more correct design of the delivery arrangement.

The frequency of premature births and births of newborns weighing less than 2500gr. remains high despite the systematic application of tocolytic preparations and the restriction of activity until complete multiple immobility of pregnant women.

Regarding the way of arranging births in multiple pregnancies, a particularly statistically significant increase in the frequency of caesarean sections was observed in the last 5 years, amounting to 97.1% for the same reasons as described by internationally renowned researchers [65–74]. Regarding the application of biophysical methods of monitoring prenatal control in twin pregnancies of our study we found increased frequency of cardiotocographic lesions in the form of predominantly varying decelerations especially in the 2nd twin fetus and the above finding can be explained by the relatively high frequency of false positive cardiotocographic findings observed internationally.

The Apgar rating of twin pregnancies, as well as between 1st and 2nd newborn twins, clearly showed that the perinatal condition, especially of the 2nd newborn, was slightly aggravated. This finding contradicts that of many researchers, although many agree with our results without a satisfactory interpretation, possibly due to the frequently changing abnormal projection of the latter. We did not find a statistically significant difference in gender [65–74]. The perinatal mortality of twin pregnancies in our study did not differ significantly from that of the international literature, which confirms the significant improvement in recent years in the application of modern and accurate methods of diagnosis, monitoring of pregnancy and childbirth.

6. Conclusions

In conclusion, in terms of the frequency of multiple pregnancies, perinatal mortality in our region did not differ significantly from that of other advanced countries in Western Europe and North America.

Increased vigilance and care is required in the arrangement of childbirth and the resuscitation of the second newborn because we found that his perinatal condition is significantly lower than that of the first. Significant effort should be made to extend the time of twin pregnancies which would effectively help reduce the frequency of preterm births and caesarean sections.

Although twins appear to be at higher risk for perinatal neonatal outcomes than single pregnancies, they are better when they are born at a mature gestational week and close to the expected due date. To date, however, the optimal delivery time of the duo although still controversial, based on current results, is 37^{+3} weeks of gestation. Regarding the manner and time of termination of labor beyond 35 weeks of gestation is determined according to the literature by many factors gestational age of the two fetuses estimated weight projection twins experience of the obstetrician.

Author details

Panagiotis Tsikouras[1]*, Anna Chalkidou[1], Anastasia Bothou[1], Angeliki Gerede[1], Xanthoula Anthoulaki[1], Spyridon Michalopoulos[1], Ioannis Tsirkas[1], Fotini Gaitatzi[1], Irene Babageorgaka[1], Apostolos Lazarou[1], Natalia Sachnova[1], Michael Koutsogiannis[1], Konstantinos Nikolettos[1], Theopi Nalbanti[1], Eythimios Demosthenous[1], Georgios Dragoutsos[1], Ifigenia Apostolou[2], Alexios Alexiou[1], Panagiotis Petsidis[3], Stefanos Zervoudis[3], George Iatrakis[4], Werner Rath[1], George Galazios[1] and Nikolaos Nikolettos[1]

1 Department of Obstetrics and Gynecology, Democritus University of Thrace, Greece

2 Neonatal Unit Intensive Care of University Hospital of Alexandroupolis, Greece

3 National and Kapodistrian University of Athens and Rea Maternity Hospital, Athens, Greece

4 Technological Educational Institute of Athens and Rea Maternity Hospital, Athens, Greece

*Address all correspondence to: tsikouraspanagiotis@gmail.com

References

[1] Ben-Nun, Twin Pregnancy, 54th Book, 2015, https://www.researchgate.net/publication/280591548_TWIN_PREGNANCY

[2] Vintzileos AM, Ananth CV, Smulian JC, Scorza WE. The impact of prenatal care on preterm births among twin gestations in the United States, 1989-2000. Am J Obstet Gynecol. 2003 Sep;189(3):818-23.

[3] Joaquin Santolaya, Revital Faro Twins--twice more trouble? Clin Obstet Gynecol 2012 Mar;55(1):296-306. doi: 10.1097/GRF.0b013e3182446f51. PMID: 22343246

[4] Vintzileos AM, Ananth CV, Smulian JC, Scorza WE, Knuppel RA. The impact of prenatal care in the United States on preterm births in the presence and absence of antenatal high-risk conditions. Am J Obstet Gynecol. 2002 Nov;187(5):1254-7. doi: 10.1067/mob.2002.127140. PMID: 12439515

[5] Kogan MD, Alexander GR, Kotelchuck M, MacDorman MF, Buekens P, Martin JA, Papiernik E. Trends in twin birth outcomes and prenatal care utilization in the United States, 1981-1997. JAMA. 2000 Jul 19;284(3):335-41. doi: 10.1001/jama.284.3.335. PMID: 10891965

[6] Alexander GR, Slay Wingate M, Salihu H, Kirby RS. Fetal and neonatal mortality risks of multiple births. Obstet Gynecol Clin North Am. 2005 Mar;32(1):1-16, vii. doi: 10.1016/j.ogc.2004.10.005. PMID: 15644285 Review.

[7] Upadhyay K, Pourcyrous M, Dhanireddy R, Talati AJ Outcomes of neonates with birth weight⩽500 g: a 20-year experience. J Perinatol. 2015 Sep;35(9):768-72. doi: 10.1038/jp.2015.44. Epub 2015 May 7. PMID: 25950920

[8] Glass HC, Costarino AT, Stayer SA, Brett CM, Cladis F, Davis PJ. Outcomes for extremely premature infants. Anesth Analg. 2015 Jun;120(6):1337-51. doi: 10.1213/ANE.0000000000000705. PMID: 25988638

[9] Ananth CV, Chauhan SP. Epidemiology of twinning in developed countries. Semin Perinatol. 2012 Jun;36(3):156-61. doi: 10.1053/j.semperi.2012.02.001. PMID: 22713495 Review

[10] Ananth CV, Joseph KS, Demissie K, Vintzileos AM. Trends in twin preterm birth subtypes in the United States, 1989 through 2000: impact on perinatal mortality. Am J Obstet Gynecol. 2005 Sep;193(3 Pt 2):1076-82. doi: 10.1016/j.ajog.2005.06.088. PMID: 16157115

[11] Lisonkova S, Hutcheon JA, Joseph KS. Temporal trends in neonatal outcomes following iatrogenic preterm delivery. BMC Pregnancy Childbirth. 2011 May 25;11:39. doi: 10.1186/1471-2393-11-39. PMID: 21612655

[12] Jauniaux E, Ben-Ami I, Maymon R Do assisted-reproduction twin pregnancies require additional antenatal care? Reprod Biomed Online. 2013 Feb;26(2):107-19. doi: 10.1016/j.rbmo.2012.11.008. Epub 2012 Nov 24. PMID: 23273753

[13] Ananth CV, Vintzileos AM. Epidemiology of preterm birth and its clinical subtypes. J Matern Fetal Neonatal Med. 2006 Dec;19(12):773-82. doi: 10.1080/14767050600965882. PMID: 17190687

[14] Deng C, Dai L, Yi L, Li X, Deng K, Mu Y, Wang K, Tao J, Li Q, Xu L. Temporal trends in the birth rates and perinatal mortality of twins: A population-based study in China. PLoS One. 2019 Jan 16;14(1):e0209962. doi: 10.1371/journal.pone.0209962. eCollection 2019. PMID: 30650106

[15] Matijasevich A, Victora CG, Silveira MF, Wehrmeister FC, Horta BL, Barros FC; Pelotas Cohorts Study Group. Maternal reproductive history: trends and inequalities in four population-based birth cohorts in Pelotas, Brazil, 1982-2015. Int J Epidemiol. 2019 Apr 1;48(Suppl 1):i16-i25. doi: 10.1093/ije/dyy169. PMID: 30883655

[16] Shinwell ES. Neonatal morbidity of very low birth weight infants from multiple pregnancies. Obstet Gynecol Clin North Am. 2005 Mar;32(1):29-38, viii. doi: 10.1016/j.ogc.2004.10.004. PMID: 15644287

[17] Chauhan SP, Scardo JA, Hayes E, Abuhamad AZ, Berghella V Twins: prevalence, problems, and preterm births. Am J Obstet Gynecol. 2010 Oct;203(4):305-15. doi: 10.1016/j.ajog.2010.04.031. Epub 2010 Aug 21.

[18] Yang H, Choi YS, Nam KH, Kwon JY, Park YW, Kim YH. Obstetric and perinatal outcomes of dichorionic twin pregnancies according to methods of conception: spontaneous versus in-vitro fertilization. Twin Res Hum Genet. 2011 Feb;14(1):98-103. doi: 10.1375/twin.14.1.98. PMID: 21314262

[19] Geisler ME, O'Mahony A, Meaney S, Waterstone JJ, O'Donoghue K Obstetric and perinatal outcomes of twin pregnancies conceived following IVF/ICSI treatment compared with spontaneously conceived twin pregnancies. Eur J Obstet Gynecol Reprod Biol. 2014 Oct;181:78-83. doi: 10.1016/j.ejogrb.2014.07.033. Epub 2014 Aug 1. PMID: 25129152

[20] Bensdorp AJ, Hukkelhoven CW, van der Veen F, Mol BWJ, Lambalk CB, van Wely M. Dizygotic twin pregnancies after medically assisted reproduction and after natural conception: maternal and perinatal outcomes. Fertil Steril 2016;106:371-377

[21] Mateizel I, Santos-Ribeiro S, Done E, et al. Do ARTs affect the incidence of monozygotic twinning? Hum Reprod 2016;31:2435-41

[22] Busnellli A, Dallagiovana C, Reschini M, Paffoni A, Fedele L, Somigliana E. Risk factors for monozygotic twinning after in vitro fertilization: a systematic review and meta-analysis. Fertil Steril 2018;111:302-314

[23] Corcoran S, Breathnach F, Burke G, McAuliffe F, Geary M, Daly S, Higgins J, Hunter A, Morrison JJ, Higgins S, Mahony R, Dicker P, Tully E, Malone FD. Dichorionic twin ultrasound surveillance: sonography every 4 weeks significantly underperforms sonography every 2 weeks: results of the Prospective Multicenter ESPRiT Study. Am J Obstet Gynecol. 2015 Oct;213(4):551.e1-5. doi: 10.1016/j.ajog.2015.07.049. Epub 2015 Aug 7. PMID: 26259909

[24] Barrett JF, Ritchie WK. Twin delivery. Best Pract Res Clin Obstet Gynaecol. 2002 Feb;16(1):43-56. doi: 10.1053/beog.2002.0254. PMID: 11866496

[25] Lee YM. Delivery of twins. Semin Perinatol. 2012 Jun;36(3):195-200. doi: 10.1053/j.semperi.2012.02.004. PMID: 22713501

[26] Mazher SB, Kanwal S. J Coll Twin birth weight discordance: associated factors and outcome. Physicians Surg Pak. 2010 Jun;20(6):391-4. PMID: 20642969

[27] Newman RB, Unal ER. Multiple gestations: timing of indicated late preterm and early-term births in uncomplicated dichorionic, monochorionic, and monoamniotic twins. Semin Perinatol. 2011 Oct;35(5):277-85. doi: 10.1053/j.semperi.2011.05.005. PMID: 21962627

[28] Sfakianaki AK, Han CS. Ultrasound in the evaluation of twin pregnancy. Minerva Ginecol. 2009 Apr;61(2):127-39. PMID: 19255560 Review.

[29] D'Alton ME, Dudley DK. Ultrasound in the antenatal management of twin gestation. Semin Perinatol. 1986 Jan;10(1):30-8. PMID: 3532340 Review. No abstract available.

[30] Simpson LL What you need to know when managing twins: 10 key facts. Obstet Gynecol Clin North Am. 2015 Jun;42(2):225-39. doi: 10.1016/j.ogc.2015.01.002. Epub 2015 Mar 9. PMID: 26002163 Review.

[31] Hartley RS, Emanuel I, Hitti J.Perinatal mortality and neonatal morbidity rates among twin pairs at different gestational ages: optimal delivery timing at 37 to 38 weeks' gestation. Am J Obstet Gynecol. 2001 Feb;184(3):451-8. doi: 10.1067/mob.2001.109399. PMID: 11228502

[32] Bamberg C, Hecher K. Update on twin-to-twin transfusion syndrome. Best Pract Res Clin Obstet Gynaecol. 2019 Jul;58:55-65. doi: 10.1016/j.bpobgyn.2018.12.011. Epub 2019 Jan 5. PMID: 30850326 Review.

[33] Kontopoulos E, Chmait RH, Quintero RA. Twin-to-Twin Transfusion Syndrome: Definition, Staging, and Ultrasound Assessment. Twin Res Hum Genet. 2016 Jun;19(3):175-83. doi: 10.1017/thg.2016.34. PMID: 27203605

[34] Wohlmuth C, Boudreaux D, Moise KJ Jr, Johnson A, Papanna R, Bebbington M, Gardiner HM. Cardiac pathophysiology in twin-twin transfusion syndrome: new insights into its evolution. Ultrasound Obstet Gynecol. 2018 Mar;51(3):341-348. doi: 10.1002/uog.17480. Epub 2018 Feb 8. PMID: 28370497

[35] Yoda H Fetal and Neonatal Circulatory Disorders in Twin to Twin Transfusion Syndrome (The Secondary Publication). J Nippon Med Sch. 2019;86(4):192-200. doi: 10.1272/jnms.JNMS.2019_86-301. PMID: 31484880

[36] Richard P Dickey Embryonic loss in iatrogenic multiples Obstet Gynecol Clin North Am 2005 Mar;32(1):17-27, vii-viii. PMID: 15644286

[37] Pharoah PO Risk of cerebral palsy in multiple pregnancies. Obstet Gynecol Clin North Am. 2005 Mar;32(1):55-67, viii. doi: 10.1016/j.ogc.2004.10.002. PMID: 15644289 Review.

[38] Colver A, Fairhurst C, Pharoah PO Cerebral palsy. Lancet. 2014 Apr 5;383(9924):1240-9. doi: 10.1016/S0140-6736(13)61835-8. Epub 2013 Nov 20. PMID: 24268104 Review.

[39] Guzman ER, Mellon R, Vintzileos AM, Ananth CV, Walters C, Gipson K. Relationship between endocervical canal length between 15-24 weeks' gestation and obstetrichistory. JMatern Fetal Med 1998; 7: 269-272.

[40] Iams JD, Johnson FF, Sonek J, Sachs L, Gebauer C, Samuels P. Cervical competence as a continuum: a study of ultrasonographic cervical length and obstetric performance. AmJObstetGynecol1995;172:1097-1103.

[41] Heath VC, Southall TR, Souka AP, Elisseou A, Nicolaides KH. Cervical length at 23 weeks of gestation: prediction of spontaneous preterm delivery. Ultrasound Obstet Gynecol1998.

[42] Sananes N, Meyer N, Gaudineau A, Aissi G, Boudier E, Fritz G, Viville B, Nisand I, Langer B, Favre R. Prediction of spontaneous preterm delivery in the first trimester of pregnancy. Eur J Obstet Gynecol Reprod Biol. 2013 Nov;171(1):18-22.

[43] Zalar RW Early cervical length, preterm labor and gestational age at delivery. Is there a relationship?. J Reprod Med 1998; 43: 1027-1033.

[44] Tsikouras P1, Galazios G, Zalvanos A, Bouzaki A, Athanasiadis A.

Transvaginal sonographic assessment of the cervix and preterm labor. Clin Exp Obstet Gynecol. 2007;34(3):159-62.

[45] Tsikouras P, Anastasopoulos G, Maroulis V, Bothou A, Chalkidou A, Deuteraiou D, Anthoulaki X, Tsatsaris G, et al. Comparative Evaluation of Arabin Pessary and Cervical Cerclage for the Prevention of Preterm Labor in Asymptomatic Women with High Risk Factors. Int J Environ Res Public Health. 2018 Apr 18;15(4). pii: E791. doi:10.3390/ijerph15040791.

[46] Shepherd E, Salam RA, Middleton P, Han S, Makrides M, McIntyre S, Badawi N, Crowther CA. Neonatal interventions for preventing cerebral palsy: an overview of Cochrane Systematic Reviews Cochrane Database Antenatal and intrapartum interventions for preventing cerebral palsy: an overview of Cochrane systematic reviews Syst Rev. 2017 Aug 8;8:CD012077. doi: 10.1002/14651858. CD012077.pub2.

[47] Parkinson JR, Hyde MJ, Gale C, Santhakumaran S, Modi N. Preterm birth and the metabolic syndrome in adult life: a systematic review and meta-analysis. Pediatrics 2013; 131:e1240-63

[48] Onland W, De Jaegere AP, Offringa M, van Kaam A. Systemic corticosteroid regimens for prevention of bronchopulmonary dysplasia in preterm infants. Cochrane Database Syst Rev. 2018 Jun 20;6:CD012409. doi: 10.1002/14651858.CD012409.pub2.

[49] Practice Bulletin. Committee Opinions. Practice Bulletin No. 171: Management of Preterm Labor. Obstet Gynecol 2016;128:155-164

[50] Jaroslaw J Oleszczuk, Louis G Keith, Agnieszka K Oleszczuk The paradox of old maternal age in multiple pregnancies Obstet Gynecol Clin North Am 2005 Mar;32(1):69-80, ix. PMID: 15644290

[51] Yang M, Xiao LL, Wang JM. Zhongguo Dang Dai Er Ke Za Zhi. Association between maternal age and adverse pregnancy outcome in twin pregnancy 2020 Mar;22(3):238-244. doi: 10.7499/j.issn.1008-8830.2020.03.011. PMID: 32204760

[52] Coates D, Homer C, Wilson A, Deady L, Mason E, Foureur M, Henry A. Induction of labour indications and timing: A systematic analysis of clinical guidelines. Women Birth. 2020 May;33(3):219-230. doi: 10.1016/j.wombi.2019.06.004. Epub 2019 Jul 6. PMID: 31285166

[53] Woolcock JG, Grivell RM, Dodd JM. Regimens of ultrasound surveillance for twin pregnancies for improving outcomes. Cochrane Database Syst Rev. 2017 Nov 7;11(11):CD011371. doi: 10.1002/14651858.CD011371.pub2. PMID: 29108135 Free PMC article. Review.

[54] D'Antonio F, Odibo A, Berghella V, Khalil A, Hack K, Saccone G, Prefumo F,et al. Perinatal mortality, timing of delivery and prenatal management of monoamniotic twin pregnancy: systematic review and meta-analysis. Ultrasound Obstet Gynecol. 2019 Feb;53(2):166-174. doi: 10.1002/uog.20100. PMID: 30125418

[55] Morin L, Lim K; Ultrasound in twin pregnancies. Diagnostic imaging committee; special contributor; genetics committee; maternal fetal medicine committee. J Obstet Gynaecol Can. 2011 Jun;33(6):643-656. doi: 10.1016/S1701-2163(16)34916-7. PMID: 21846456

[56] Zaretsky MV, Tong S, Lagueux M, Lim FY, Khalek N, Emery SP, Davis S,et al Moon-Grady AJ, Drennan K, Treadwell MC, Petersen E, Santiago-Munoz P, Brown R; North American Fetal Therapy Network. North American Fetal Therapy Network: Timing of and indications for delivery following laser ablation for twin-twin

transfusion syndrome. Am J Obstet Gynecol MFM. 2019 Mar;1(1):74-81. doi: 10.1016/j.ajogmf.2019.02.001. Epub 2019 Mar 27. PMID: 32832884

[57] Barrett JF. Twin delivery: method, timing and conduct. Best Pract Res Clin Obstet Gynaecol. 2014 Feb;28(2):327-38. doi: 10.1016/j.bpobgyn.2013.12.008. Epub 2014 Jan 8. PMID: 24445020

[58] Ganchimeg T, Morisaki N, Vogel JP, Cecatti JG, Barrett J, Jayaratne K, Mittal S, et al Mode and timing of twin delivery and perinatal outcomes in low- and middle-income countries: a secondary analysis of the WHO Multicountry Survey on Maternal and Newborn Health. WHO Multicountry Survey on Maternal and Newborn Health Research Network. BJOG. 2014 Mar;121 Suppl 1:89-100. doi: 10.1111/1471-0528.12635. PMID: 24641539

[59] Ezra O, Lahav-Ezra H, Zemet R, Mazaki-Tovi S, Barzilay E The effect of mode of delivery in twin pregnancies on the latency period between diagnosis of preterm labor and birth. J Matern Fetal Neonatal Med. 2020 Mar 26:1-7. doi: 10.1080/14767058.2020.1743659. Online ahead of print. PMID: 32212937

[60] Dodd JM, Crowther CA, Haslam RR, Robinson JS. Timing of birth for women with a twin pregnancy at term: a randomised controlled trial. BMC Pregnancy Childbirth. 2010 Oct 25;10:68. doi: 10.1186/1471-2393-10-68. PMID: 20973989

[61] Hack KE, Derks JB, Elias SG, van Mameren FA, Koopman-Esseboom C, Mol BW, Lopriore E, Schaap AH, Arabin B, et al. Perinatal mortality and mode of delivery in monochorionic diamniotic twin pregnancies 32 weeks of gestation: a multicentre retrospective cohort study. BJOG. 2011 Aug;118(9):1090-7. doi: 10.1111/j.1471-0528.2011.02955.x. Epub 2011 May 18. PMID: 21585638

[62] Dodd JM, Deussen AR, Grivell RM, Crowther CA. Elective birth at 37 weeks' gestation for women with an uncomplicated twin pregnancy. Cochrane Database Syst Rev. 2014 Feb 10;(2):CD003582. doi: 10.1002/14651858.CD003582.pub2. PMID: 24510739

[63] De Silva DA, Lisonkova S, von Dadelszen P, Synnes AR; Canadian Perinatal Network (CPN) Collaborative Group, Magee LA. Timing of delivery in a high-risk obstetric population: a clinical prediction model. BMC Pregnancy Childbirth. 2017 Jun 29;17(1):202. doi: 10.1186/s12884-017-1390-9. PMID: 28662632

[64] Dodd JM, Crowther CA. Elective delivery of women with a twin pregnancy from 37 weeks' gestation. Cochrane Database Syst Rev. 2003;(1):CD003582. doi: 10.1002/14651858.CD003582. PMID: 12535480

[65] Dodd JM, Crowther CA, Haslam RR, Robinson JS; Elective birth at 37 weeks of gestation versus standard care for women with an uncomplicated twin pregnancy at term: the Twins Timing of Birth Randomised Trial. Twins Timing of Birth Trial Group. BJOG. 2012 Jul;119(8):964-73. doi: 10.1111/j.1471-0528.2012.03356.x. Epub 2012 Jun 13. PMID: 22691051

[66] Dias T, Thilaganathan B. Elective birth at 37 weeks of gestation versus standard care for women with an uncomplicated twin pregnancy at term: the Twins Timing of Birth Randomised Trial. BJOG. 2012 Dec;119(13):1676; author reply 1676-7. doi: 10.1111/1471-0528.12000. PMID: 23164122

[67] Welsh A, Clements S, Henry A, Bisits A. Elective birth at 37 weeks of gestation versus standard care for women with an uncomplicated twin pregnancy at term: the Twins Timing of Birth Randomised Trial. BJOG. 2012

Dec;119(13):1675-6; author reply 1676-7. doi: 10.1111/1471-0528.12001. PMID: 23164120

[68] Yamazaki H, Torigoe K, Numata O, Nagai S, Haniu H, Uchiyama A, Ogawa Y, Imamura M, Hasegawa S. Neonatal clinical outcome after elective cesarean section before the onset of labor at the 37th and 38th week of gestation. Pediatr Int. 2003 Aug;45(4):379-82. doi: 10.1046/j.1442-200x.2003.01751.x. PMID: 12911470

[69] Han BR, Park KH, Lee SY, Jung EY, Park JW Prediction of the risk of cesarean delivery after labor induction in twin gestations based on clinical and ultrasound parameters. J Obstet Gynaecol Res. 2016 Sep;42(9):1125-31. doi: 10.1111/jog.13038. Epub 2016 May 16. PMID: 27199212

[70] Williams KP, Galerneau F. Intrapartum influences on cesarean delivery in multiple gestation. Acta Obstet Gynecol Scand. 2003 Mar;82(3):241-5. doi: 10.1034/j.1600-0412.2003.00098.x. PMID: 12694120

[71] Aviram A, Weiser I, Ashwal E, Bar J, Wiznitzer A, Yogev Y Combined vaginal-cesarean delivery of twins: risk factors and neonatal outcome--a single center. experience. J Matern Fetal Neonatal Med. 2015 Mar;28(5):509-14. doi: 10.3109/14767058.2014.927430. Epub 2014 Jun 18. PMID: 24853342

[72] Aviram A, Weiser I, Ashwal E, Bar J, Wiznitzer A, Yogev Y Intrapartum management of multiple gestations. Houlihan C, Knuppel RA. Clin Perinatol. 1996 Mar;23(1):91-116. PMID: 8689804 Review.

[73] Saccone G, Berghella V. .Planned delivery at 37 weeks in twins: a systematic review and meta-analysis of randomized controlled trials. J Matern Fetal Neonatal Med. 2016 Mar;29(5):685-9. doi: 10.3109/14767058.2015.1016423. Epub 2015 Feb 26. PMID: 25716078 Review.

[74] Inde Y, Satomi M, Iwasaki N, Ono S, Yamashita E, Igarashi M, Hiraizumi Y, Murata T, Miyake H, Suzuki S. Maternal risk factors for small-for-gestational age newborns in Japanese dichorionic twins. J Obstet Gynaecol Res. 2011 Jan;37(1):24-31. doi: 10.1111/j.1447-0756.2010.01301.x. Epub 2010 Nov 18.

Chapter 3

Cesarean Section and Breastfeeding Outcomes

Angeliki Antonakou and Dimitrios Papoutsis

Abstract

The cesarean section rates in the developed countries are well above the 5% to 15% rate of all births as suggested by the World Health Organization (WHO) in 2009 and currently range widely between 25% and 50%. Moreover, the WHO guidance promotes early breastfeeding initiation during the first hour postpartum, exclusive breastfeeding up until the 6th month and maintaining breastfeeding at least up to the second year of the infant's life. In this review, we discuss the current evidence on whether a cesarean section interferes with the initiation and the long-term duration of breastfeeding practice among new mothers. The literature shows that a cesarean birth does have a detrimental effect on breastfeeding outcomes, however it is not per se a negative factor. It rather seems that infants who have feeding difficulties in the immediate postpartum period may experience long term problems. Therefore, interventions are discussed to promote breastfeeding after cesarean section for health professionals. Emphasis is given on promoting early skin-to-skin contact and on counseling new mothers about the advantages of breastfeeding as well as providing practical support and guidance throughout the early postpartum period.

Keywords: breastfeeding, cesarean section, cesarean birth, outcomes, interventions, neonate, mode of birth

1. Introduction

Even though there is no global consensus on the optimal rate of cesarean section (CS), nevertheless the World Health Organization (WHO) advocates that this should be approximately 15% of all live births [1]. Many developed countries over the past 30 years are well in excess of this rate, without there being any significant improvement in either maternal or neonatal outcomes [2]. A study conducted on a worldwide scale using country-level data has found that as CS rates exceed 10% and increase up to 30% there is no essential effect on reducing maternal and neonatal morbidity or mortality rates. Moreover, the initial inverse relationship observed between CS rates and morbidity or mortality appears to be explained by socioeconomic factors [3].

The latest epidemiological data from Western countries has placed Greece among those with the highest CS rates reaching 54% for the year 2018 [4]. This rising CS trend however is not uncommon and represents a universal finding over the past decades [5]. The CS rate for 2019 in Canada was 29.1% [6] and for 2018 in the United States of America was 31.9% [7], whereas in the United Kingdom was 26.1% (**Figure 1**). Since an increasing number of women delay their first pregnancy

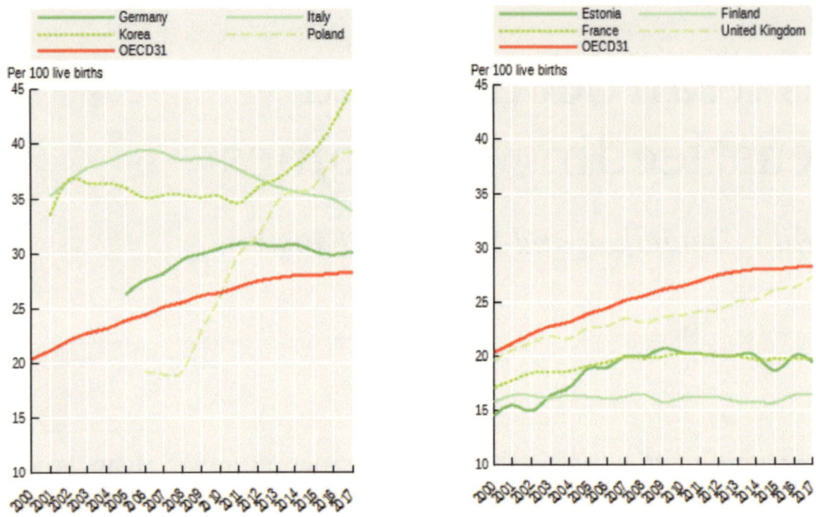

Figure 1.
Cesarean section trends in selected OECD countries for the time period between 2000 and 2017. (Source: OECD Health Statistics 2019. Access: https://DOI.org/10.1787/888934017937).

until after the third decade of their life and as the percentage of women with obesity is getting higher, this constitutes a high-risk environment for more CS births in the future [8]. At present, it is contemplated that one in three newborns are born with a CS worldwide.

2. Mode of birth and the neonate

2.1 Neonatal outcomes

Cesarean birth has been associated with a variety of adverse neonatal outcomes in the literature. Fetal and neonatal complications include the increased risk for neonatal intensive care unit admission, respiratory morbidity, and mother-infant separation with all its consequences [9]. While CS delivery has been regarded as a method to reduce the risk of neonatal asphyxia, Kupari et al. [10] in their review found that the rate of neonatal intensive care admissions is higher after a cesarean birth. A recent study at a university based-tertiary hospital in Jordan showed that 50.5% of all deliveries were by CS, and from those 72% were performed at term. However, 30% of the newborns with a cesarean birth were admitted to the neonatal intensive care unit (NICU). The rate of NICU admissions was 23% among the elective ceserean births when compared to 43% among the emergency ceserean births. It is noteworthy that among the term neonates who were admitted to the NICU almost two thirds were born by elective CS between 37 and $38^{6/7}$ weeks of gestation. Moreover, an estimated 18% of NICU admissions were complicated by sepsis and the mortality rate was 5% [11]. An earlier study also showed that an elective CS is associated with an almost two-fold increase in the rate of newborn transfers to the neonatal intensive care unit, and in the diagnosis of transient tachypnea of the newborn when compared with a planned vaginal birth [12].

Recent studies have highlighted the close interplay between host genetics, the prenatal environment and the route of birth on determining the newborn's microbiome at birth. There is emerging evidence that neonates born by CS have different hormonal, physical, bacterial, and medical exposures, and that these exposures can subtly alter their physiology. The short-term risks of CS include the altered immune system development, the increased likelihood of allergy, atopy and asthma, and the reduced diversity of the intestinal microbiome. It is not clear in the literature how these alterations might affect the children's health later on in life as young adults, although there is accumulating evidence of long-term effects. In the literature it is quoted that we have just started to realize the importance of the developing neonatal microbiome for the future health outcomes of the individual [13].

Formation of the microbiome begins *in utero* and the resulting disturbances may lead to changes in the fetal epigenetic programming [14]. Factors related to the labor and birth environment have been shown to influence the initial colonization process of the newborn microbiome. Studies have shown that there are distinct differences in the microbiome profiles of newborns born vaginally when compared to those born by CS [15]. The microbiome signature of pregnancy is dynamic and it changes throughout gestation even though the factors that regulate such changes are not yet fully understood [16]. It is possible that gestational changes in the microbiome may occur as a natural mechanism to prepare for the initial transfer of microbes to the newborns [15].

There is evidence showing that children born by a CS versus those born vaginally are more likely to develop immune-related disorders such as asthma and allergies [17], inflammatory bowel disease [17], and obesity [18]. These findings have led some researchers to suggest that the association between chronic disease and route of birth may be caused by alterations in the microbiome seeding of the neonate following the cesarean birth [19]. The hypothesis is that the mode of delivery affects the epigenetic state of the stem cells of the newborn, thus impacting on their plasticity and responsiveness later on in life [14]. It is important to note that neonates born to a CS when compared to neonates born vaginally have a smaller degree of similarity to the intestinal microbiome of their mother, which includes skin and oral cavity microbes, and bacteria from the operating room [18]. Furthermore, it has been shown that children with a slight exposure to their mother's vaginal microbiome during labor, even if they were delivered by a CS, have a reduced risk of developing asthma than those born with an elective CS [17].

There is evidence that the previously described differences in the microbiome remain long term, and the adults who were born with a CS have fecal microbiota that are distinctly different from those of adults who were born vaginally [20].

2.2 Alterations to the neonatal microbiome

It has been shown that for neonates born with a CS, their microbiome consists of different maternal microbiota than in neonates born vaginally. Bacteria from the operating room [18] have also been found to be present, while the antibiotics that women receive intrapartum to reduce the risk of post-operative infection may also affect the newborn's microbiome [21]. The question that has been raised in the literature is how the neonate can counter these alterations in its microbiome. An intervention that has been proposed involves the medical, midwifery and nursing personnel adopting a mother-friendly, family-centered approach in the operating room during the cesarean birth [15]. Early skin-to-skin contact with the neonate, early initiation of breastfeeding and support in a maternal-focused environment with a concurrent reduction of the time-spams of separation between the mother and the newborn while the neonate is hosted in the nursery, may also result in minimal disturbances to the neonatal microbiome. Breastfeeding after a cesarean birth may potentially be the way to minimize the adverse effects of the mode of delivery on the neonate's microbiome by promoting optimal early newborn microbiota formation. This may occur despite the effect of the antibiotics given to the mother during the CS, which have been found to lower the counts of *Bifidobacterium* species in breast milk that are known to prevent infection and to provide anticarcinogenic capacities to the newborn [22].

Epigenetic programming during the perinatal period may induce very important physiological changes to the neonate. Potential adverse events may lead to epigenetic changes with serious implications for health and disease. There are studies as discussed earlier that suggest that epigenetic alterations are linked to early life environmental stressors such as the mode of delivery. However, it seems that epigenetic modifications due to perinatal environmental exposures can be potentially reversible [14]. It seems that during the first 3 years of life starting from conception to the second birthday of the child, there is a high turnover of the different types of colonizing bacteria, after which the microbiome is more stable [23].

3. CS and breastfeeding

3.1 The benefits of breastfeeding to the neonate and the mother

Among the postnatal factors that may contribute to lifelong health and disease through epigenetic mechanisms, infant feeding seems to play a key role (**Table 1**) [23]. Maternal breast milk is universally considered to be the normative standard for infant feeding, as it confers unique nutritional and non-nutritional benefits that could in some extent be explained through epigenetics [24]. WHO promotes early breastfeeding initiation during the first hour postpartum, exclusive breastfeeding up until the 6th month and maintaining breastfeeding up to the second year of the infant's life or more in order to optimize its growth, development and good health [25]. The special content of breast milk with long chain poly-unsaturated fatty acids [26], oligosaccharides [27], lactoferrin [28] and other important nutrients makes it the ideal nutrition for newborns and infants.

A meta-analysis on the short-term effects of breastfeeding has indicated that breastfeeding reduces the severity of diarrhea and the risk of hospitalization and mortality due to respiratory infections by 72% and 77%, respectively [29]. With regards to the long-term effects of breastfeeding, another meta-analysis was performed by the World Health Organization in 2007 and was updated in 2013. The most recent meta-analysis suggests that a causal association exists between

Nutrition			
Maternal nutrition	**Neonatal & infant nutrition**	**Microbiome**	**Epigenome**
Over-/ under-nutrition	Breast milk	Maternal microbiota	Human genome
Vitamin D status	Formula milk	Mode of delivery	Environmental factors
Dietary methyl donors	Prebiotics/probiotics	Maternal & infant diet	
LCPUFA* intakes		Antenatal & post-natal antibiotic exposure	
Food pollutants		Urban/rural environment	

Data from Ref. [23].
**Long chain polyunsaturated fatty acids.*

Table 1.
Significant factors affecting the long term health outcomes over the first 1,000 days of life.

breastfeeding and the increased performance in intelligence (IQ) tests during childhood and adolescence, and has been estimated to lead to an average increase of 3.5 points of IQ score. Though the maternal intelligence scoring (IQ) was acknowledged as an important confounder, nevertheless it accounted for a small part of this association. The practical implications of this finding of the small increase of performance in intelligence tests are not yet clear [30].

The meta-analysis of 2013 also found a small reduction of about 10% in the prevalence of overweight or obese children exposed to longer durations of breastfeeding. However, there were confounding factors related to this finding since in the majority of study settings the duration of breastfeeding was higher in families with a higher educational and economic status. Breastfeeding was also found to have a protective effect against type-2 diabetes particularly among adolescents. Furthermore, a small protective effect of breastfeeding against systolic blood pressure was found, however as the authors state, residual confounding cannot be ruled out [30]. Finally, the American Association of Pediatrics [31] states that breastfeeding plays a protective role against the sudden infants death syndrome.

Breastfeeding confers numerous short-term and long-term benefits to the mother [25]. Women who do not breastfeed are in a greater risk of developing breast cancer and ovarian cancer [32, 33]. The protective role of breastfeeding is even greater among mothers with the BRCA1 mutation, and it has been estimated that those who breastfeed for at least one year have a 37% lower risk of breast cancer [34]. There is growing evidence indicating that breastfeeding seems to have a protective role against obesity later on in the mother's life [35]. Breastfeeding also confers a lower risk of developing diabetes mellitus [36] and hyperlipidemia [37]. Studies have shown that even a single month of breastfeeding significantly reduces the risk of developing diabetes in later life [38]. Finally, it seems that breastfeeding and especially long term with a duration of more than 7 months, reduces the maternal risk of hypertension and cardiovascular disease [39, 40].

3.2 Cesarean birth and the initiation of breastfeeding

Though the importance of breastfeeding is well established in the literature, the way by which the mode of delivery interferes with breastfeeding is still obscure. A systematic review and meta-analysis has shown that newborns born with a CS are almost half as likely to initiate breastfeeding before hospital discharge when compared to newborns born vaginally [41]. There is an abundance of literature reports since the late 1990's showing that women who deliver by CS are less likely to breastfeed and most probably will delay breastfeeding initiation. A recent study in Canada found that women planning to have a cesarean birth had no intention to breastfeed or did not initiate breastfeeding (7.4% and 4.3%, respectively) when compared to women with vaginal births (3.4% and 1.8%, respectively) [42]. This finding is further supported in the literature by a study from Ohio in the United States of America indicating that women who underwent a scheduled repeat cesarean delivery were less likely to initiate breastfeeding than those having a successful vaginal birth after a previous CS and those who ultimately delivered by cesarean birth after an unsuccessful trial of labor [43]. It seems that maternal choice for the mode of delivery may also influence her decision to breastfeed. This is a key element that needs to be thoroughly addressed by health care professionals, since to date the motivation of mothers to breastfeed is the most important determining factor for the success of breastfeeding. Another recent study in China calculated that the unadjusted odds ratio [OR] for lower breastfeeding rates associated with CS was 2.11 [95%CI: 1.58–2.81] and 1.36 [95%CI: 1.01–1.83] at the 5th day and 6th month post delivery. After adjusting for early breastfeeding behaviors, it is interesting that the negative effect of CS on long term breastfeeding was attenuated and was no longer significant. In fact, the authors of this study noted that although cesarean birth had a detrimental effect on early breastfeeding behaviors and long-term breastfeeding outcomes, it is not *per se* a negative factor. It rather seems that infants who have feeding difficulties in the immediate postpartum period may experience long-term feeding problems [44].

The main question therefore is whether being born with a CS increases the difficulties in breastfeeding. There is evidence that a CS can act as an independent risk factor for reduced breastfeeding rates due to the difficulties of early lactation for the mother and baby. In a recent study, women having a CS experienced more difficulties with breastfeeding, while those having an emergency CS were more likely to have an unsuccessful first breastfeeding attempt and were unable to breastfeed their baby within the first 24 h and upon leaving the hospital, than those having a vaginal birth [42]. These difficulties might originate from maternal reasons such as the adverse effect of the administered anesthesia drugs [45], postpartum maternal fatigue after a long eventful labor, or due to postpartum wound pain after the surgery [46]. Mothers after cesarean birth report greater pain scores when compared to those women having a vaginal birth, and more problems with latching on and positioning of the baby during breastfeeding [47]. Mothers after a cesarean birth need to deal with some practical difficulties, such as having to try to breastfeed with a drip in their arm, or not being able to move around easily and pick up their babies as easily as mothers after a vaginal birth. These minor issues can enhance maternal fatigue and postpartum depressive feelings following the birth [46].

Moreover, there has been fair discussion in the literature about the hormonal impact of cesarean birth on lactogenesis. Lactogenesis is the process of developing the ability to secrete milk and involves the maturation of alveolar cells. Stage I lactogenesis takes place during the second half of pregnancy whereas stage II lactogenesis starts with copious milk production after delivery. As the placenta detaches after the delivery of the neonate, there is a rapid drop in progesterone which enables the other hormones that are present in high levels such as prolactin, cortisol and insulin, to stimulate breast milk production. It has been noted that in primiparous women, stage II is slightly delayed and early milk volume is lower. A lower milk volume was also observed in women who had cesarean births compared with those who delivered vaginally [48]. It is postulated that the hormonal pathway that stimulates lactogenesis is disrupted by a CS delivery, either because of maternal stress or decreased oxytocin secretion, and can hinder the milk production [49]. This means that mothers following a cesarean birth may encounter more practical difficulties while trying to breastfeed than mothers after a vaginal birth [50].

Another issue is the breastfeeding difficulties of the new-born after the CS delivery. It has been noted that neonates after a cesarean birth are more likely to display poorly coordinated tongue movements and to perform unsatisfactory infant sucking activity [51] due to drug exposure or to a long tiring labour. Neonates born by CS are more likely to have mucus secretions, which can affect how interested they are in feeding [52]. Intravenous fluids administered during labour can cause mothers' breasts to become swollen, making it harder for the newborn to latch on properly [53].

Another important inhibiting factor to breastfeeding after a CS is the psychological factor, namely the loss of confidence. Mothers and especially those after an emergency CS might be less likely to believe in their ability to nurture and feed their baby as they experience increased feelings of failure. In addition, their family members are usually more likely to suggest offering formula milk to the newborns so they could rest after the surgery [52]. This suggestion may sometimes also originate from the health care personnel along with the advice to keep the newborn at the nursery for long periods of time or overnight in order for the mother to sleep. Long separation periods between the mother and newborn make lactation establishment more difficult. It is a vicious circle where mothers do not trust their body to produce enough milk, those around them make them feel that they are not capable of feeding their offspring and that leads mothers quitting breastfeeding before practically ever starting it [54].

One of the major factors that has been acknowledged for its contribution to breastfeeding success is the early onset of lactation. Unfortunately, it has been proven that cesarean birth neonates have a delay in their onset of lactation as in many cases mother to baby contact inside the operating theatre is delayed, and when offered it is usually shorter in duration than recommended or even absent [55, 56]. Skin-to-skin contact begins ideally at birth and should last continuously until the end of the first breastfeeding [57]. This practice involves placing the dried, naked newborn in a prone position on the mother's bare chest, and sometimes can be covered with a warm blanket. Women and newborns that practice skin-to-skin contact immediately after birth have been proven to show increased rates of breastfeeding at hospital discharge and up to six months postpartum [57].

3.3 Skin-to-skin contact after a cesarean birth

As mentioned above, early skin-to-skin contact is a key element for the success of breastfeeding as it leads to early initiation of breastfeeding and to the maternal hormonal response, that is the secretion of oxytocin and endorphins which are important to establish lactation [57]. Skin-to-skin contact provides however far more benefits for the mother and baby. This intimate contact evokes neurobehaviors that ensure the fulfillment of basic biological needs and affects the future programming of the infant's physiology and behavior [57]. It is beneficial for the newborns by improving their cardio-respiratory stability [57], their thermo- and glucose regulation [57, 58], and it also reduces the stress of birth while facilitating a smooth transition to extrauterine life [59]. Moreover, since newborns born by CS do not acquire maternal vaginal microbes, skin-to-skin contact immediately after birth permits the microbial colonization of the newborn with maternal skin microbiota [60]. Mothers after a cesarean birth also benefit by appropriate skin-to-skin contact with their newborns, since due to the boost in oxytocin secretion it has been found that the risk of postpartum hemorrhage is ameliorated [61]. In addition, it reduces maternal stress, anxiety, and pain during and after the CS delivery [57]. Long term, it seems that skin-to-skin contact has significant positive effects on reducing the maternal depressive symptoms and the physiological stress she experiences during the postnatal period [62].

Although the WHO guidelines [25] state that keeping the mother and baby together for at least the first hour after birth leads to an improved initiation and duration of breastfeeding, however it is not always as easy to apply for women having a CS and especially an emergency CS [63]. Nevertheless, skin-to-skin contact is recommended by the relevant health authorities such as the National Institute for Health and Care Excellence (NICE) [50] and the Pan American Health Organization [64]. It has been reported that early initiation and a long duration of skin-to-skin contact when compared to a short time duration, has a dose–response effect on breastfeeding [65]. A recent study has shown that for infants after vaginal delivery, the average time from birth to first breastfeeding was 40.91 minutes, while for CS newborns the average time was 74.54 minutes. The duration of the first breastfeeding was maintained for 18.33 minutes for babies after a vaginal delivery, and only 14.98 minutes for those after cesarean birth ($p = 0.00$). Newborns after a vaginal delivery maintained a longer sucking duration for the first ($p = 0.000$) and second ($p = 0.008$) day postpartum. Correspondingly, cesarean birth newborns were more frequently ($p = 0.000$) supplied with formula, and they consumed more volumes ($p = 0.000$) of formula within the first 72 hours after birth [44]. In another quasi-experimental feasibility study in the United States of America, it was shown that women who practiced immediate skin-to-skin contact with their newborns during their CS surgery (within one minute after birth) were more satisfied with the experience and had lower levels of salivary cortisol across time ($p = 0.015$ and $p = 0.003$ respectively) than those who practiced early skin-to-skin contact (within the first hour after birth) [66]. It has been reported in the literature that in those cases where the mother is not capable of performing skin-to-skin contact during the surgery then the father can hold the baby [66, 67]. Although this can be a reliable alternative, a recent study found a statistically significant association between skin-to-skin contact with the mother and the exclusive breastfeeding rates upon discharge, which was maintained at three- and six-months postpartum, when compared to the groups that had paternal skin-to-skin contact or no skin-to-skin contact at all [67].

3.4 Cesarean birth and the duration of breastfeeding

As already mentioned, there is scientific evidence showing that a CS can lead to the early discontinuation of breastfeeding [68]. On the other hand, there are earlier studies showing that cesarean birth does not affect the duration of breastfeeding if women initiate breastfeeding from the time point of birth and maintain it for at least four weeks postpartum [69]. In a recent prospective cohort study of 3,021 women in Canada, it was shown that the mode of birth is a significant independent predictor for breastfeeding cessation at or prior to 12 weeks postpartum ($p = 0.014$). In the adjusted multivariable logistic regression model, women who had a planned CS were more likely to have early cessation of breastfeeding [≤12 weeks] [OR = 1.61; 95%CI: 1.14-2.26; $p = 0.006$] when compared to those who

Independent variable	Unadjusted OR (95% CI)	Adjusted OR [95% CI]
Mode of birth[d]		--[b]
Emergency cesarean	1.35 (1.03-1.76)[b]	1.22 (0.91-1.62)[a]
Planned cesarean	1.33 (0.97-1.82)[a]	1.61 (1.14-2.26)[b]
Low income	1.61 (1.25-2.06)[c]	1.58 (1.19-2.09)[b]
Lower education	2.14 (1.61-2.85)[c]	1.82 (1.31-2.53)[c]
No previous birth	1.38 (1.13-1.68)[b]	1.42 (1.13-1.77)[b]
Preterm birth	1.66 (1.18-2.33)[b]	1.54 (1.06-2.23)[b]
Maternal physical health	0.96 (0.95-0.98)[c]	0.96 (0.94-0.98)[c]
Maternal mental health	0.99 (0.98-1.00)[b]	0.99 (0.97-0.99)[b]
Caucasian	1.49 (1.14-1.95)[b]	1.67 (1.25-2.22)[c]
≥ 1 breastfeeding difficulty	2.09 (1.67-2.61)[c]	1.82 (1.43-2.31)[c]

Reproduced from Hobbs et al. [42].
[a]*≥0.05.*
[b]*<0.05.*
[c]*<0.001.*
[d]*Reference group set as vaginal delivery.*

Table 2.
Unadjusted and adjusted logistic regression model of mode of delivery on the duration of breastfeeding up to 12-weeks postpartum.

delivered vaginally. There was no significant difference in breastfeeding cessation between women who had an emergency CS and women who delivered vaginally in the adjusted analysis [42] (**Table 2**).

Another study found that cesarean births were associated with lower rates of exclusive breastfeeding at 6 months, with no difference found between planned versus emergency CS [70].

There is a large systematic review and meta-analysis on breastfeeding outcomes after cesarean birth that included data of 53 studies from 33 different countries. Prior and colleagues (2012) identified lower rates of any breastfeeding and exclusive breastfeeding at 6 months among women who had a cesarean birth (planned or unplanned) when compared with a vaginal birth (normal or instrumental). However, based on a subgroup analysis they found that although cesarean birth was associated with lower rates of initiation, those mothers who did initiate successfully were as likely to exclusively breastfeed at 6 months with those who had a vaginal birth. This important finding suggests that early interventions could be very effective following a cesarean birth in terms of establishing lactation and continuation of breastfeeding for a long period of time [41].

4. Effective interventions to promote early breastfeeding initiation following a cesarean birth

4.1 Prenatal preparation

Decisions about infant feeding are determined by a range of complex factors including the woman's socio-demographic background, age, ethnicity, and peer support network [71]. To date, the most important factor for the success of breastfeeding is the mother's motivation. As it has been commented earlier, mothers planning to have a cesarean birth report lower level of willingness to breastfeed their offspring [42, 43]. It has been reported in the literature that all health professionals need to look closely into this fact and identify the reasons that drive women to this decision. Antenatal programs addressing the importance of breastfeeding both for mothers and babies, with emphasis to the key effects on CS newborns' health need to be implemented. There is a false impression that women after a CS are not able to breastfeed adequately their offspring and this involves the women themselves, their families and exists even among health professionals. As mentioned above, women after a CS may face more difficulties than women following a vaginal birth but with adequate help and consultation from health professionals and their family, they are able to provide the best nourishment to their newborns. The women themselves express lack of knowledge and skills about breastfeeding after the CS birth [54]. During the antenatal courses, midwives have the opportunity and ability to provide this knowledge in a secure relaxed environment and demonstrate coping strategies that women can easily rehearse and learn prior to their birth. This way their confidence will increase, and they will feel more confident and ready to breastfeed their newborns after their CS.

4.2 The importance of adequate bonding time

We know from the neuroendocrine mechanisms involved in the initiation and maintenance of lactogenesis that the mother-to-newborn contact is the most effective and powerful stimulus to milk production. Health professionals need to ensure undisturbed immediate or early skin-to-skin contact for mothers and their newborns after a cesarean birth. Skin-to-skin contact is a practice that requires minimal organizational effort or costs for the hospitals that offer it [67]. Numerous studies show that skin-to-skin contact is an easy to apply, low-cost and safe intervention that can have important health benefits both for the mother and newborn, as described in the previous sections. There are studies that prove the feasibility of applying this method to women undergoing an uncomplicated CS, and even on an emergent basis, while skin-to-skin contact can safely begin during surgery and continue uninterrupted for an extended time duration [66]. As an alternative, when the mother is not capable or willing to provide skin-to-skin contact, then the partner can assist and hold the newborn [67]. Furthermore, the health professionals need to ensure that the mother and newborn will have undisturbed time to bond by minimizing the separation time spams. This can be achieved with performing the clinical examination while the newborn is on the mother's arms, delaying the first newborn bath for after the first 24 hours, and by delaying the transfer of the mother while she is breastfeeding [50]. Rooming-in should be offered to all mothers as well as reassurance that the health professionals will be present to provide their assistance if needed, as the Family-Centered Care and the Baby-Friendly Hospital Initiative (BFHI) recommends [72]. Mothers following a cesarean birth will require more help handling their newborn, so the hospital policies should allow for a family member to be present or additional helping staff to be allocated. On the other hand, undisturbed bonding time with the newborn means that there should be a minimum number of visitors and in specified time frames during the hospital stay. Moreover, while breastfeeding there should be an indication on the door to keep people away from entering so as to preserve privacy and comfort.

4.3 Dealing with practical difficulties after a cesarean birth

In a recent qualitative study exploring the breastfeeding behavior of mothers following a cesarean birth, some of the main reported challenges for breastfeeding after a CS included the physical discomfort and the lack of knowledge and coping skills in managing their depressive mood after a CS [54]. It is important to realize that health professionals need to provide extra care and consultation to women after a CS. Women that feel greater levels of pain and discomfort are usually more easily to quit breastfeeding, as they feel that they are not able to do it properly. Health professionals need to provide encouragement, emotional support and empowerment to these women to adopt their nourishing role. They also need to provide adequate analgesia for mothers so as not to feel sore while breastfeeding [50]. It needs to be explicit that there are numerous analgesic and antibiotic drugs that are compatible with breastfeeding and women and their families need to be aware of that. At this point, it is important to comment that mothers who require anesthesia or sedation sometimes may receive inconsistent information from health care professionals regarding the passage of drugs into their breast milk. This can potentially lead to the interruption of feeding, discarding of their breast milk or early cessation of breastfeeding. A recent consensus document launched by the Association of Anesthetists and endorsed by the Royal College of Midwives and the Royal College of Obstetricians and Gynecologists clearly states that '*breastfeeding is acceptable to continue after anesthesia and should be supported as soon as the woman is alert and able to breastfeed, and that breast milk should not be discarded*' [73].

Health professionals need to provide consultation and guidance on a more practical level such as advising on different breastfeeding positions that women may find useful and comfortable after the surgery [50]. Midwives need to assist newborns to latch on effectively, especially if they are drowsy from medication or if the mothers' breasts are engorged after having intravenous fluids. They also need to ensure that the newborn is feeding frequently. In case the newborn cannot breastfeed directly, they should assist the mother to express her milk and provide it to her newborn, so that the milk supply will be maintained and promoted.

Another very important element for health professionals is to provide the accurate birth weight to CS newborns. Researchers propose that using newborns' weight at 24 hours rather than the immediate weight after birth, could be a more accurate reference for weight loss and in turn could support breastfeeding by reducing supplementation rates in the absence of a clinical need. We know that fluids administered intravenously during labor due to the transplacental passage could lead to the newborn's weight inflation immediately after a cesarean birth [74]. In a recent study, it was noted that when the 24-hour weight was used as a reference among healthy full-term newborns delivered by CS, the overall supplementation rate decreased from 43.6% pre-intervention to 27.4% post-intervention, and in first-time mothers from 51.9% to 31.0% [75]. Thus, health professionals need to take under consideration these findings and not easily attribute any newborn's loss of weight to the lack of adequate milk supply which in turn can easily enhance maternal stress and lead to formula supplementation and no or less breastfeeding.

Women following a cesarean birth tend to face more practical difficulties with breastfeeding than women following a vaginal birth. Therefore, midwives and health professionals will need to offer ongoing support providing necessary advice and consultation on practical issues such as breastfeeding positions. Some comfortable breastfeeding positions for mothers after a cesarean birth include the following:

a. Lying down on the side position: This position keeps pressure away from the CS scar and is quite restful for the mother and baby, and the hand with the cannula does not pose any extra difficulties. However, the mother might need some extra help to roll over and breastfeed from the other side.

b. Lying back breastfeeding position: The mother is not sitting upright as she is laying backwards, and her body is supporting the baby's weight. The baby can be put diagonally so it does not apply pressure on the wound.

c. Rugby ball or under the arm position: The mother uses pillows to support her back and her baby under her arm. This position also keeps the baby away from the wound.

There are many different breastfeeding positions that a mother after a cesarean birth can try while breastfeeding. The most important element is to find a comfortable position for her that she can maintain for as long as her baby wants to feed. She also needs to feel free to ask for assistance from the health personnel while in hospital and from her family members while at home. It has been mentioned in the literature that women following a cesarean birth were not feeling comfortable asking for help from the health professionals as they considered it being a sign of failure, so they tried to endure as long as they could. This eventually led to exhaustion, frustration and the decision to quit breastfeeding quite early [54].

4.4 The significance of peer support and the partner's role

There is a growing trend on the use of social media and mothers' support groups among new mothers to find support and guidance while breastfeeding. The WHO has recently commented in a positive manner on their effectiveness to encourage women while breastfeeding. A recent Cochrane database systematic review on interventions for promoting the initiation of breastfeeding included 107,362 women from seven countries and found low-quality evidence that healthcare professional-led breastfeeding education and non-healthcare professional-led counseling and peer support interventions can result in some improvements in the number of women beginning to breastfeed [76]. Another systematic review that tried to identify effective interventions for women having a cesarean birth to increase uptake and duration of breastfeeding, identified a limited number of effective interventions such as immediate or early skin-to-skin contact, parent education, the provision of side-bed bassinets when rooming-in, and the use of breast pumps. However, there was one study that tested a bundle intervention consisting of parent education and targeted breastfeeding support and found an increased initiation and continuation of breastfeeding [77]. Both of the above mentioned systematic reviews conclude that more research is needed to explore the effectiveness of several interventions that are initiated prior to conception or during pregnancy and postpartum.

The role of the father or partner during breastfeeding has also been supported in the literature. A quasi-experimental study in China has shown that families where fathers in the antenatal period were specifically informed about ways to support their wives with breastfeeding, maintained exclusive breastfeeding at four and six months postpartum in a larger proportion than families who received standard antenatal care [78]. A recent systematic review highlighted the value of including fathers or partners in interventions to support breastfeeding. The review showed that the inclusion of fathers or partners in breastfeeding interventions improves breastfeeding initiation, duration, and exclusivity rates. Interventions that include face-to-face information delivery, that are designed in a culturally appropriate manner, and provide information on how partners can support breastfeeding are more likely to have a beneficial effect [79]. In a recent qualitative study from Canada, it was shown that fathers themselves perceived their role as much more complex than the limited role of a breastfeeding facilitator that is usually attributed to them. They see themselves as stakeholders in decision-making on how their child is to be fed and they react to the imbalance created by breastfeeding. They want to be considered as partners during the decision-making and they acknowledge the importance of providing emotional and practical support to their breastfeeding spouses. The researchers of this study comment that health professionals need to include fathers in the parental preparation programs and should find ways to support them effectively in managing their various roles [80].

5. Conclusion

Cesarean births represent almost one third of all births globally. There is evidence showing that this medical intervention has an impact on women's infant feeding decision and leads to important breastfeeding difficulties that involve mainly the initiation and duration of breastfeeding. The WHO promotes breastfeeding as the ideal nutrition for all newborns and infants up to the sixth month of their life, and at least up to the second year supplemented with solid foods. Health professionals can play an important role on promoting women's breastfeeding behaviors after a cesarean section. Through high quality antenatal education programs they can assist women to change their attitudes and beliefs concerning the feasibility of breastfeeding after a CS and help them become more confident and committed. The preparation for breastfeeding after a CS should ideally start in the antenatal period. Health professionals can also implement immediate and uninterrupted skin-to-skin contact and minimize separation as the standard of care during and after an uncomplicated cesarean birth. They can also provide advice and important guidance and practical support after the birth to mothers and their family members to create a strong support network. The network of family members alongside allocated health professionals can effectively assist during the lactation process in order to ensure that both the mother and infant receive the benefits of long-term breastfeeding.

Conflict of interest

The authors declare no conflict of interest.

Author details

Angeliki Antonakou[1*] and Dimitrios Papoutsis[2]

1 Midwifery Department, School of Health Science, International Hellenic University, Greece

2 Midwifery Department, School of Health Science, University of Western Macedonia, Greece

*Address all correspondence to: angelantonakou@gmail.com

References

[1] Monitoring emergency obstetric care: A handbook, Geneva: World Health Organization; 2009.

[2] WHO statement on cesarean section rates: WHO; 2019. Available from: https://www.who.int/reproductivehealth/publications/maternal_perinatal_health/cs-statement/en/ [Accessed 2021-01-02]

[3] Ye J, Zhang J, Mikolajczyk R, Torloni MR, Gülmezoglu AM, Betrán AP. Association between rates of cesarean section and maternal and neonatal mortality in the 21st century: a worldwide population-based ecological study with longitudinal data. BJOG. 2016 Apr;123(5):745-753. DOI: 10.1111/1471-0528.13592.

[4] WHO Greece commits to addressing excessive reliance on cesarean sections. Available from http://www.euro.who.int/en/countries/greece/news/news/2016/11/greece-commits-to-addressing-excessive-reliance-on-cesarean-sections [Accessed 2021-01-02]

[5] Betrán AP, Ye J, Moller AB, Zhang J, Gülmezoglu AM, Torloni MR. The Increasing Trend in cesarean Section Rates: Global, Regional and National Estimates: 1990-2014. PLoS One. 2016;11(2):e0148343. DOI:10.1371/journal.pone.0148343.

[6] Gu J, Karmakar-Hore S, Hogan ME, Azzam HM, Barrett JFR, Brown A, Cook JL, Jain V, Melamed N, Smith GN, Zaltz A, Gurevich Y. Examining cesarean Section Rates in Canada Using the Modified Robson Classification. J Obstet Gynaecol Can. 2020 Jun;42(6):757-765. DOI: 10.1016/j.jogc.2019.09.009.

[7] CDC – Methods of delivery. Available from https://www.cdc.gov/nchs/fastats/delivery.html [Accessed 2021-01-02]

[8] Papoutsis D, Antonakou A, Gornall A, Tzavara C, Mohajer M. The SaTH risk-assessment tool for the prediction of emergency cesarean section in women having induction of labor for all indications: a large-cohort based study. Arch Gynecol Obstet. 2017;295(1):59-66. DOI: 10.1007/s00404-016-4209-4.

[9] Gould JB, Danielsen B, Korst LM, Phibbs R, Chance K, Main E, et al. cesarean delivery rates and neonatal morbidity in a low-risk population. Obstet Gynecol. 2004;104(1):11-19. DOI: 10.1097/01.AOG.0000127035.64602.97.

[10] Kupari M, Talola N, Luukkaala T, Tihtonen K. Does an increased cesarean section rate improve neonatal outcome in term pregnancies? Arch Gynecol Obstet. 2016;294(1):41-46. DOI: 10.1007/s00404-015-3942-4

[11] Khasawneh W, Obeidat N, Yusef D, Alsulaiman J. The impact of cesarean section on neonatal outcomes at a university-based tertiary hospital in Jordan. BMC Pregnancy Childbirth 2020; 20, 335 DOI.org/10.1186/s12884-020-03027-2.

[12] Kolas T, Saugstad OD, Daltveit AK, Nilsen ST, Oian P. Planned cesarean versus planned vaginal delivery at term: Comparison of newborn infant outcomes. American Journal of Obstetrics and Gynecology. 2006;195(6):1538-1543. DOI: 10.1016/j.ajog.2006.05.005.

[13] Sandall J, Tribe RM, Avery L, Mola G, Visser GH, Homer CS et al. Short-term and long term effects of cesarean section on the health of women and children. Lancet. 2018;392(10155):1349-1357. DOI: 10.1016/S0140-6736[18]31930-5.

[14] Linnér A, Almgren M. Epigenetic programming-The important first 1000

days. Acta Paediatr. 2020;109(3):443-452. DOI: 10.1111/apa.15050

[15] Dunn AB, Jordan S, Baker BJ, Carlson NS. The Maternal Infant Microbiome: Considerations for Labor and Birth. MCN Am J Matern Child Nurs. 2017;42(6):318-325. DOI: 10.1097/NMC.0000000000000373.

[16] Aagaard K, Riehle K, Ma J, Segata N, Mistretta TA, Coarfa C, et al. A metagenomic approach to characterization of the vaginal microbiome signature in pregnancy. PLoS One. 2012;7(6):e36466. DOI: 10.1371/journal.pone.0036466.

[17] Kristensen K, Henriksen L. cesarean section and disease associated with immune function. Journal of Allergy and Clinical Immunology. 2016;137(2):587-590. DOI: 10.1016/j.jaci.2015.07.040

[18] Bernardi JR, Pinheiro TV, Mueller NT, Goldani HA, Gutierrez MR, Bettiol H et al. cesarean delivery and metabolic risk factors in young adults: A Brazilian birth cohort study. American Journal of Clinical Nutrition. 2015;102(2)1:295-301. DOI: 10.3945/ajcn.114.105205.

[19] Dominguez-Bello MG, De Jesus-Laboy KM, Shen N, Cox LM, Amir A, Gonzalez A, Clemente JC. Partial restoration of the microbiota of cesarean-born infants with a vaginal microbial transfer. Nature Medicine. 2016;22(6):250-253. DOI: 10.1038/nm.4039.

[20] Goedert JJ, Hua X, Yu G, Shi J. Diversity and composition of the adult fecal microbiome associated with history of cesarean birth or appendectomy: Analysis of the American Gut Project. EBioMedicine. 2014;1(2-3):167-172. DOI: 10.1016/j.ebiom.2014.11.004.

[21] Smaill FM, Grivell RM. Antibiotic prophylaxis versus no prophylaxis for preventing infection after cesarean section. Cochrane Database Systematic Reviews. 2014;(10):CD007482. DOI: 10.1002/14651858.CD007482.pub3.

[22] Quigley L, O'Sullivan O, Stanton C, Beresford TP, Ross RP, Fitzgerald GF, et al. The complex microbiota of raw milk. FEMS Microbiology Reviews. 2013;37(5):664-698. DOI: 10.1111/1574-6976.12030.

[23] Indrio F, Martini S, Francavilla R, Corvaglia L, Cristofori F, Mastrolia SA et al. Epigenetic Matters: The Link between Early Nutrition, Microbiome, and long term Health Development. Front Pediatr. 2017;5:178. DOI: 10.3389/fped.2017.00178.

[24] Koletzko B, Brands B, Poston L, Godfrey K, Demmelmair H. Early Nutrition Project. Early nutrition programming of long term health. Proc Nutr Soc. 2012; 71(3):371-378.

[25] World Health Organization. Protecting, promoting and supporting breastfeeding in facilities providing maternity and newborn services Guideline. Geneva 2017. ISBN 978-92-4-155008-6 Available from https://www.who.int/nutrition/publications/guidelines/breastfeeding-facilities-maternity-newborn/en/ [Accessed 2021-01-02]

[26] Antonakou A, Skenderi KP, Chiou A, Anastasiou CA, Bakoula C, Matalas AL. Breast milk fat concentration and fatty acid pattern during the first six months in exclusively breastfeeding Greek women. Eur J Nutr. 2013;52(3):963-973. DOI: 10.1007/s00394-012-0403-8.

[27] Weng M, Walker WA. The role of gut microbiota in programming the immune phenotype. J Dev Orig Health Dis. 2013;4(3):203-214. DOI: 10.1017/S2040174412000712.

[28] Minekawa R, Takeda T, Sakata M, Hayashi M, Isobe A, Yamamoto T et al.

Human breast milk suppresses the transcriptional regulation of IL-1beta-induced NF-kappaB signaling in human intestinal cells. Am J Physiol Cell Physiol. 2004;287(5):C1404-C1411. DOI: 10.1152/ajpcell.00471.2003.

[29] Horta B, Victora C. Short-term effects of breastfeeding: a systematic review on the benefits of breastfeeding on diarrhea and pneumonia mortality. WHO Library Cataloguing-in-Publication Data. ISBN 978 92 4 150612 0

[30] Horta B, Victora C. long term effects of breastfeeding: a systematic review. WHO Library Cataloguing-in-Publication Data. ISBN 978 92 4 150530 7

[31] AAP TASK FORCE ON SUDDEN INFANT DEATH SYNDROME. SIDS and Other Sleep-Related Infant Deaths: Updated 2016 Recommendations for a Safe Infant Sleeping Environment. Pediatrics. 2016;138(5):e20162938. DOI: 10.1542/peds.2016-2938

[32] Schwarz E, Nothnagle M. The Maternal Health Benefits of Breastfeeding. Am Fam Physician. 2015;91(9):602-604. PMID: 25955734.

[33] Luan NN, Wu QJ, Gong TT, Vogtmann E, Wang YL, Lin B. Breastfeeding and ovarian cancer risk: a meta-analysis of epidemiologic studies. Am J Clin Nutr. 2013;98(4):1020-1031. DOI: 10.3945/ajcn.113.062794.

[34] Pan H, He Z, Ling L, Ding Q, Chen L, Zha X et al. Reproductive factors and breast cancer risk among BRCA1 or BRCA2 mutation carriers: results from ten studies. Cancer Epidemiol. 2014;38(1):1-8. DOI: 10.1016/j.canep.2013.11.004.

[35] Bobrow KL, Quigley MA, Green J, Reeves GK, Beral V; Million Women Study Collaborators. Persistent effects of women's parity and breastfeeding patterns on their body mass index: results from the Million Women Study. Int J Obes (Lond). 2013;37(5):712-717. DOI: 10.1038/ijo.2012.76.

[36] Jäger S, Jacobs S, Kröger J, Fritsche A, Schienkiewitz A, Rubin D et al. Breast-feeding and maternal risk of type 2 diabetes: a prospective study and meta-analysis. Diabetologia. 2014;57(7):1355-1365. DOI: 10.1007/s00125-014-3247-3.

[37] StuebeAM,KleinmanK,GillmanMW, Rifas-Shiman SL, Gunderson EP, Rich-Edwards J. Duration of lactation and maternal metabolism at 3 years postpartum. J Womens Health (Larchmt). 2010;19(5):941-950. DOI: 10.1089/jwh.2009.1660.

[38] Schwarz EB, Brown JS, Creasman JM, Stuebe A, McClure CK, Van Den Eeden SK, et al. Lactation and maternal risk of type 2 diabetes: a population-based study. Am J Med. 2010;123(9):863.e1-6. DOI: 10.1016/j.amjmed.2010.03.016

[39] Schwarz EB, Ray RM, Stuebe AM, Allison MA, Ness RB, Freiberg MS et al. Duration of lactation and risk factors for maternal cardiovascular disease. Obstet Gynecol. 2009;113(5):974-982. DOI: 10.1097/01.AOG.0000346884.67796.ca.

[40] Stuebe AM, Schwarz EB, Grewen K, Rich-Edwards JW, Michels KB, Foster EM et al. Duration of lactation and incidence of maternal hypertension: a longitudinal cohort study. Am J Epidemiol. 2011;174(10):1147-1158. DOI: 10.1093/aje/kwr227.

[41] Prior E, Santhakumaran S, Gale C, Philipps LH, Modi N, Hyde MJ. Breastfeeding after cesarean delivery: A systematic review and meta-analysis of world literature. The Am J Clin Nutr. 2012;95(5):1113-1135. DOI: 10.3945/ajcn.111.030254.

[42] Hobbs AJ, Mannion CA, McDonald SW, Brockway M,

Tough S. The impact of cesarean section on breastfeeding initiation, duration and difficulties in the first four months postpartum. BMC Pregnancy Childbirth 2016;16(90). DOI:10.1186/s12884-016-0876-1

[43] Regan J, Thompson A, DeFranco E. The influence of mode of delivery on breastfeeding initiation in women with a prior cesarean delivery: a population-based study. Breastfeed Med. 2013;8(2):181-186. DOI: 10.1089/bfm.2012.0049.

[44] Zhang F, Cheng J, Yan S, Wu H, Bai T. Early feeding behaviors and breastfeeding outcomes after cesarean section. Breastfeed Med 2019;(5):325e33. DOI:10.1089/bfm.2018.0150.

[45] Cobb B, Liu R, Valentine E, Onuoha O. Breastfeeding after Anesthesia: A Review for Anesthesia Providers Regarding the Transfer of Medications into Breast Milk. Transl Perioper Pain Med. 2015;1(2):1-7. PMID: 26413558; PMCID: PMC4582419.

[46] Lai YL, Hung CH, Stocker J, Chan TF, Liu Y. Postpartum fatigue, baby-care activities, and maternal-infant attachment of vaginal and cesarean births following rooming-in. Appl Nurs Res. 2015;28(2):116-120. DOI: 10.1016/j.apnr.2014.08.002.

[47] Brown A, Jordan S. Impact of birth complications on breastfeeding duration: an internet survey. J Adv Nurs. 2013;69(4):828-839. DOI: 10.1111/j.1365-2648.2012.06067.x.

[48] Pillay J, Davis TJ. Physiology, Lactation. [Updated 2020 Jul 26]. In: StatPearls [Internet]. Treasure Island [FL]: StatPearls Publishing; 2020 Jan-. Available from: https://www.ncbi.nlm.nih.gov/books/NBK499981/ [Accessed 2021-01-05]

[49] Hyde MJ, Mostyn A, Modi N, Kemp PR. The health implications of birth by cesarean section. Biol Rev. 2012;87(1):229-243. DOI: 10.1111/j.1469-185X.2011.00195.x

[50] NICE. [2019] cesarean section [CG132]. Published date: 23 November 2011 Last updated: 04 September 2019 Available from: https://www.nice.org.uk/guidance/cg132 [Accessed 2021-01-05]

[51] Sakalidis V, Williams T, Hepworth A, Garbin C, Hartmann P, Paech M, et al. A Comparison of Early Sucking Dynamics During Breastfeeding After cesarean Section and Vaginal Birth. Breastfeeding Medicine. 2013;(1)79-85. DOI:10.1089/bfm.2012.0018

[52] Tully KP, Ball HL. Maternal accounts of their breast-feeding intent and early challenges after cesarean childbirth. Midwifery. 2014;30(6):712-719. DOI: 10.1016/j.midw.2013.10.014.

[53] Genna C. Supporting sucking skills in breastfeeding infants. 3rd ed. Jones and Bartlett Learning, Burlington; 2017 p.65-88. ISBN-13: 978-1284093919

[54] Wen J, Yu G, Kong Y, Liu F, Wei H. An exploration of the breastfeeding behaviors of women after cesarean section: A qualitative study. Int J Nurs Sci. 2020;7(4):419-426. DOI: 10.1016/j.ijnss.2020.07.008.

[55] Cadwell K, Brimdyr K, Phillips R. Mapping, Measuring, and Analyzing the Process of Skin-to-Skin Contact and Early Breastfeeding in the First Hour After Birth. Breastfeed Med. 2018;13(7):485-492. DOI: 10.1089/bfm.2018.0048.

[56] Brimdyr K, Cadwell K, Stevens J, Takahashi Y. An implementation algorithm to improve skin-to-skin practice in the first hour after birth. Matern Child Nutr. 2018;14(2):e12571. DOI: 10.1111/mcn.12571.

[57] Moore ER, Bergman N, Anderson GC, Medley N. Early skin-to-skin contact for mothers and their healthy newborn infants. Cochrane Database of Systematic Reviews 2016, Issue 11. Art. No.: CD003519. DOI: 10.1002/14651858.CD003519.pub4. Accessed 03 January 2021.

[58] Safari K, Saeed AA, Hasan SS, Moghaddam-Banaem L. The effect of mother and newborn early skin-to-skin contact on initiation of breastfeeding, newborn temperature and duration of third stage of labor. Int Breastfeed J 2018;13 (32). DOI: 10.1186/s13006-018-0174-9

[59] Takahashi Y, Tamakoshi K, Matsushima M, Kawabe T. Comparison of salivary cortisol, heart rate, and oxygen saturation between early skin-to-skin contact with different initiation and duration times in healthy, full-term infants. Early Hum Dev. 2011;87(3):151-157. DOI: 10.1016/j.earlhumdev.2010.11.012.

[60] Dominguez-Bello MG, Costello EK, Contreras M, Magris M, Hidalgo G, Fierer N et al. Delivery mode shapes the acquisition and structure of the initial microbiota across multiple body habitats in newborns. Proc Natl Acad Sci U S A. 2010;107(26):11971-11975. DOI: 10.1073/pnas.1002601107.

[61] Karimi FZ, Heidarian Miri H, Salehian M, Khadivzadeh T, Bakhshi M. The Effect of Mother-Infant Skin to Skin Contact after Birth on Third Stage of Labor: A Systematic Review and Meta-Analysis. Iran J Public Health. 2019;48(4):612-620. PMID: 31110971; PMCID: PMC6500522

[62] Bigelow A, Power M, MacLellan-Peters J, Alex M, McDonald C. Effect of mother/infant skin-to-skin contact on postpartum depressive symptoms and maternal physiological stress. J Obstet Gynecol Neonatal Nurs. 2012;41(3):369-382. DOI: 10.1111/j.1552-6909.2012.01350.x.

[63] Gouchon S, Gregori D, Picotto A, Patrucco G, Nangeroni M, di Giulio P. Skin-to-skin contact after cesarean delivery: an experimental study. Nursing Research. 2010; 59(2):78– 84. DOI: 10.1097/NNR.0b013e3181d1a8bc

[64] Stevens J, Schmied V, Burns E, Dahlen H. Immediate or early skin-to-skin contact after a cesarean section: a review of the literature. Matern Child Nutr. 2014; 10(4):456-473. DOI: 10.1111/mcn.12128.

[65] Bramson L, Lee JW, Moore E, Montgomery S, Neish C, Bahjri K, et al. Effect of early skin-to-skin mother--infant contact during the first 3 hours following birth on exclusive breastfeeding during the maternity hospital stay. J Hum Lact. 2010;26(2):130-137. DOI: 10.1177/0890334409355779.

[66] Crenshaw JT, Adams ED, Gilder RE, DeButy K, Scheffer KL. Effects of Skin-to-Skin Care During cesareans: A Quasiexperimental Feasibility/Pilot Study. Breastfeed Med. 2019;14(10): 731-743. DOI: 10.1089/bfm.2019.0202.

[67] Guala A, Boscardini L, Visentin R, Angellotti P, Grugni L, Barbaglia M et al. Skin-to-Skin Contact in cesarean Birth and Duration of Breastfeeding: A Cohort Study. ScientificWorldJournal. 2017;2017:1940756. DOI: 10.1155/2017/1940756.

[68] Brown A, Jordan S. Impact of birth complications on breastfeeding duration: an internet survey. J Adv Nurs. 2013;69(4):828-839. DOI: 10.1111/j.1365-2648.2012.06067.x.

[69] Pérez-Escamilla R, Maulén-Radovan I, Dewey KG. The association between cesarean delivery and breast-feeding outcomes among Mexican women. Am J Public Health. 1996

Jun;86(6):832-836. DOI: 10.2105/ajph.86.6.832.

[70] Zanardo V, Pigozzo A, Wainer G, Marchesoni D, Gasparoni A, Di Fabio S et al. Early lactation failure and formula adoption after elective cesarean delivery: Cohort study. Archives of Disease in Childhood: Fetal and Neonatal Edition. 2013;98(1). DOI:10.1136/archdischild-2011-301218

[71] McAndrew F, Thompson J, Fellows L, Large A, Speed M, Renfrew M. Infant feeding survey 2010: Summary. Health and Social Care Information Centre. Available at http://www.hscic.gov.uk/catalogue/PUB08694 [Accessed 2021-01-05]

[72] Theo LO, Drake E. Rooming-In: Creating a Better Experience. J Perinat Educ. 2017;26(2):79-84. DOI:10.1891/1058-1243.26.2.79

[73] Mitchell J, Jones W, Winkley E, Kinsella SM. Guideline on anaesthesia and sedation in breastfeeding women 2020. Anaesthesia 2020;75: 1482-1493. DOI:10.1111/anae.15179.

[74] Chantry CJ, Dewey KG, Peerson JM, Wagner EA, Nommsen-Rivers LA. In-hospital formula use increases early breastfeeding cessation among first-time mothers intending to exclusively breastfeed. J Pediatr. 2014;164(6):1339-45.e5. DOI: 10.1016/j.jpeds.2013.12.035.

[75] Deng X, McLaren M. Using 24-Hour Weight as Reference for Weight Loss Calculation Reduces Supplementation and Promotes Exclusive Breastfeeding in Infants Born by cesarean Section. Breastfeed Med. 2018;13(2):128-134. DOI: 10.1089/bfm.2017.0124.

[76] Balogun OO, O'Sullivan EJ, McFadden A, Ota E, Gavine A, Garner CD, et al. Interventions for promoting the initiation of breastfeeding. Cochrane Database Syst Rev. 2016 Nov 9;11(11):CD001688. DOI: 10.1002/14651858.CD001688.pub3.

[77] Beake S, Bick D, Narracott C, Chang YS. Interventions for women who have a cesarean birth to increase uptake and duration of breastfeeding: A systematic review. Matern Child Nutr. 2017;13(4):e12390. DOI:10.1111/mcn.12390

[78] Su M, Ouyang YQ. Father's Role in Breastfeeding Promotion: Lessons from a Quasi-Experimental Trial in China. Breastfeed Med. 2016;11:144-149. DOI: 10.1089/bfm.2015.0144.

[79] Abbass-Dick J, Brown HK, Jackson KT, Rempel L, Dennis CL. Perinatal breastfeeding interventions including fathers/partners: A systematic review of the literature. Midwifery. 2019;75:41-51. DOI: 10.1016/j.midw.2019.04.001.

[80] De Montigny Fr, Gervais Ch, Larivière-Bastien D, St-Arneault K. The role of fathers during breastfeeding. Midwifery. 2018; 58: 6-12 DOI:10.1016/j.midw.2017.12.001

Chapter 4

VTE Prophylaxis in Cesarean Section

Frederico José Amédeé Péret and Liv Braga de Paula

Abstract

Venous thromboembolism (VT is a major cause of maternal mortality and severe morbidity. Pharmacological and non-pharmacological methods of prophylaxis are therefore often used for women considered to be a risk including women who have given birth by cesarean section. The risk is potentially increased in women with a personal or family history of VTE, women with genetic or acquired thrombophilia, and another risk factors like sickle cell disease, inflammatory bowel disease, active cancer, obesity, preeclampsia·and SARS COVID 19 infection. However, a specific score in obstetrics has not yet been well defined. Recommendations from major society guidelines for post-cesarean section (C/S) thromboprophylaxis differ greatly; the safety and efficacy of drug prophylaxis - mainly low molecular weight heparins - has been demonstrated, but large scale randomized trials of currently-used interventions should be conducted. The purpose of this chapter is to discuss the indications and contraindications for VTE prophylaxis in cesarean sections, prophylaxis regimens and potential adverse events.

Keywords: VTE, DVT, cesarean section, thromboprophylaxis, heparin

1. Introduction

Venous thromboembolism (VTE) is a major cause of maternal morbidity and mortality. The risk of VTE is particularly elevated during the postpartum period and especially after cesarean section (CS) delivery. The risk of VTE was fourfold greater following CS than following vaginal delivery; seemed independent of other VTE risk factors; and was greater following emergency CS than following elective procedures [1].

Although a number of risk factors have been identified, the size of the increases in risk attributable to these factors is generally poorly quantified and there is considerable variation in the approach to prophylaxis of venous thromboembolism after CS [2–5].

In women with risk factors a combination of pharmacological and non-pharmacological methods are recommended. There is limited literature on the effect of mechanical methods for postpartum thromboprophylaxis, however benefit has been shown in other clinical areas [2, 4].

Antithrombotic prophylaxis are based on unfractionated heparin (UFH), low-molecular weight heparin (LMWH). LMWH was associated with fewer adverse effects when compared with UFH. Therefore, LMWH is considered to be a safe and effective in for postpartum thromboprophylaxis, although high-quality evidence is not available [1, 2].

 IntechOpen

In this chapter we will discuss the risk factors for VTE, their interactions and potential risk scores, as well as the prophylaxis alternatives and international guidelines for the prevention of VTE.

2. Epidemiology of VTE in pregnancy and puerperium

Women during pregnancy and the immediate puerperal period are considered at risk for VTE and there is a substantially higher prevalence that in non-pregnant women of the same age. A case-control study reported that compared with non-pregnant women, the risk of VTE was increased five-fold during pregnancy, and by 60-fold during the first three months after birth. However the absolute risk remains low, estimated at around one to two in 1000 pregnancies [6, 7].

The incidence of VTE, especially Pulmonary Embolism (PE), is believed to be much higher during the immediate puerperal period - mostly associated with cesarean section - with between 40% and 60% of all acute PE cases reported to occur postpartum(with a estimated 15-fold increased risk of PE postpartum compared with during pregnancy). In a systematic review the risk of VTE was fourfold greater following CS than following uncomplicated vaginal delivery; and was greater following emergency CS than following elective CS. On average, was estimated that three in 1,000 women will develop a VTE following CS [6, 7].

However a decline overall in deaths associated with VTE in recent years has been observed since publication and more adherence to prevention guidelines for obstetric population [2, 6].

Currently there one reported study on incidence of Deep venous thrombosis (DVT) in women receiving thromboprophylaxis using heparin after CS. This study found that the incidence of asymptomatic DVT among women at high risk of VTE was 3.9%. In patients without thromboprophylaxis symptomatic DVT was detected in 0.04% and 0.5% [7–9].

3. Risk factors for VTE in pregnancy and puerperium

Some groups of women have a higher risk of developing VTE. The most important individual risk factor for VTE in pregnancy is a personal history of thrombosis without a trigger factor and/or following use of estrogen-based hormonal therapy. For women who have had a previous thrombosis in pregnancy, the risk of VTE increases considerably in subsequent pregnancies if antenatal thromboprophylaxis is not used, with an estimated increased risk of recurrence of three- to four-fold [1–4].

Another important individual risk factor for VTE in pregnancy is the presence of an inherited or acquired thrombophilia (a condition that predisposes individuals to developing thromboses) [2–4].

The risk of a thromboembolic event occurring during pregnancy has been shown to differ according to the nature of the thrombophilia, with estimates of risk varying from 5–33% (Homozygotic mutations or multiple thrombophilias) [3, 7, 8].

Other pregnancy-related factors shown to increase the risk of VTE include multiple gestation, pregnancy induced hypertension, prolonged active fase of labour and cesarean section (mainly in the emergency and or after labor). In a case–control study the overall risk of VTE was 0.09%, with a higher risk of events in the postnatal period following cesarean birth; and the authors verified that the risk in the antenatal period was estimated as 0.18% following cesarean section compared with 0.03% without cesarean section [2, 6, 7].

Obesity, smoking, advanced maternal age, severe heart disease, sickle cell disease, inflammatory bowel disease, active cancer, family history of VTE, and prolonged immobilization are other commonly reported risk factors [2].

VTE risk factors vary in their association with but appear to be common. In a recently published cross-sectional study of prospectively collected data from 21 019 sequential postpartum VTE risk assessments in a hospital setting the most prevalent VTE risk factors related to maternal and delivery characteristics included overweight and obesity (36%), age ≥ 35 (35%) and cesarean section (32%). Over three-quarters of women had at least 1 VTE risk factor (78%), and over 40% had multiple (2 or more) VTE risk factors. An important finding is the fact that in 19% of women all VTE risk developed during delivery or in the post-partum period (and were not present prior to the peripartum period) highlighting the critical importance of performing continuos VTE risk assessment even after delivery [8, 9].

COVID-19 is new disease with potentially impact in pregnancy and pueperium. The evidence addressing the issues of coagulopathy and thrombosis in pregnancy in association with COVID-19 is sparse and so far, there is no available high-quality studies at this moment. However, given the possible association between the hypercoagulability characteristic of pregnancy and the risk increase in COVID-19-related VTE, the International Society of Thrombosis and Haemostasys (ISTH), as well as the Ministry of Health in Brazil, suggest that all pregnant and postpartum women admit had at the hospital for COVID-19 (i.e., severe and moderate cases) receiving pharmacological prophylaxis [10, 11].

4. Interaction of VTE risk factors and potencial risk scores

The interaction of VTE risk factors remains an important knowledge gap. However in a large hospital- based case–control study, including 559 women with objectively verified VTE during pregnancy or the postpartum period and 1229 controls, some risk factors exhibited additive interaction (as observed with the combination of assisted reproductive technology with multiple pregnancy, and emergency cesarean section with infection), while others appeared to act as multipliers, as with the combination of antepartum immobilization and elevated body mass index [12, 13].

In particular, understanding how these VTE risk factors translate into absolute PA-VTE is essential. A risk prediction model for postpartum VTE was recently developed using large data on 433 353 deliveries. This model was externally validated using another data sets of 662 387 deliveries. Emergency cesarean section, stillbirth, varicose veins, preeclampsia/eclampsia, infection, and medical comorbidities were the strongest VTE predictors in the final multivariable model. The risk prediction model was able to discriminate postpartum women with and without VTE with statistical significance [C statistic of 0.70 (95% CI, 0.67-0.73)] [13].

The risk assessment models in surgical patients (e.g., Caprini and Padua) to predict VTE after cesarean delivery has not been adequately studied suggesting the establishment of a maternal clinical registry and more extensive research to identify optimal models with which to predict VTE risk in the obstetrical population [4, 13].

At the Maternity Hospital of the Hospital das Clínicas, Universidade de São Paulo in Brazil – a tertiary referral service provider for obstetric pathologies - a risk score for VTE was developed since 2014. Since the establishment of this risk score, there have been no more maternal deaths from PE during hospitalization or up to three months postpartum. Among patients who received prophylaxis with enoxaparin, 0.4% had VTE (failure of treatment); in the untreated (that is, low risk) group had 0.06% of VTE. In our institution we have adapted this score since

3 points High risk factors	2 points Moderate risk factors	1 point Low risk factors
Previous VTE associated with pregnancy and or hormonal treatment	Previous VTE with a trigger factor	—
High Risk Thrombophilia	Low risk Thrombophilia	—
Covid 19 severe cases Sickle cell anemia Severe cardiovascular disease Active Cancer	Previous cancer Severe infections Obesity Severe bleeding with transfusion of blood products	Preeclampsia Multiple pregnancy C-Section or any surgical procedure Massive varicose veins
Obesity with Imobilization >4 days Inflammatory Bowel Disease Nephrotic Proteinuria		Severe hyperemesis Severe smoking

Adapted from: [14].

Table 1.
Risk factors for VTE in hospitalization of pregnant women and puerperal women.

2020 and The National Specialized Commission on Thromboembolism of the Febrasgo (CNE-TEV), based on this national experience proposes the risk score for pregnant women and hospitalized mothers in Brazil. The risk factors were divided into high, medium and low risks, which score, respectively, 3, 2 or 1 point. The fine score occurs by the sum of the values attributed to each factor present in the patient. Pharmacological anticoagulation with is indicated for patients with a score risk of VTE greater than or equal to three [14, 15].

The score is summarized in **Table 1**.

5. Considerations for VTE prophylaxis in cesarean section

A Cochrane's systematic review concluded that there is insufficient evidence of post-cesarean thromboprophylaxis due to the small number of studies and different comparison criteria. Although the risk of VTE associated with cesarean section is low, when there is a relationship with other risk factors, the occurrence of VTE becomes significant and the institution of thromboprophylaxis should be indicated [1, 2].

Based on observational data, some authors have attempted to calculate the number needed to treat (NNT) to prevent 1 episode of VTE during the postpartum period, and reported that among women deemed at high risk for VTE postpartum, 640 as high as 4000 would require prophylaxis to prevent 1 episode of VTE [13].

The potential benefit of pharmacologic prophylaxis needs to be weighed against the potential for adverse outcomes associated with the intervention. The use of pharmacologic VTE prophylaxis after cesarean delivery has been associated with increased rates of wound morbidity. The number needed to harm (NNH) with the use of pharmacologic VTE prophylaxis after cesarean delivery has been reported to be as low as 200. Due to inadequate sample calculation in the available studies the optimal risk threshold for initiating pharmacological thromboprophylaxis in the antepartum and postpartum periods, particularly in women with lower-risk thrombophilic traits and multiple (common) VTE risk factors remains to be established [16].

Another question is optimal optimal time to start and duration of thromboembolism prophylaxis after a cesarean delivery. Recent guidelines have addressed the optimal interval between neuraxial anesthesia and initiation of pharmacologic VTE prophylaxis to prevent the development of spinal or epidural hematomas take in consideration the time of insert and removal of epidural catheter [5, 15, 16]. Prophylactic doses of enoxaparin (40 mg subcutaneously every day) may be started postoperatively as early as 4 hours after catheter removal but not earlier than 12 hours after the block was performed [4, 15, 17]. Another complication to be considered is iatrogenic postoperative bleeding. The risk of bleeding with prophylactic doses are usually mild, such as wound hematomas, and rarely life-threatening hemorrhagic complications [16–21]. In cases with significant intraoperative bleeding complications, the decision of when to start pharmacologic prophylaxis (if indicated) must be individualized according with the clinical and surgical scenarios [2, 3, 21].

Although the evidence is scarce Women with risk factors should receive thromboprophylaxis at minimum for 6 weeks postpartum; women with transient risk factors in the antepartum and intrapartum should receive thromboprophylaxis until hospital discharge or up to 2 weeks after delivery [2–5].

In SARS COVID-19 given the potential increase in VTE risk a weight-adjusted VTE prophylaxis with low molecular weight heparin (LMWH) should be considered in all pregnant and post partum women admitted to hospital (in the absence of active bleeding and with a platelet count above 30 × 109/L or indication for immediate delivery). In case of indicated or emergency delivery VTE prophylaxis should be evaluated individually [10, 11].

6. Pharmacologic agents for prophylaxis of VTE

The 2 most common agents used for prophylaxis of VTE are LMWH and Unfractionaded Heparin (UFH). Recent guidelines recommend LMWH (most recomended enoxaparin) as the first-line pharmacologic agent. Enoxaparin has a half-life of 4 to 6 hours and is eliminated by the kidney and it is not recommended in patients with significant impaired renal function but has the advantage of better bioavailability, longer half-life, more predictable anticoagulation effect, less bleeding risks, and less risk of heparin-induced thrombocytopenia and osteopenia [2–5, 17, 18].

The recommended dose of enoxaparin is typically 40 mg subcutaneously once a day. Obese women may require higher doses; some evidence supports the use of intermediate doses of enoxaparin (40 mg subcutaneously every 12 hours) for obese women or a weight-based prophylactic dose of 0.5 mg/kg subcutaneously every 12 hours of enoxaparin in morbidly obese women after cesarean delivery [2, 17].

UFH has a shorter half-life than LMWH of 60 to 90 minutes and is mostly cleared by the reticuloendothelial system, rendering it a good choice in women with renal disease. Recommended prophylactic dosages in the postpartum period is 5000 units subcutaneously every 8 to 12 hours [17].

Fondaparinux is a completely synthetic pentasaccharide heparin analog and the first of a new class of selective indirect antithrombin-dependent factor Xa inhibitors, which inhibits thrombin generation, has some benefit for thromboprophylaxis. Heparin-induced thrombocytopenia (HIT) is an extremely rare situations of fondaparinux in comparison with the UFH and LMWH, suggesting that fondaparinux is an alternative for the treatment of thrombosis associated with HIT [22]. In a small study in Japan short term fondaparinux (2,5 mg/day)appears to be an adequate and safe method for prevention of symptomatic VTE in women at risk after cesarean section [22, 23].

There are insufficient safety and efficacy data to recommend the use of new oral anticoagulants (e.g., apixaban, rivaroxaban, dabigatran) during the postpartum period [24, 25].

7. Contraindications and patient risks for pharmacological prophylaxis

a. Potential contraindications to prescribing enoxaparin or heparin.

Thrombocytopaenia - Low platelet count (<100.000 ui/ml)
High risk of uncontrolled hemorrhage or current bleeding
Adverse reaction/allergy to enoxaparin or heparin
Acute bacterial endocarditis [2]

b. Patient related risk factors for bleeding:

Current active major bleeding with need for transfusion
Current chronic bleeding over 48 hours
Bleeding disorders (e.g. hemophilia)
Recent central nervous system bleeding
Intracranial or spinal lesion
Current renal impairment with secondary coagulation did
Underlying coagulopathy or coagulation factor abnormalities
Thrombocytopaenia.- a platelet count <50000/uL
Severe platelet dysfunction
Active peptic ulcer or active ulcerative gastrointestinal disease
Obstructive jaundice or cholestasis
Recent major surgical procedure with a high bleeding risk [2, 3].

8. Summary of the recommendations

To date, guideline recommendations are mainly based on expert opinion rather than high-quality evidence and provide conflicting recommendations (**Table 2**).

Recently The Society of Maternal Fetal Medicine published a evidence based guideline summarized in **Table 3** [17].

9. Electronic medical records and improvements in the prevention of VTE

Predicting individual VTE risk is extremely challenging because no single variable is strongly predictive, and we are investing on systems that incorporate multiple variables to produce significant predictive values for VTE. The medical records waistband Electronics (EMR) Scoring systems with use of artificial intelligence should be seen as an opportunity to support clinical decision. Some studies indicate that computer alert interventions may increase the adherence to appropriate risk stratification for VTE, reduce costs and avoiding unnecessary thromboprophylaxis in low-risk patients [15].

10. Conclusions

VTE remains an important and preventable cause of maternal morbidity and mortality during the postpartum period [26–29]. Despite absence or robust evidence use of mechanical prophylaxis sequential compression devices is an inexpensive, safe intervention and should be used in all women undergoing

Organization	Recommendation	Risk stratification
American College of Obstetricians and Gynecologists [4]	• Pneumatic compression for all • Women with additional risk factors for VTE may benefit from pharmacologic prophylaxis	A risk scoring system is not endorsed
American College of Chest Physicians [3]	• Early mobilization is recommended in absence of risk factors. Prophylaxis with heparin is suggested when 1 major or 2 or more minor risk factors are present or when 1 minor risk factor is associated with emergent cesarean section In women at very high risk, we suggest ad pharmacologic to mechanical prophylaxis After delivery, prophylaxis is suggested for up to 6 weeks postpartum in the presence of risk factors	Major risk factors for VTE: Immobility(for at least 7 days antepartum) Postpartum hemorrhage with surgical intervention Previous history of VTE Pregnancy induced hypertension with fetal growth restriction Antithrombin deficiency Factor V Leiden or Prothrombin gen mutations Blood transfusion Puerperal infection Active Systemic lupus erythematosus Severe Heart disease Sickle cell disease Minor risk factors: Obesity Multiple pregnancy Postpartum hemorrhage Smoking Pregnancy induced hypertension Protein C or S deficiency
Royal College of Obstetricians and Gynecologists [2]	Women at high risk should receive pharmacologic prophylaxis for 6 weeks after delivery; women at intermediate risk for VTE should receive pharmacologic prophylaxis for at least 10 days after delivery. For women at low risk for VTE, we recommender early mobilization and adequated hydratation	**High-risk patients** Any previous VTE, any woman requiring antenatal LMWH, high-risk thrombophilia, low-risk thrombophilia with family history of thrombosis **Intermediate-risk** Cesarean delivery after labor, Obesity, postpartum hospital readmission, surgical procedures during the puerperium, Maternal diseases - cancer, heart failure, active lupus, nephrotic syndrome, sickle cell disease, type 1 diabetes with nephropathy, inflammatory bowel disease, or Two or more of the following: Age > 35 years, parity 3, obesity, smoker, elective cesarean delivery, family history of VTE, low-risk thrombophilia, varicose veins, current systemic infection, pregnancy induced hypertension, immobility, multiple pregnancy, preterm delivery, stillbirth, operative vaginal delivery, prolonged labor >24 hours, postpartum hemorrhage

Adapted from [17].

Table 2.
Current guidelines on prophylaxis of thromboembolism after C/S.

cesarean delivery until the woman is fully ambulatory [1, 2, 4, 17]. The decision to add pharmacologic prophylaxis depends on the presence or absence of risk factors [2–4, 15, 17]. Women with a previous personal history of deep venous thrombosis or pulmonary embolism and women with a personal history of an inherited thrombophilia (either high-risk or low-risk), and should receive pharmacologic prophylaxis after cesarean delivery [3, 4, 27, 29]. Another risk factors like obesity

	Recommendation	Grade
1	All women who undergo cesarean sectionreceive sequential compression devices starting before surgery and that the compression devices be used continuously until discharge	1C
2	Women with a previous personal history of DVT venous thrombosis or PE submitted to cesarean section receive both mechanical and pharmacologic prophylaxis. Pharmacological must be maintained for up to 6 weeks postpartum	2C
3	Women with a personal history of an inherited thrombophilia (high-risk or low-risk) but no previous thrombosis submitted to cesarean section receive both mechanical and pharmacologic prophylaxis. Pharmacological must be maintained for up to 6 weeks postpartum	2C
4	Low-molecular-weight heparin is the preferred thromboprophylactic agent in pregnancy and the postpartum period	1C
5	We suggest the use of intermediate doses of enoxaparin in pharmacologic thromboprophylaxis for pregnant women with class III obesity,	2C
6	A patient safety bundle with an institutional protocol for venous thromboembolism prophylaxis must be developed for women who undergo cesarean delivery	Best Practice

Adapted from [17].

Table 3.
SMMF summary of recommendations.

and clinical complications (Sickle cell disease, Hypertension, COVID 19 infections) should be considered. The use of universal or near-universal pharmacological prophylaxis for low risk women undergoing cesarean delivery, cannot be recommended until further studies demonstrate that such a strategy is beneficial [14]. At present, the available VTE risk stratification tools used to decide for or against pharmacologic prophylaxis have not been validated in women undergoing cesarean delivery being a good opportunity for research and development. Individualization of care is recommended for women at very high risk for VfE and institucional safety bundles are recommended as a best practice [14, 15, 17]. In the last half-century, we have made tremendous progress in understanding the epidemiology and prevention of VTE, and it is imperative that these advances be studied and implemented in obstetric care [26].

Conflict of interest

"The authors declare no conflict of interest."

Author details

Frederico José Amédeé Péret[1*] and Liv Braga de Paula[2]

1 Unimed BH Coop/Maternal Fetal Medicine – Hospital Vila da Serra, Belo Horizonte, Minas Gerais, Brazil

2 Department of Gynecology and Obstetrics, Faculdade de Ciências Médicas de Minas Gerais (FCMMG), Belo Horizonte, Minas Gerais, Brazil

*Address all correspondence to: fredperet@gmail.com

References

[1] Bain E, Wilson A, Tooher R, Gates S, Davis LJ, Middleton P. Prophylaxis for venous thromboembolic disease in pregnancy and the early postnatal period. Cochrane Database of Systematic Reviews 2014, Issue 2. Art. No.: CD001689. DOI: 10.1002/14651858. CD001689.pub3. Accessed 15 February 2021.

[2] Royal College of Obstetricians and Gynaecologists. Reducing the risk of venous thromboembolism during pregnancy and the puerperium (Green top guideline 37a April 2015 Available https://www.rcog.org.uk/globalassets/documents/guidelines/gtg-37a.pdf. Access in 16 february 2021

[3] Bates SM, Greer IA, Middeldorp S, Veenstra DL, Prabulos AM, Vandvik PO. VTE, thrombophilia, antithrombotic therapy, and pregnancy: Antithrombotic Therapy and Prevention of Thrombosis, 9th ed: American College of Chest Physicians Evidence-Based Clinical Practice Guidelines. Chest 2012;141 (2 Suppl):e691S–736S.

[4] American College of Obstetricians and Gynecologists. ACOG practice bulletin no. 196: thromboembolism in pregnancy. Obstet Gynecol 2018;132:e1-17

[5] Palmerola KL, D'Alton ME, Brock CO, Friedman AM. A comparison of recommendations for pharmacologic thromboembolism prophylaxis after caesarean delivery from three major guidelines. BJOG 2016;123: 2157-62

[6] O'Shaughnessy F, Donnelly JC, Bennett K, Damkier P, Ainle FN, Cleary BJ. Prevalence of postpartum venous thromboembolism risk factors in an Irish urban obstetric population. J Thromb Haemost. 2019;17(11):1875-85

[7] Blondon M, Casini A, Hoppe KK, Boehlen F, Righini M, Smith NL. Risks of Venous Thromboembolism After Cesarean Sections: A Meta-Analysis. Chest. 2016 Sep;150(3):572-96

[8] Ewins K, Ní Ainle F. VTE risk assessment in pregnancy. Res Pract Thromb Haemost. 2020;4:183-192

[9] Jacobsen AF, Skjeldestad FE, Sandset PM. Ante- and postnatal risk factors of venous thrombosis: a hospital-based case-control study. J Thromb Haemost. 2008;6(6):905-12

[10] Kadir RA, Kobayashi T, Iba T, Erez O, Thachil J, Kazi S, Malinowski AK, Othman M. COVID-19 coagulopathy in pregnancy: Critical review, preliminary recommendations, and ISTH registry-Communication from the ISTH SSC for Women's Health. J Thromb Haemost. 2020 Nov;18(11): 3086-3098.

[11] Brasil. Ministério da Saúde. Secretaria de Atenção Primária à Saúde. Departamento de Ações Programáticas e Estratégicas. Manual de Recomendações para a Assistência à Gestante e Puérpera frente à Pandemia de COVID-19. Brasília (DF):Ministério da Saúde; 2020

[12] Sultan AA, West J, Grainge MJ, Riley RD, Tata LJ, Stephansson O, et al. Development and validation of risk prediction model for venous thromboembolism in postpartum women: multinational cohort study. BMJ. 2016;355:i6253

[13] Tran JP, Stribling SS, Ibezim UC, et al. Performance of risk assessment models for peripartum thromboprophylaxis. Reprod Sci 2019;26:1243-8.

[14] Barros V, Igai A, Fernanda B, Bortolotto M, Francisco R, Zugaib M. Preventing maternal death and morbidity from venous thromboembolism (VTE): results from

a VTE risk score trial during hospitalization. Res Pract Thromb Haemost.2020;4 (Suppl 1):PB2280. [cited 2020 Nov 4]. Available from: https://abstracts.isth.org/abstract/preventing-maternal-death-and-morbidity-from-venous thromboem bolism- vte-results-from-a-vte-risk-score-trial-during-hospitalization/

[15] Comissão Nacional Especializada em Tromboembolismo Venoso. Protocolo FEBRASGO de Obstetrícia, n. 58. : https://www.febrasgo.org.br/

[16] Society for Maternal-Fetal Medicine (SMFM). Electronic address: pubs@smfm.org, Pacheco LD, Saade G, Metz TD. Society for Maternal-Fetal Medicine Consult Series #51: Thromboembolism prophylaxis for cesarean delivery. Am J Obstet Gynecol. 2020 Aug;223(2):B11-B17.

[17] Kotaska A. Postpartum venous thromboembolism prophylaxis may cause more harm than benefit: a critical analysis of international guidelines through an evidence-based lens. BJOG 2018;125:1109-16

[18] Goto M, Yoshizato T, Tatsumura M, Takashima T, Ogawa M, Nakahara H, Satoh S, Sanui A, Eguchi F, Miyamoto S. Safety and efficacy of thromboprophylaxis using enoxaparin sodium after cesarean section: A multi-center study in Japan. Taiwan J Obstet Gynecol. 2015 Jun;54(3):248-52

[19] Côté-Poirier G, Bettache N, Côté AM, Mahone M, Morin F, Cumyn A, Bureau YA, Malick M, Sauvé N. Evaluation of Complications in Postpartum Women Receiving Therapeutic Anticoagulation. Obstet Gynecol. 2020 Aug;136(2):394-401

[20] Limmer JS, Grotegut CA, Thames E, Dotters-Katz SK, Brancazio LR, James AH. Postpartum wound and bleeding complications in women who received peripartum anticoagulation. Thromb Res. 2013 Jul;132(1):e19-23

[21] Yang R, Zhao X, Yang Y, Huang X, Li H, Su L. The efficacy and safety of pharmacologic thromboprophylaxis following caesarean section: a systematic review and meta-analysis. PLoS One 2018;13:e0208725.

[22] Knol HM, Schultinge L, Erwich JJ, Meijer K. Fondaparinux as an alternative anticoagulant therapy during pregnancy. J Thromb Haemost 2010;8:1876-9

[23] Kawaguchi R, Haruta S, Kobayashi H. Efficacy and safety of venous thromboembolism prophylaxis with fondaparinux in women at risk after cesarean section. Obstet Gynecol Sci. 2017 Nov;60(6):535-541

[24] Lameijer H, Aalberts JJJ, van Veldhuisen DJ, Meijer K, Pieper PG. Efficacy and safety of direct oral anticoagulants during pregnancy; a systematic literature review. Thromb Res. 2018 Sep;169:123-127

[25] Sessa M, Mascolo A, Callréus T, Capuano A, Rossi F, Andersen M. Direct-acting oral anticoagulants (DOACs) in pregnancy: new insight from VigiBase®. Sci Rep. 2019 May 10;9(1):7236-7241

[26] Kourlaba, G.; Relakis, J.; Kontodimas, S.; Holm, M.V.; Maniadakis, N. A systematic review and meta-analysis of the epidemiology and burden of venous thromboembolism among pregnant women. Int. J. Gynecol. Obs. 2016, 132, 4-10.

[27] Nicholson M, Chan N, Bhagirath V, Ginsberg J. Prevention of Venous Thromboembolism in 2020 and Beyond. J Clin Med. 2020 Aug 1;9(8):2467-2478

[28] D'Souza R, Malhamé I, Teshler L, Acharya G, Hunt BJ, McLintock C.

A critica lreview of the pathophysiology of thrombotic complications and clinical practice recommendations for thromboprophylaxis in pregnant patients with COVID-19. Acta Obstet Gynecol Scand. 2020;99(9):1110-20.

[29] Nichols KM, Henkin S, Creager MA. Venous Thromboembolism Associated With Pregnancy: JACC Focus Seminar. J Am Coll Cardiol. 2020;76(18):2128-41.

Chapter 5

Caesarean Section

Tshililo J. Mashamba

Abstract

Caesarean section is a procedure performed to save the life of the fetus and sometime to save the life of the woman. Although risks are low, affected women suffer from severe complications. The first caesarean section performed has a bearing on management of subsequent pregnancies. It is crucial that the procedure is performed when necessary. The evolution of caesarean section has shown marked improvement in maternal outcome especially after the introduction of antibiotics. The resistance of bacteria to antibiotics may lead to rethinking about the procedure performed long ago to try and minimised complications related to sepsis. Complications of caesarean sections are common in patients who have had a previous caesarean section. Training in previous caesarean sections will be vital in preventing these complications.

Keywords: ruptured membranes, preterm, prelabour

1. Introduction

Caesarean section is a procedure to deliver the baby though the incision made on the uterus. Ideally this is to deliver a viable fetus which is of 22 weeks or fetal weight of 500 g. Contrary to repeated use of caesarean section referring to the laparotomy to have access to perform a hysterotomy. The objective of caesarean section is to save the life of the mother and fetus. The origin of caesarean is section is somehow not clear as it was believed that Julius Caesar was born following this procedure but the Latin word "caedare" refers to cut.

2. Epidemiology

Caesarean section is the most common surgical procedure. The rapid increase in caesarean deliveries without clear evidence of concomitant decreases in maternal or neonatal morbidity and mortality is a significant concern that the procedure may be overused [1]. Caesarean section rate is defined as the number of caesarean deliveries over the total number of live births and is expressed as a percentage. This is obviously the definition used which does not follow the statistical guideline, as the number the denominator should pregnancy that have reached 22 weeks and not live births as some would have had stillborns but are not included in this definition. Majority of caesarean sections are emergencies compared to elective caesarean sections. In South Africa emergency caesarean sections accounted for 80.9% of total caesarean sections [2] while in the United States of America 63% were emergencies [3].

3. Classification of caesarean sections

Classification relates to the degree of urgency to save the mother's life or the fetus and the mother's life should be always a priority over the fetal life, accept in a situation that the mother's life cannot be modified by the surgical procedure. The word emergency may comprise of many components within which the extent of urgency differs. Once the decision to deliver has been taken, delivery should be carried out with the urgency appropriate to the risk to the baby and the safety of the mother. The objective should be to shorten the decision to delivery time in such circumstances [4] (**Table 1**).

Category	Description
1	Immediate threat to the life of the mother or fetus
2	No immediate threat to the life of the mother or the fetus, has maternal or fetal compromise
3	No maternal or fetal compromise but require early delivery
4	Elective –delivery at a time that suit maternity services and the mother

Table 1.
Classification of caesarean sections.

4. Indications for caesarean sections

See **Table 2** indications for caesarean sections [5].

Urgent caesarean	Elective caesarean
1. Poor progress of labour	1. 2 Previous caesarean section
2. Cephalopelvic disproportion	2. Macrosomia
3. Fetal compromise	3. Transverse lie/unstable lie
4. Abuptio placentae	4. Placenta previa
5. Placenta previa with hemodynamic instability or placenta previa major	5. Previous major shoulder dystocia
6. Cord prolapse with live fetus	6. Active genital Herpes infection
7. Transverse lie in labour	7. Cardiomyopathy with EF < 45%
8. Footling breech in labour	8. Breech presentation at term
9. Uterine rupture	9. Multiple pregnancy with leading twin no-vertex
10. 2 Previous caesarean in labour	10. Previous pelvic fracture
11. Prolonged second stage	11. Previous 3rd/4th degree perineal tear
12. Failed assisted delivery, etc	12. High HIV viral load
	13. Transverse lie not in labour
	14. Preterm rupture of memebranes in a previous caesarean
	15. Pelvic tumour obstructing pelvic inlet
	16. Intrauterine growth restriction
	17. Decreased fetal movements
	18. Contracted pelvis
	19. Recurrent intrauterine fetal death late in third trimester
	20. Previous repair of vesico vaginal fistula,etc

Table 2.
Indications for caesarean sections.

5. Preoperative management

Preoperative discussion should take place to assess the disciplines involved [6, 7].

5.1 Objectives

1. To identify medical and obstetric comorbidities that may increase anaesthetic and surgical risks

2. To establish the urgency of the caesarean section

3. To obtain anaesthetic and surgical informed consent

4. To enable patient preparation

The above objectives may require multidisciplinary team management in certain cases like, cardiac disease, respiratory diseases, concurrent surgical conditions, endocrine conditions and others. It is important that the patient has a full understanding of the procedure and its anticipated complications. In case of emergencies the discussion with the patient should be carried out in a best shortest time not to jeopardise the objective of the procedure. Blood products should be organised if deemed necessary.

The person performing the surgical procedure is responsible for checking that the written consent has been signed and explain the need for the operation again. Risks and complications should be clearly communicated with the patient and care must be taken when explaining the frequency of the complications and those that are less likely.

5.2 Preoperative procedure principles

There is evidence abdominal shave if done should be performed in the operating room just before applying the antiseptic preparation and not a night before. Prolonged shave to operating time increases the bacterial count on the abdomen. The abdomen is scrubbed with alcohol containing solution or nonorganic iodide solution.

Nonparticulate antacid should be given orally before transferring patient to operating table. In some instances, long acting antacid could be given a night before like Ranitidine 150 mg orally. Metoclopramide is given to increase the tone of lower oesophageal sphincter, preferably after oxygenation [6, 7].

Patient should be placed in the 15 degree left lateral tilt position to minimise uterine compression of inferior vena cava [8]. Urinary catheter should be placed to allow the bladder to drain during the operation keeping the operative field clear.

The principle should be to have adequate exposure but not excessive. Gentle handling of tissues with attention to haemostasis.

5.3 Different abdominal incisions

5.3.1 Transverse abdominal incisions

The full thickness abdominal wall incision should be adequate to allow easy delivery of the fetus. At least a minimum incision of 15 cm to allow bladder retractor with ease.

1. Pfannensteil incision is made transversely on the suprapubic area approximately 2-3 cm above the symphysis pubis and should be curvilinear, with the lateral apices of the incision curved slightly up toward the anterior superior iliac spines. The incision is performed sharply to the level of the rectus fascia. The fascia is incised with the scalpel in the transverse manner to expose the muscles. The incision in the anterior rectus fascia may be extended laterally

using the scalpel or dissecting scissors. Watch out for the superficial epigastric and superficial circumflex iliac veins. It is important to minimise the risk of haematoma. After the is incised, the anterior rectus sheath is then dissected from the underlying rectus muscle both in the cephalic and caudal direction using blunt and sharp dissection. Care must be taken to identify perforating vessels between the rectus muscles and the anterior fascia. Peritoneum should be exposed staying in the midline and avoid hooking fingers under the rectus muscles which can damage the underlying vessels. The entry through the peritoneum should be made high in the operative field to avoid injury to the bladder. The peritoneum should be elevated using artery forceps and palpate the intended entry point to exclude small bowel that may be trapped.

2. Joel-Cohen incision is performed in a transverse manner above the location of a Pfannesteil incision and is linear. Once the fascia is incised the rest of the dissection is performed bluntly. There are no maternal or fetal advantages over Pfannensteil incision, but may be quicker.

3. Misdav Ladach incision is based on Joel Cohen incision introduced for hysterectomy. This is a straight transverse incision somewhat higher than the Pfannesteil. The subcutaneous tissue is left undisturbed apart from the midline. The rectus sheath is separated, and the muscles are separated by pulling [9].

5.3.2 Vertical abdominal incisions

Midline vertical incision was the preferred incision for caesarean section because is faster and ease of entry into the peritoneal cavity with minimal dissection required (**Figure 1**). The incision is useful in situation where high peritoneal access is needed. The incision is made vertically just below the umbilicus to at least 1 cm above the symphysis pubis. The advantage is that it can be extended above the umbilicus if necessary if exposure in the upper part of the abdomen is required. The procedure is undertaken by sharp dissection to the level of the rectus sheath (**Figure 2**).

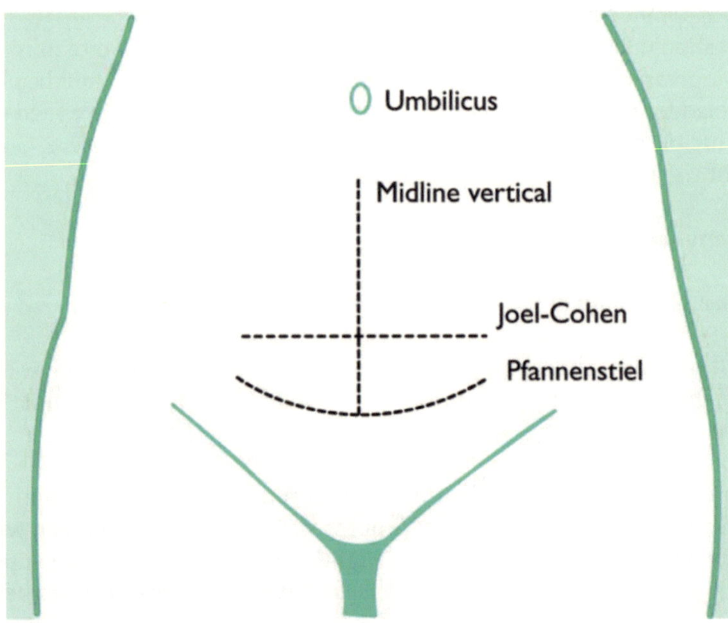

Figure 1.
Abdominal wall incisions.

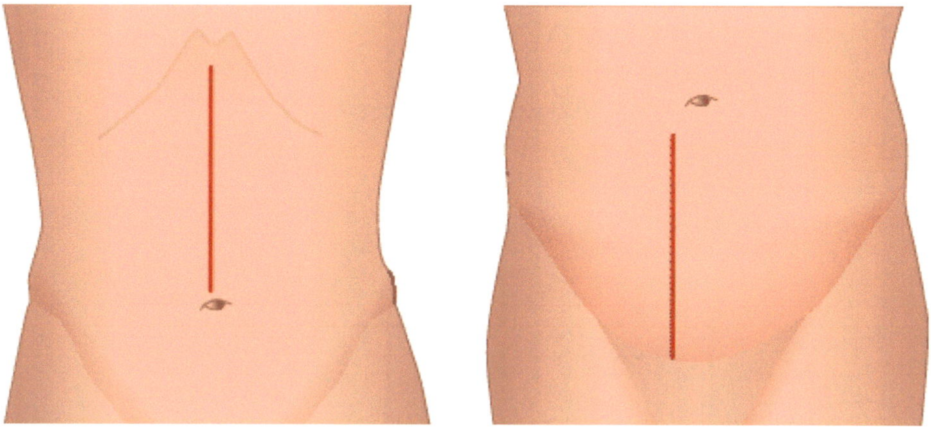

Figure 2.
Midline subumbilical incision (left) and paramedian subumbilical incision (right).

Paramedian incisions are made to serve the purpose of the procedure. For caesarean sections paramedian incisions are made 2-5 cm lateral to the midline over the median aspect of bulging convexity of rectus muscles. Closure is theoretically more secure because rectus muscle can act as buttress between the re-approximated posterior and anterior fascial planes (**Figure 2**).

In obese patients the challenges are anaesthetic with difficult intubation [10], extensive subcutaneous tissue leading to prolonged entry time, obscured vision, difficult delivery, increased bleeding, etc. whether a transverse or midline incision is superior for the obese patient remains controversial, but a larger incision is advisable. Retractors should be used to aid with exposure (**Figure 3**).

Bladder flap reflection is not universally as the creation of the flap was not associated with any increase of complications like bladder injury, increased blood loss or prolonged hospital stay [10]. Non flap reflection was associated with reduced operation time [11]. Situation when bladder flap may be advisable is when the fetal head is impacted and in previous caesarean section. The location of the bladder is best delineated by palpating the bladder catheter (**Figure 4**).

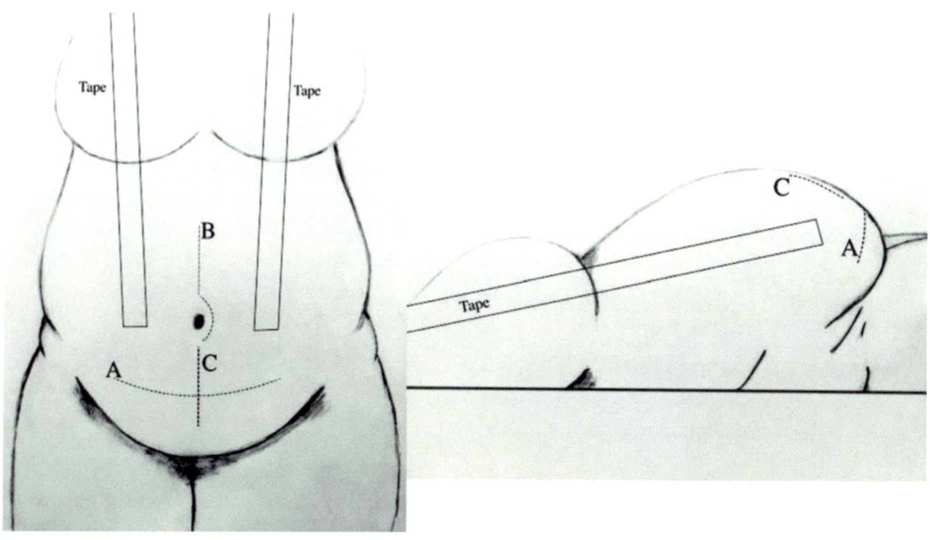

Figure 3.
A = Transverse subumbilical incision; B = Midline incision extending above the umbilicus; C = Midline subumbilical incision.

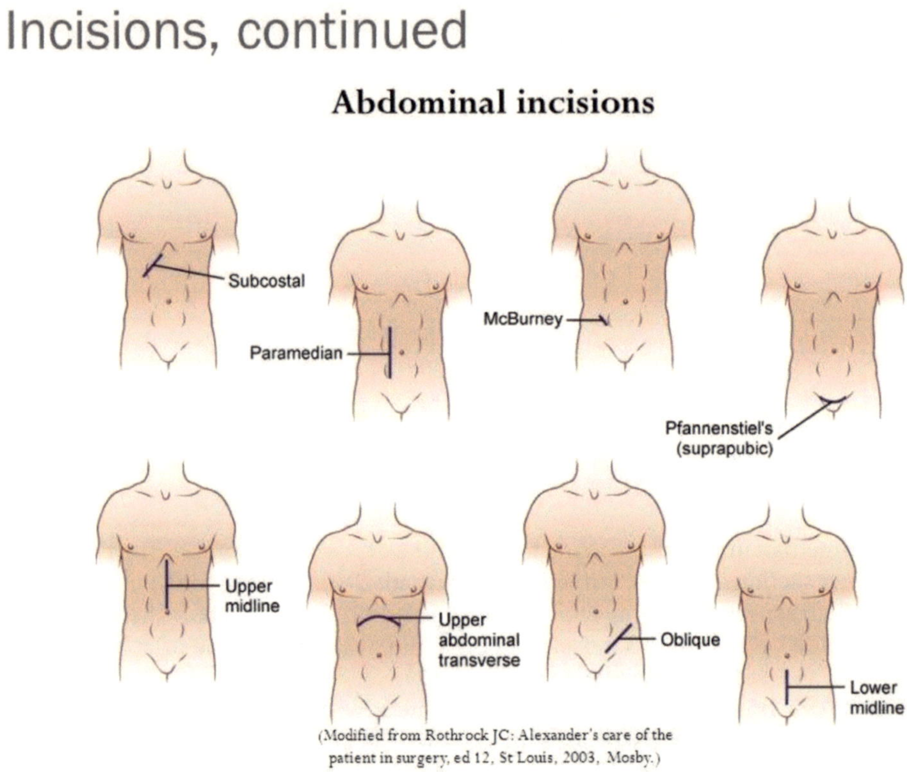

Figure 4.
Different abdominal wall incisions.

5.4 Uterine incisions

The uterine incision is usually transverse but may be vertical. The incision should be large enough to allow atraumatic delivery of the fetus. Factors to consider before a uterine incision is made are

1. Position of the uterus

2. Size of the uterus

3. Location of the placenta

4. Presence of uterine tumours

5. Accessible and developed lower segment

6. Future pregnancy plans

5.4.1 Transverse uterine incision

This is the incision recommended for most patients unless there is a contraindication. For the term pregnancies the incision is made 2-3 cm below the upper edge of the uterovesical fold of the peritoneum [12, 13].

Advantages of lower segment incision:

1. Less blood loss because it is less vascular

2. Less risks of uterine rupture

3. Less subsequent adhesions to the bowel and omentum

4. Reduced risk of ileus and peritonitis

5. Rapid healing

There are different types of incisions on the uterus to deliver the fetus [14], but Kerr incision is the one performed commonly in uncomplicated cases.

1. Kerr incision

2. Kronig incision

3. Sanger high classical incision

4. Delee lower segment vertical incision

5. Kerr transverse lower uterine segment incision

If there is a need to extend the incision this should be done with blunt dissection as sharply extending the uterine incision significantly increases intraoperative blood loss and the need for blood transfusion [12].

The incision to delivery intervals does not significantly contribute to Apgar scores and cord blood gases, but the maternal status prior to caesarean section and optimal anaesthetic management are the most important factors for good neonatal outcome [13, 15].

Lower vertical uterine incision are of 2 types which is either on the lower segment or on the upper segment. The lower segment vertical incision is as strong as the lower segment transverse incision. The major disadvantage of the low vertical incision is likelihood of extension cephalad into the uterine fundus or caudally into the bladder, cervix or vagina.

The classical incision is rarely performed at or near term because of its likelihood to rupture spontaneously antenatally or early in labour. It also associated with increased maternal morbidity [16] (**Figures 5–8**).

Indications for vertical uterine incision are [17]:

1. Poorly developed lower segment like in preterm pregnancies

2. Anterior morbidly adherent placenta

3. Anterior lower segment uterine tumours

4. Dense lower segment adhesions involving the bladder adhesions

5. Delivery of a marked macrosomia

6. Transverse lie

7. Gross congenital anomaly to minimise uterine incision extension and trauma to the fetus

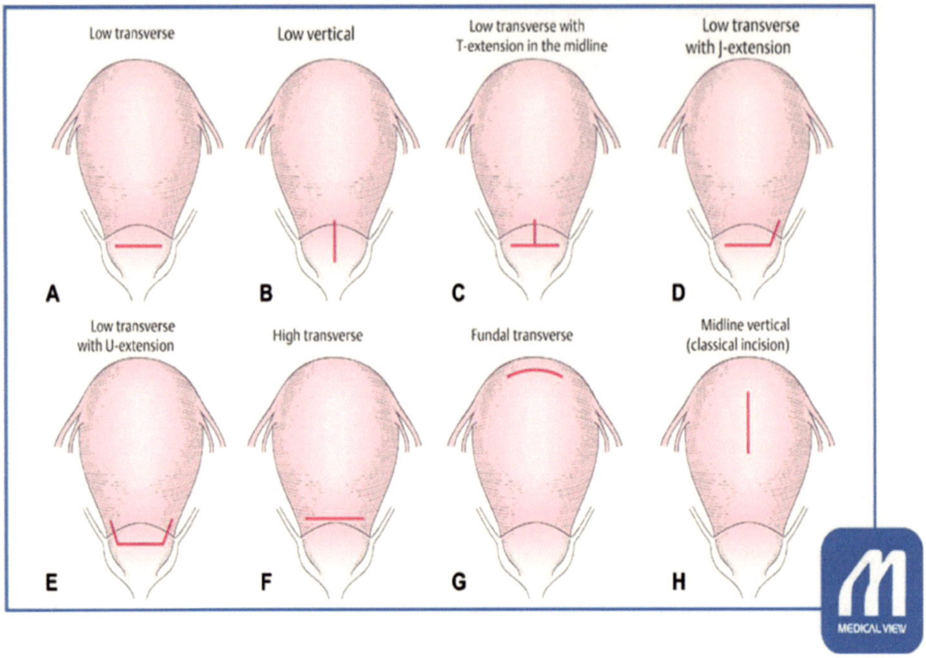

Figure 5.
Different types of uterine incisions.

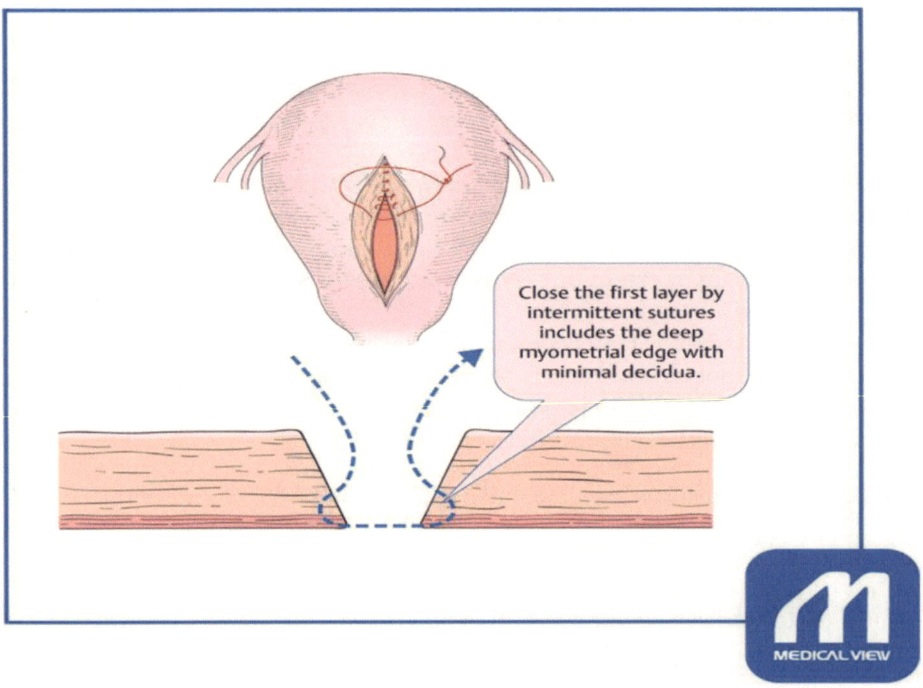

Figure 6.
First layer for uterine closure.

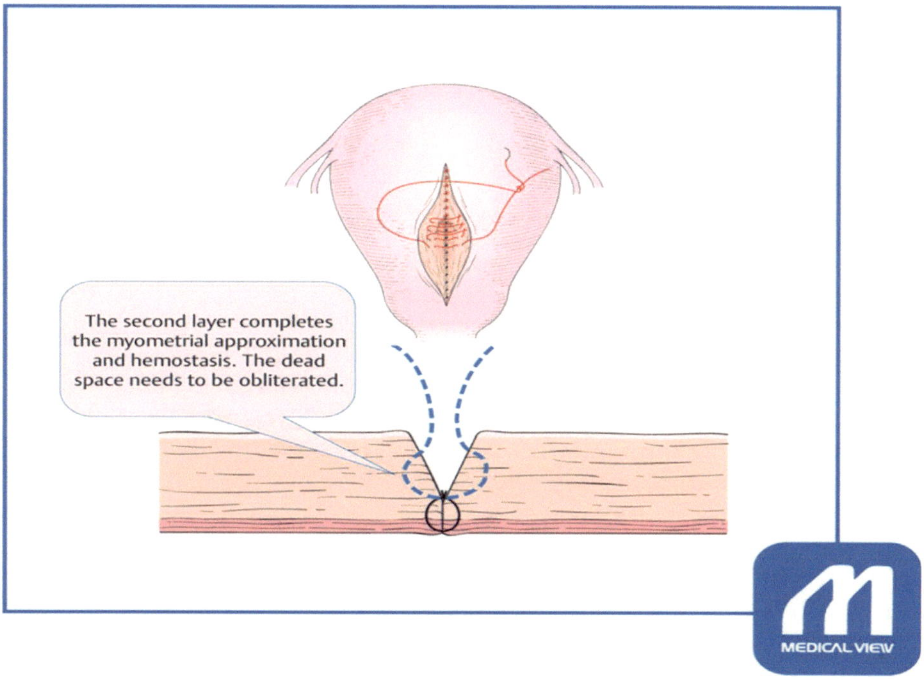

Figure 7.
Second layer closure technique.

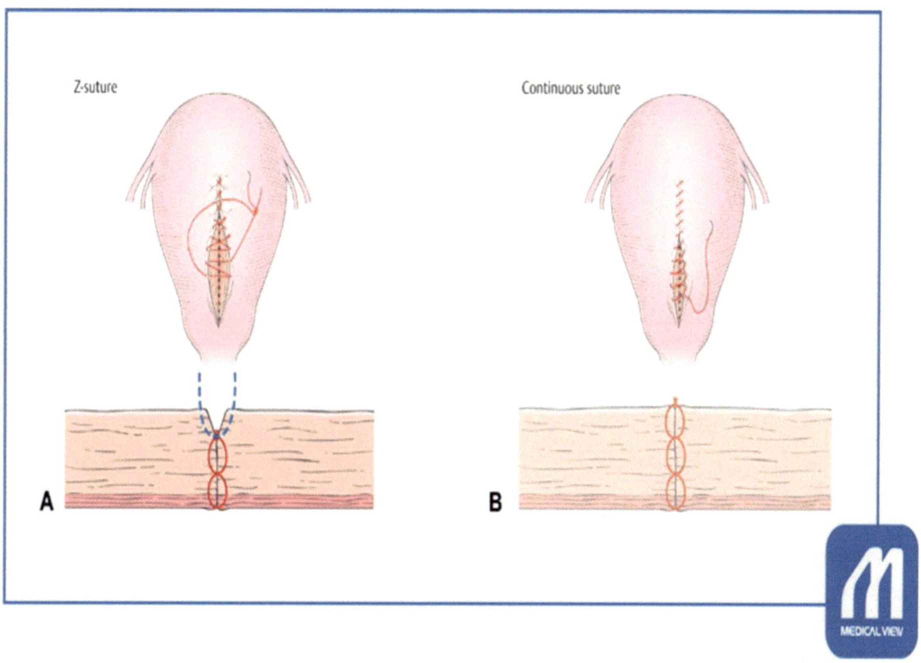

Figure 8.
Abdominal closure techniques.

8. Breech
9. Cervical malignancy
10. Conjoined twins
11. Uterine anomaly

5.5 Extraction of the fetus

The fetus should be extracted expeditiously and in a non-traumatic way. The delay in delivery after a uterine incision with contractions following leads to decreased uteroplacental blood flow and compromise the fetus [15]. Fingers are put around the curvature of the fetal head for leverage, lifting without overly flexing the wrist not using the lower segment and symphysis pubis as a fulcrum, to avoid extensions of the incision. The head is gently elevated and flexed to bring the occiput into incision, with the aid of modest fundal pressure. The shoulders are then delivered transversely along the largest diameter of the incision. Of note that there are conditions that may make this process difficult like impacted head and abnormal lie [16, 17]. Instrumental delivery has been suggested to assist delivery of the fetal head when is found to be difficult and forceps are preferred. The objective should be to carry out an atraumatic fetal delivery as possible.

5.6 Cord clamping

For newborns who do not require resuscitation delayed cord clamping for 30-60 seconds is recommended. Clamping should be done following onset of respiration.

Delivery of the placenta should be by cord traction as this has many benefits compared to manual removal and the use of oxytocin [18].

Advantages are:

1. Less blood loss
2. Less endometritis
3. Shorter hospital stay
4. Slightly shorter duration of surgery

5.7 Closure of uterine incision

After the delivery of the placenta is exteriorized onto the abdominal wall although this kinks the uterine vessels and may seem like there is no bleeding which may occur when replaced back in the pelvis. It is therefore advisable that when replaced haemostasis is verified by checking with systolic blood pressure of 100 mmHg or more. Non exteriorization is challenging but reassures for the achievement of haemostasis. The benefits of exteriorization found was only shorter surgical time [19, 20].

Uterine incision closure technique is the most important factor for good healing to minimise complications later. The assistant should compress the uterus to assist in approximation of the wound edges. Dead spaces need to be obliterated to achieve haemostasis. The angles of the incision should be secured and a full thickness needle bite 1 cm away from the margin of the incision and coming out at the junction of the myometrium and decidua using polyglactin, poliglecaprone or catgut 1 sutures to avoid endometrial inversion at the scar site as this may delay healing. The type of a suture is largely based on personal preference with no statistical difference in maternal outcome [21, 22]. Double uterine incision closure with continuous locked or unlocked suture [23]. Two layer rather than a single layer is preferred but in a patient performing tubal ligation single layer can be done as there is no concern of subsequent uterine rupture.

Closure of the classical incision has no consensus as interrupted or continuous sutures have been used but the important objective is to obliterate all dead spaces. Approximation of the edges is important to minimise the tension when sutures are placed. The thick myometrium should have a separate layer of suture.

Abdominal irrigation with the use of prophylactic antibiotics seems not to reduce the maternal morbidity but also has not been found to be harmful.

Peritoneal closure has been found to be associated with adhesion formation, but personal experience is different. This may be due to marked tissue handling rather than washing. Re-operating on the patients self-operated before can clarify this issue. The lesser the tissue handling the lesser the adhesion formation.

There is no need for rectus muscle re-approximation unless in cases if rectus diasthesis to minimise visceral injury in subsequent abdominal surgical procedures. It is recommended that subcutaneous tissue with a depth of 2 cm or more should be closed to obliterate dead spaces using interrupted suture.

Skin closure can done with fine sutures like rapidly absorbable continuous or interrupted sutures unless in septic cases where interrupted non absorbable suture closure is mandatory. Absorbable suture give the best aesthetic outcome especially post caesarean section [24].

The challenge for performing caesarean section is when there is prolonged rupture of membranes as this may be associated with severe infections. Before the era of effective antibiotics extra-peritoneal caesarean section was advised. The skill to perform such a procedure has disappeared as effective antibiotics became available. Though the procedure had advantages like less postoperative pyrexia, less hospital stay, less incidence of pelvic abscesses and septic shock, less wound sepsis, lower incidence of secondary post-partum haemorrhage and need for further surgery, it had a prolonged anaesthetic time to delivery [25]. This was a way of minimising complications associated with caesarean section in the presence of infection.

5.8 Complications of caesarean section

In comparison with vaginal delivery caesarean section delivery is associated with increased morbidity and mortality [26].

5.8.1 Operative

1. Anaesthetic complications which related failure to intubate with associated aspiration leading to Mendelson syndrome

2. Extension of uterine incision laterally to involve the uterine vessels and inferiorly to the bladder and vagina

3. Massive intraoperative haemorrhage leading to hypovolaemic shock with associated coagulopathy. Uterine atony is common in caesarean delivery compared to vaginal delivery

4. Bowel injuries especially in patients who had previous laparotomy

5. Urological injuries in patients in prolonged second stage of labour and previous caesarean section

6. Fetal injuries In emergencies to salvage the fetal life

5.8.2 Post operative

1. Paralytic ileus and vomiting

2. Respiratory infections especially following general anaesthesia. This has been reduced to a minimal by the frequent utilisation of regional anaesthesia

3. Puerperal pelvic sepsis

4. Wound infection

5. Thromboembolism, this is even increased in the HIV era as antiretroviral drugs have effect on the functionality of the liver. This also increase the occurrence of pulmonary embolism

6. Fistulae formation in cases where bladder or ureter were injured

7. Rupture of the scar in subsequent pregnancies

8. Incisional hernia which is common in midline incisions compared to transverse incisions

5.9 Counselling for caesarean delivery

Caesarean delivery is the most common abdominal surgical procedure on women of reproductive age. Majority of patients present in a healthy physical state, so the outcome of pregnancy is expected to be a joyful one. Most nulliparous women have a strong preference for vaginal delivery. Women should be encouraged to attend child birth classes to prepare them for the labour and delivery experience. Interventions that decrease the chance of especially the first caesarean delivery include avoidance of non-medical indication for induction of labour. The woman experiences pain after caesarean delivery which limit the welcoming experience of the newborn. The techniques to improve the outcome of caesarean delivery should be developed and minimise the complications following this procedure. The procedure, intraoperative and post-operative complications should be discussed in detail. The unexpected outcome should be emphasised.

6. Conclusion

Caesarean section is the most common surgical procedure in women of reproductive age. Though it seems like a safe procedure it may have devastating consequences for the mother and the fetus. Pregnancy is a results of normal physiology and not a disease as most patients present with no complaints, but coming ambulating. The common complications occur when the labour is prolonged which presents with difficulty in delivery resulting in serious morbidity and/or death. Maternal death rate is high in underdeveloped countries as a result of inadequate facilities and equipment to look after pregnant patients and monitor labour.

Author details

Tshililo J. Mashamba
Sefako Makgatho Health Sciences University, Pretoria, South Africa

*Address all correspondence to: tjmashamba@yahoo.com

References

[1] Hedwige Saint Louis. Caesarean delivery: Medscape, Dec 2018

[2] Magwede TY, Mashamba TJ, Mavukani MP; Clinical audit of caesarean sections performed at Dr George Mukhari Academic Hospital. Obstetrics and Gynaecology Forum, 29: 4, 20-24, 2019.

[3] Clark SC, Taffel SM: Stae variation in rates of caesarean and VBAC delivery; 1989 and 1993. Sta Bull Metrop Insur Co 77:28-29, 1996

[4] Royal College of Obstetricians and Gynaecologists. Good practice no. 11: April 2010

[5] Phaneuf LE. Cesarean section: Indications and technique. The American journal of surgery, 1937, 35(2): 446-456

[6] Mcauley DM, Moore J, McCaughey W, Donnelly BD, Dundee JW: Ranitidine as an antacid before Caesarean section. Anaesthesia 1983; 38, 108-114

[7] Sui An Lie, May Un Sam Mok. Peri-operative management of caesarean section for the occasional obstetric anaestheist-an aide memoire: Proceedings of Singapore Healthcare, Review article, 2017 .1-.9

[8] Lee AL, Landau R, Mattingly JL, Meenan MM, Corradini B, Wang S, Goodman SR: Left lateral table tilt for Elective Cesarean delivery under Spinal Anaesthesia has no effect on neonatal acid-base status. Anaesthesiology 2017; 127: 241-249.

[9] Gunnar Holmgren, Lennart Sjoholm, Michael Stark: The Misgav Ladach method for caesarean section: method description. Acta Obstet Gynecol Scand 1999;78:615-621

[10] Tingting Wang, Shen Sun, Shaoqiang Huang: The association of body mass index with difficult tracheal intubation management by direct laryngoscopy; a meta-analysis; BMC Anesthesiology (2018) 18:79

[11] O'Neill HA, Egan G, Walsh CA. et al. Omission of the bladder flap at caesarean section reduces delivery time without increased morbidity, a meta-analysis of randomized controlled trials. Eur J Obstet Gynecol Reprod Biol 2014, 174:20

[12] Peleg d, Burke Y Z, Solt I, Fisher M. the history of the low transvers cesarean section: The pivotal role of Munro Kerr. IMAJ 2018,20:316-319

[13] Magann EF, Chauhan SP, Bufkin L. intra-operative haemorrhage by blunt versus sharp expansion of the uterine incision at caesarean delivery: a randomized clinical trial, BJOG 2002; 94:735

[14] Wood RM, Simon H, Oz AU. Pelosi type vs traditional caesarean delivery. A prospective comparison. The Journal of Reproductive Medicine 1999, 44(9): 788-795

[15] Andersen HF, Auster GH, Marx GF, Merkatz IR. Neonatal status in relation to incision intervals, obstetric factors, and anesthesia at cesarean section. Am J Perinatology 1987;4:279

[16] Patterson LS, O'Connell CM, Baskett TF. Maternal and perinatal morbidity associated with classic and inverted T cesarean incisions. Obstet Gynecol 2002; 100:633.

[17] FontanarosA m, Fontanarosa N. incision to delivery interval and neonatal wellbeing during cesarean section. Minerva Ginecol 2008;60:23

[18] Cochrane update. Methods of delivering the placenta at caesarean section. Obstet Gynecol 2008; 112(5): 1173-1174

DOI: http://dx.doi.org/10.5772/intechopen.97290

[19] Kan A. classical cesarean section. Surg J (N Y) 2020 Jul; 6 (suppl 2)

[20] Bolla D, Schoning A, Drack G. technical aspects of the cesarean section. Gynecol Surg (2010) 7:127-132

[21] CORONIS collaborative group, Abalos E, Addo V, et al. Cesarean section surgical techniques(CORONIS): a fractional, factorial, unmasked, randomized controlled trial. Lancet 2013; 382:234

[22] CORONIS collaborative group, Abalos E, Addo V, et al. Ceasarean section surgical techniques; 3 year follow-up of the CORONIS fractional, factorial, unmasked, randomized controlled trial. Lancet 2016; 388:62

[23] Stegwee SI, Jordans IPM, van der Voet LF, de Groot CJM et al. Single versus double-layer closure of the caesarean(uterine) scar in the prevention of gynaecological symptoms in relation to niche development-The 2Close study: a multicenter randomized controlled trial. BMC Pregnancy and childbirth (2019)19:85

[24] de Lima RJ, Schnaider TB, Francisco AMC, FrancescatoVeiga D. Absorbable suture. Best aesthetic outcome in cesarian scar. Acta Cir Bras 2018; 33(11) 1027-1036

[25] Mokgokong ET, Crichton D. Exptraperitoneal lower segment caesarean section for infected cases. S Afr Med J 1974;48 788

[26] Landon MB. Vaginal birth after cesarean delivery. Clin Perinatol 2008 Sep. 35(3);491-504

Chapter 6

Magnitude, Factors Associated with Cesarean Delivery and Its Appropriateness

Awoke Giletew Wondie

Abstract

Inappropriate use of CS can have profoundly negative consequences for women and the broader community. A recent meeting of the International Confederation of Midwifes, the International Federation of Gynecologists and Obstetrics and the Gates Foundation to discuss the impact of rising CS rates on maternal and infant mortality in LMICs highlights the international importance of the issue. Knowledge of CS determinants is a first step in the effort to define strategies to reduce unnecessary CSs. Previous studies showed that the main reasons for performing CS are clinical factors. However, non-clinical factors such as demographic, health system factors, organizational variables were overlooked determinants that best predicted which women have a higher risk of CS.

Keywords: Caesarean delivery, appropriateness, low income countries

1. Introduction

Worldwide, 830 women die every day due to pregnancy or childbirth-related complications, and almost all maternal deaths (99%) occur in developing countries [1]. In Africa and South Asia, it is the leading cause of death for women of reproductive age. Another 5.7 million suffer severe or long-lasting illnesses or disabilities caused by complications during pregnancy or childbirth every year globally [1, 2]. Half of the world's maternal, newborn, and child deaths occur in sub-Saharan countries. The maternal mortality ratio in developing countries is 240 per 100,000 births versus 16 per 100,000 in developed countries [1, 2]. The risk of a woman dying in sub-Saharan Africa as a result of pregnancy or childbirth is 1 in 39, as compared to 1 in 4,700 in industrialized countries. In sub-Saharan Africa, children under the age of five are 15 times more likely to die than in high-income countries [1]. However, an estimated 74% of maternal deaths could be averted if all women had access to emergency obstetric care [2, 3]. The consequences of maternal mortality have a ripple effect in families, communities and nations. Children without mothers are less likely to receive proper nutrition, health care and education. The implications for girls tend to be even greater, leading to a continued cycle of poverty and poor health. And every year, over $15 billion in productivity is lost due to maternal and newborn death, placing a huge burden on developing nations [2].

Preventable maternal morbidity and mortality is associated with the absence of timely access to quality care, defined as too little, too late (TLTL) which refers

IntechOpen

to either inadequate access to services, resources, care that is unavailable until too late to help or a combination of these factors [4]. Caesarean section (CS) is the most common obstetric intervention designed to prevent or treat life-threatening pregnancy or childbirth-related complications [5]. When it is done on a timely basis CS provides an appropriate opportunity to prevent adverse obstetric outcomes, including maternal death, stillbirth and neonatal death [6–8]. According to World Health Organization (WHO), a maximum of 15% of births have a medical justification for a caesarean section, rates above this do not improve maternal and fetal outcomes and are considered inappropriate and unnecessary [9].

However, CS used inappropriately is an obstetric intervention described as too much, too soon (TMTS) which refers the over-medicalisation of normal pregnancy and birth. TMTS includes unnecessary use of non-evidence-based interventions, as well as use of interventions that can be lifesaving when used appropriately, but harmful when applied routinely or overused [4]. CS carries risks for both the mother and her child and therefore the reason for conducting the surgery must outweigh any potential adverse outcome [10]. Maternal deaths and perinatal deaths following caesareans sections are disproportionately high in lower and middle income countries (LMIC) [11]. The maternal mortality after caesarean birth in Africa is 50 times higher than that of high-income countries [10]. Mothers in Sub-Saharan countries are 37 times more likely to die than those from LMIC in European and Central Asia after caesarean section, and the risk is high in countries with low caesarean section rates. The rates of stillbirths and perinatal deaths in caesarean section births were 56.6 and 84.7 per 1000 CS procedures respectively [11]. Compared to vaginal birth CS has an eightfold higher mortality risk for the mother with increased risk of infection and bleeding, and similarly, CS is associated with a high risk of infant death, preterm birth, breathing difficulties and iatrogenic injury [9, 12–15]. Other complications believed to contribute to mortality were intraoperative hypotension (75%), operative hemorrhage (53%), ventilation difficulty (14%), regurgitation of stomach contents (13%), pre-eclampsia (8%), and difficult intubation (1%) [10]. Furthermore, CS is associated with post-surgical complications such as postpartum hemorrhage and deep vein thrombosis which are major contributors to maternal mortality worldwide. CS is also a profitable surgical procedure for physicians and hospitals, despite the high cost of caesarean birth resulting in significantly increased health expenditure for individuals and families [16, 17]. In comparison, vaginal birth is associated with fewer risks, fewer interventions such as anesthesia pose a lower potential for postpartum morbidity, involves a shorter hospital stay, is more affordable, and encourages earlier and better bonding between mother and infant [18]. The inappropriate use of CS is likely to contribute to the disease burden of poor obstetric outcome rather than improve it [10].

2. Prevalence and factors associated with CS

Low-income countries (LICs) especially sub-Saharan Africa have historically had very low CS rates, probably reflecting inadequate availability [19–21], whereas high income countries (HICs) generally have higher CS rates, indicating overuse [22]. In 2010, an estimated 3.5–5.7 million unnecessary caesarean sections were done in high and middle income countries (HMICs), whereas 1–3.5 million caesarean sections were needed, but not performed in LICs which is an indication of global extremes [23]. However, the burden of maternal mortality was high in countries with low caesarean section rates. In regions such as Sub-Saharan Africa, despite only 3.5% of all pregnant women delivering by caesarean section, 20% of all who died from any cause were delivered by caesarean section [11, 24]. The very high rates of stillbirths and perinatal deaths in caesarean section births are of concern, particularly in Sub-Saharan region where up to one in ten babies delivered by caesarean section are stillborn. When the fetus is no longer alive, caesarean section is considered only if the birth needs to be rapidly expedited to avoid complications, or when vaginal birth is not appropriate. The high stillbirth and perinatal mortality may reflect conditions where caesarean sections were carried out despite a diagnosis of stillbirth or when the procedure was done far too late to save the baby [11]. Evidence shows increasing overuse of potentially harmful interventions especially caesarean section in facility births and one of the critical knowledge gaps identified for research priority in LMIC is over-medicalization of birth leading to increased rates of unnecessary CS [4, 25]. Overall, CS rates are lower in poorer women and tend to increase with rising economic status [26]. Disparities within countries and hospital-level variations in CS rates even within the same socio-demographic or economic groups, implied that TLTL and TMTS can coexist within countries and facilities [27, 28]. These indicates that, some women might be exposed to unnecessary CS while others do not get the CS they need [29]. Therefore, optimizing and ensuring the availability of a CS service while reducing the unnecessary CS for women is a global concern [30].

In Ethiopia physician-led obstetric care is provided by a four-tier healthcare system organized as primary health care units or health centers, district hospitals, general hospitals, and specialized hospitals. Ethiopia is one of the countries where CS practice is rising and reached 46% in the private for-profit sector and 18% in government institutions [31, 32]. The population-based CS rate of Ethiopia is still one of the lowest in the world (2%), since many women in need of CS never reach facilities (institutional delivery rate of 26%) and the disparities within a country might masked the national averages [29, 33]. This overall low coverage of CS indicates TLTL, however, a stark disparities with higher rates in private practice and higher wealth quintiles, suggesting TMTS for wealthy women [4, 29]. These differences have been linked to insufficient adherence to, or absence of, clear evidence-based guidelines and reflect weak regulatory capacity especially in the private sector [4, 34–36]. Previous research undertaken by the applicant in support of this proposal reported a higher CS rate (47.6%) in Dessie town, Ethiopia with a significant discrepancy between public (18.2%) and private (76.1%) sectors. Fetal distress was the leading cause of caesarean birth possibly due to over-diagnosis of abnormal fetal heart rate patterns in the absence of an electronic fetal monitoring system. Additionally, mothers having a history of previous caesarean birth had higher odds of having caesarean birth which may be associated with the obstetrician's fear of attempting a trial of vaginal birth in facilities with limited fetal monitoring capabilities. Furthermore, mothers whose labour was not monitored using partograph (a labour monitoring tool used to identify and intervene abnormal labour) had higher odds of CS as most of these women were referred from the primary health care facility to the nearby hospitals with a labour complication where emergency CS would be done without further monitoring of progress [37].

Evidences have shown the contribution of non-clinical factors to the rising trend of CS and suggested that identifying the determinants of caesarean birth is the priority to improve the efficacy of this obstetric intervention [38]. However, the determinants of CS are very complex and include not only clinical indications, but also multiple factors: demographic, economic, social, logistical, and health system affect CS rates. On the other hand, most of the clinical indications are not absolute and very subjective, and disagreement sometimes exists between clinicians about when to use CS. This nature of clinical factors coupled with multiple non clinical factors including providers' practice differences at facility and individual levels, financial incentives (private providers), and inadequate adherence to clear evidence-based guidelines contributes to significant variability among hospitals and countries concerning CS rates for particular medical indications [27, 39]. This, in turn, leads to inequities in the use of the procedure, not only between countries but also within countries with an additional financial burden upon the overstretched health system particularly in LMIC [40, 41]. Therefore, rising trends of caesarean birth impose an inappropriate allocation of scarce resources in the poor economy countries [40, 41].

3. Optimizing the use of caesarean section

To rationalize the use of this major procedure in obstetrics practice, individual providers, professional associations, facilities, and health-care systems should seek a path beyond TLTL and TMTS, which means reducing unnecessary CS while ensuring the availability of caesarean birth for women who required it [4]. However, the challenge is to keep CS rates low while maintaining safe outcomes for the mother and infant. This requires continuous auditing of CS and increasing adherence to guidelines [4, 42].

For such endeavor identifying the clinical and non-clinical factors contributing to caesarean birth and the appropriate consideration of risks and alternatives used in the decision to undertake a CS is an important activity. This is supported by evidence that indicates the main reasons for performing a CS were clinical factors and the doctor's role in decision making [43]. Other non-clinical factors may also contribute, though these are more challenging to identify. For example, studies conducted to evaluate the appropriateness of decisions made for CS in Tehran and Uganda hospitals showed that more than half of CS performed was considered inappropriate with a significant difference between public and private hospitals. Conducting clinical audit would examine in more detail the clinical conditions for which they need for CS is questionable or inappropriate [39, 44, 45].

Therefore, auditing the clinical factors related to the use of CS is strongly recommended in all hospitals to reduce unnecessary interventions, to improve decision-making and consistency of practice among care providers particularly in resource-limited countries [43]. These in turn will increase adherence to guidelines and protocols in using the procedure, and to enable the development of guidelines or protocols that consider the difference of contextual factors [4]. Even though, global organizations are creating guidelines for interventions to reduce caesarean section rates evidence is insufficient for most strategies [4, 46]. More research is urgently needed on interventions for reducing unnecessary caesarean section and increasing vaginal birth after caesarean section rates [4].

Vaginal Birth After Cesarean Section (VBAC) is another mechanism of reducing CS rates since a repeat CS after caesarean birth is the major contributor to rising trends of CS rate globally [47]. However, limited numbers of mothers with a previous CS are allowed to attempt VBAC and factors behind this and its success was not well-understood [18]. Furthermore, perinatal outcomes of children born by caesarean section in LMIC are not known and the risks of maternal death after caesarean section in countries with low and high rates of the procedure are not known. Unless the key risk factors for complications in women undergoing caesarean section are known, it is difficult to target efforts to improve pregnancy outcomes [11, 48, 49]. In Ethiopia little information is locally available regarding outcomes between vaginal, VBAC and CS birth, and most of these studies provide limited evidence on maternal and perinatal outcomes occurred before hospital discharge and use secondary data which suffers from incompleteness and unreliable information [50].

The difficulty with monitoring and comparing CS rates, as well as planning or instituting interventions to modify CS rates, requires information about the indications for CS and the appropriateness of surgical birth. A major part of the problem is that there is no agreed-upon international standard of classification of indications for CS. After conducting several systematic reviews, the WHO concluded that the Robson classification as a global standard tool for international use which is important to know which groups of women are mainly contributing to the increase in CS rate [51]. The Robson classification also called the Ten Group Classification System (TGCS), classifies women into 10 mutually exclusive and exhaustive groups based on the category of the pregnancy, the previous obstetric record of the woman, the course of labour and delivery, and the gestational age of the pregnancy [6]. Multiple studies have examined rising CS rates in high and middle-income countries using the Robson classification system, though few studies involving low-income countries have been conducted [52–56]. In Ethiopia only one study has been conducted using Robson classification among women who underwent CS. The study was limited to one public hospital site which excludes the influences of private obstetric care [29]. Therefore, a prospective study involving both women receiving both public and private hospital care is recommended to understand the proportion of CS within each Robson group. Furthermore, as TGCS is not an audit of the appropriateness of indications for CS, further research is required to assess the suitability of the clinical indications [29]. Whilst small number of studies have reported maternal and perinatal outcomes in Ethiopia [31, 32, 50] no previous research has explored the institutional and decision making factors influencing CS use despite a high rate of post-CS mortality and morbidity.

4. Conclusions

Inappropriate use of CS can have profoundly negative consequences for women and the broader community. A recent meeting of the International Confederation of Midwifes, the International Federation of Gynecologists and Obstetrics and the Gates Foundation to discuss the impact of rising CS rates on maternal and infant mortality in LMICs highlights the international importance of the issue. Knowledge of CS determinants is a first step in the effort to define strategies to reduce unnecessary CSs. Previous studies showed that the main reasons for performing CS are clinical factors. However, non-clinical factors such as demographic, health system factors, organizational variables were overlooked determinants that best predicted which women have a higher risk of CS. Therefore, auditing the clinical factors related to the use of CS is strongly recommended in all hospitals to reduce unnecessary interventions, to improve decision-making and consistency of practice among care providers particularly in resource-limited countries.

Conflict of interest

The authors declare no conflict of interest.

Author details

Awoke Giletew Wondie
Debre Tabor University, Debre Tabor, Ethiopia

*Address all correspondence to: awokegiletew@yahoo.com

References

[1] Organization WH: **Maternal mortality: fact sheet**. In. Swizerland: WHO; 2016.

[2] UNFPA: **Giving Birth Should Not Be A Matter Of Life And Death** In.; 2012.

[3] Matthew Jowett: **Safe motherhood interventions in low-income countries: an economic justification and evidence of cost-effectiveness."**. Health Policy 2000, **53**:201-228.

[4] Miller S, Abalos E, Chamillard M, Ciapponi A, Colaci D, Comandé D, et al: **Beyond too little, too late and too much, too soon: a pathway towards evidence-based, respectful maternity care worldwide**. The Lancet [Internet]. Elsevier BV; 2016 Oct;**388**(10056): 2176-92. Available from: http://dx.doi.org/10.1016/s0140-6736(16)31472-6.

[5] Ethiopian Public Health Institute and Federal Ministry of Health Addis Ababa E: **Ethiopian Emergency Obstetric and Newborn Care (EmONC) Assessment 2016, Final Report. Averting Maternal Death and Disability (AMDD)**. In. Columbia University New York, USA 2017.

[6] Organization WH: **Robson Classification: Implementation Manual**. In. Geneva; 2017.

[7] Minkoff H PK, Chervenak F, McCullough LB: **Ethical dimensions of elective primary caesarean delivery**. Obstet Gynecol 2004, **103**(2):387-392.

[8] Wu JM HA, Visco AG: **Elective primary caesarean delivery: attitudes of urogynecology and maternal-fetal medicine specialists**. Obstet Gynecol 2005, **105**(2):301-306.

[9] Fernando A JMB: **Caesarean section: the paradox**. Lancet 2006, **368**(14):72-73.

[10] David Bishop RD, Salome & Maswime etal: **Maternal and neonatal outcomes after caesarean delivery in the African Surgical Outcomes Study: a 7-day prospective observational cohort study**. Lancet Glob Health 2019, 7(e513–e522).

[11] Sobhy S, Arroyo-Manzano D, Murugesu N, Karthikeyan G, Kumar V, Kaur I, et al: **Maternal and Perinatal Mortality and Complications Associated With Caesarean Section in Low-income and Middle-income Countries: A Systematic Review and Meta-Analysis**. Obstetric Anesthesia Digest [Internet]. Ovid Technologies (Wolters Kluwer Health); 2020 Feb 26;**40**(1):16-8. Available from: http://dx.doi.org/10.1097/01.aoa.0000652820.07964.a2.

[12] Lumbiganon P LM, Gulmezoglu AM, Souza JP, Taneepanichskul S, Ruyan P, et al: **Method of delivery and pregnancy outcomes in Asia: the WHO global survey on maternal and perinatal health 2007-08**. Lancet 2010, **375**(9713):490-499.

[13] Souza JP GA, Lumbiganon P, Laopaiboon M, Carroli G, Fawole B, et al: **Caesarean section without medical indications is associated with an increased risk of adverse short-term maternal outcomes: the 2004-2008 WHO Global Survey on Maternal and Perinatal Health**. BMC medicine 2010, **8**(71).

[14] Betrán AP YJ, Moller A-B, Zhang J, Gülmezoglu AM, Torloni MR: **The Increasing Trend in Caesarean Section Rates: Global, Regional and National Estimates: 1990-2014**. PLoS ONE 2016, **11**(2).

[15] Soto-Vega E CS, Chamizo K, Flores-Hernández D, Landini V, Guillén-Florez A **Rising Trends of Caesarean**

Section Worldwide: A Systematic Review. Obstet Gynecol Int J 2015, **3**(2).

[16] Field A HR: **Complications of caesarean section**. The Obstetrician & Gynaecologist 2016, **18**(2):65-72.

[17] Haider MR RM, Moinuddin M., Rahman AE, Ahmed S, KhanMM **Ever increasing. Caesarean section and its economic burden in Bangladesh**. PLoS ONE 2018, **13**(12).

[18] George O Ugwu CA, Hyacinth EOnah, Vincent EEgwuatu, Frank O Ezugwu: **Maternal and perinatal outcomes of delivery after a previous Caesarean section in Enugu, Southeast Nigeria: a prospective observational study**. International Journal of Women's Health 2014.

[19] Betran AP TM, Zhang J, et al.: **What is the optimal rate of caesarean section at population level? A systematic review of ecologic studies**. Reprod Health 2015, **12**(57).

[20] Vogel JP BA, Vindevoghel N, et al: **Use of the Robson classifi cation to assess caesarean section trends in 21 countries: a secondary analysis of two WHO multicountry surveys**. Lancet Glob Health 2015, **3**:e260–e270.

[21] Benova L MD, Footman K, Cavallaro F, Lynch C, Campbell OMR: **Role of the private sector in childbirth care: cross-sectional survey evidence from 57 low- and middle-income countries using Demographic and Health Surveys**. Trop Med Int Health 2015, **20**(16):57-73.

[22] Souza JP P-CC: **On labor and childbirth: the importance of quaternary prevention**. Cad Saude Publica 2014, **30**(S1-S2).

[23] Pap WHRB: **The global numbers and costs of additionally needed and unnecessary caesarean sections performed per year: overuse as a barrier to universal coverage**. In., vol. 30:1-31; 2010.

[24] Betran AP YJ, Moller AB, Zhang J, Gulmezoglu AM, Torloni MR: **The Increasing Trend in Caesarean Section Rates: Global, Regional and National Estimates: 1990-2014**. PloS one 2016, **11**(2).

[25] Kendall T: **Critical Maternal Health Knowledge Gaps in Low- and Middle-Income Countries for Post-2015: Researchers' Perspectives**. Women and Health Initiative Working Paper 2015.

[26] Adeline Adwoa Boatin AS, Ana Pilar Betran and etal: **Within country inequalities in caesarean section rates: observational study of 72 low and middle income countries**. *BMJ* 2018, **360**(k55).

[27] Melman S SE, de Boer K, et al: **Development and measurement of guidelines-based quality indicators of caesarean section care in the Netherlands: a RAND-modifi ed Delphi procedure and retrospective medical chart review**. PLoS One 2016, **11**(e0145771).

[28] Bragg F CD, Edozien LC, et al: **Variation in rates of caesarean section among English NHS trusts after accounting for maternal and clinical risk: cross sectional study**. BMJ 2010, **341**(c5065).

[29] Tura AK PO, de Man M, et al: **Analysis of caesarean sections using Robson 10-group classification system in a university hospital in eastern Ethiopia: a crosssectional study**. BMJ Open 2018.

[30] Suellen Miller ea: **Beyond too little, too late and too much, too soon: a pathway towards evidence-based, respectful maternity care worldwide**. *The Lancet* 29 October–4 November 2016, **388**(10056): 2176-2192.

[31] Cordova G AS: **Caesarean section and associated factors at MizanAman General Hospital Southwest Ethiopia.** Journal of Gynecology and Obstetrics 2014, **2**(3):37-41.

[32] Y. Ali: **Analysis of caesarean delivery in Jimma Hospital, South-western Ethiopia.** *East Afr Med J* 1995, **72**(1):60-63.

[33] ICF CSACEa: **Ethiopia Demographic and Health Survey: CSA and ICF, 2016.** In. Addis Ababa, Ethiopia, and Rockville, Maryland, USA; 2016.

[34] Bollini P PS, Wanner P, Kupelnick B: **Pregnancy outcome of migrant women and integration policy: a systematic review of the international literature.** Soc Sci Med 2009, **68**(4):52-61.

[35] Carballo M GM, Hadzihasanovic A: **Women and migration: a public health issue.** World Health Stat Q 1996, **49**:158-164.

[36] Pottie K MJ, Cornish S, et al: **Access to healthcare for the most vulnerable migrants: a humanitarian crisis.** Confl Health 2015, **9**(16).

[37] Wondie AG ZA, Yenus H, Tessema GA **Caesarean delivery among women who gave birth in Dessie town hospitals, Northeast Ethiopia.** PLoS ONE 2019, **14**(5):e0216344.

[38] Elisa Stivanello PR, Jacopo Lenzi, and Maria Pia Fantini: **Determinants of caesarean delivery: a classification tree analysis.** BMC Pregnancy and Childbirth 2014, **14**(215).

[39] Alejandro Arrieta: **Health reform and caesarean sections in the private sector: The experience of Peru.** Health Policy 2010, **99**:124-130.

[40] Field A HR: **Complications of caesarean section.** *The Obstetrician & Gynaecologist* 2016, **18**(265-72).

[41] Haider MR RM, Moinuddin M., Rahman AE, Ahmed S, KhanMM **Ever increasing. Caesarean section and its economic burden in Bangladesh.** PLoS ONE 2018, **13**(12):e0208623.

[42] Stanton C RCBGoC: **Recommendations for routine reporting on indications for cesarean delivery in developing countries.** Birth 2008, **35**:204-211.

[43] Khawaja M JR, Kabakian-Khasholian T **Rising Trends in Caesarean Section Rates in Egypt.** Birth 2004, **31**(1):12-16.

[44] Ostovar R PA, Rashidian A, Hossein Rashidi B, Hantooshzadeh S, Haghollai F, Eftekhar Ardebili H, Mahmoudi M: **Appropriateness of Caesarean Sections using the RAND Appropriateness Method Criteria.** Arch Iran Med 2012, **15**(1):8-13.

[45] Nelson JP: **Indications and appropriateness of caesarean sections performed in a tertiary referral center in Uganda: a retrospective descriptive study.** The Pan African Medical Journal 2017, **26**(64).

[46] Hartmann KE AJ, Jerome RN, et al.: **Strategies to reduce cesarean birth in low-risk women.** *Rockville, MD: Agency for Healthcare Research and Quality (US)* 2012.

[47] Sabol B DM, Guise JM: **Vaginal birth after caesarean: an effective method to reduce caesarean.** Clin Obstet Gynecol 2015, **58**(2):309-319.

[48] Esteves-Pereira AP D-TC, Nakamura-Pereira M, Saucedo M, Bouvier-Colle MH, Leal Mdo C: **Caesarean Delivery and Postpartum Maternal Mortality: A Population-Based Case Control Study in Brazil.** PloS one 2016, **11**(4):e0153396.

[49] Ologunde R VJ, Cherian MN, Sbaiti M, Merialdi M, Yeats J:

Assessment of cesarean delivery availability in 26 low- and middle-income countries: a cross-sectional study. *Am J Obstet Gynecol* 2014, **211**(5):504 e501-504 e512.

[50] Fantu Abebe Eyowas, Ashebir Kidane Negasi, Gizachew Eyassu Aynalem, Abebaw Gebeyehu Worku: **Adverse birth outcome: a comparative analysis between caesarean section and vaginal delivery at Felegehiwot Referral Hospital, Northwest Ethiopia: a retrospective record review.** Pediatric Health, Medicine and Therapeutics 2016, 7.

[51] Organization WH: **WHO Statement on Caesarean Section Rates [Internet].** In.; 2015.

[52] Vogel JP BA, Vindevoghel N, Souza JP, Torloni MR, Zhang J, et al: **Use of the Robson classification to assess caesarean section trends in 21 countries: a secondary analysis of two WHO multicountry surveys.** Lancet Glob Health 2015, **3**(5):260-270.

[53] Amatya A PR, Poudyal A, Wagle RR, Singh M, Thapa S: **Examining stratified caesarean section rates using Robson classification system at Tribhuvan University Teaching Hospital.** J Nepal Health Res Counc 2013, **11**(25):255-258.

[54] Litorp H KH, Nyström L, Darj E, Essen B: **Increasing section rates among low-risk groups: a panel study classifying deliveries according to Robson at a university hospital in Tanzania.** BMC Pregnancy Childbirth 2013, **13**(107).

[55] Makhanya V GL, Moodley J: **Utility of the Robson Ten Group Classification System to determine the appropriateness of section at a rural regional hospital in KwaZulu-Natal, South Africa.** S Afr Med J 2015, **105**(4):292-295.

[56] Sorbye IK VS, Oneko O, Sundby J, Bergsjo P: **Ceserean section among referred and self-referred birthing women: a cohort study from a tertiary hospital, northeastern Tanzania.** BMC Pregnancy Childbirth 2011, **11**(55).

Chapter 7

Association of Pre-Pregnancy Body Mass Index and Gestational Weight Gain with Preterm Delivery in Pregnant Women

Bhavya Baxi and Jigna Shah

Abstract

The perinatal mortality rate, which is one of the important adverse pregnancy outcome and includes stillbirths and infant death within first week of life is estimated to be nearly 40 deaths per 1,000 pregnancies in Gujarat. Also the infant mortality rates have been estimated to be 50 deaths before age of one year per 1,000 pregnancies. It is stated that children whose mothers are illiterate or belong to low socio-economic class have two and half times more chances to die within 1 year of their birth compared to those whose mothers have completed atleast 10 years of education or belong to high socio-economic class. There are nearly 13% of women who does not receive proper antenatal care and facility during pregnancy. In India, there are nearly half of the women (52%) who possess normal BMI range: rest are either underweight or overweight. Approximately 55% of the women of total population in India are anaemic. These maternal parameters directly affect the children causing 48% of the children to be malnourished and 43% to be underweight. Therefore, it is imperative to examine the association of pre-pregnancy Body Mass Index (BMI) as well as Gestational Weight Gain (GWG) with diverse pregnancy outcomes such as gestational diabetes, gestational hypertension and also with preterm delivery, caesarean delivery, etc. The present study was designed to investigate the prevalence, GWG, various pregnancy outcomes of underweight, overweight or obese pregnant women, and to explore the relationship between pre-pregnancy BMI as well as gestational weight gain during pregnancy and adverse pregnancy outcomes. This is a prospective, multi-centric study involving pregnant women with gestation week ≤20 weeks in Ahmedabad in Gujarat region. Our study observed that out of 226 women enrolled, 44 women (19.47%) were underweight, 137 women (60.62%) were normal, 30 women (13.27%) were overweight and 15 women (6.64%) were obese. The incidence of caesarean delivery (56.92%) was found more in nuclear family as compared to joint family (46.92%). It was found that in women taking no junk food at all, the chances of LBW were 16.39%, which was less as compared to mothers who had junk food. It was also observed that amongst women taking 1 glass milk daily (42.92%), about 55.67% of had normal type of delivery. Amongst women taking 1 fruit daily (57.52%), 53% women had normal delivery. Present study spotted decrease in risk of caesarean delivery with increase in maternal haemoglobin level from 9.0 gm/dl till 12.0 gm/dl. Average weight gain observed in underweight was 12.93 ± 1.90, in normal 12.32 ± 1.71, in overweight 10.23 ± 1.28 and in obese 9.6 ± 1.50. A negative correlation was found

IntechOpen

between GWG and pre-pregnancy BMI, i.e. as pre-pregnancy BMI increase, the GWG decrease. The incidence of pre-term delivery (9.49%) was much less in normal BMI range. The average infant birth weight observed in underweight women was 2.63 ± 0.47, in normal was 2.9 ± 0.49, in overweight was 2.92 ± 0.56 and in obese was 2.95 ± 0.86. It is observed that highest birth weight is obtained in obese women, which decreases as the maternal BMI range decreases. The incidence of LBW in normal and overweight women was 15.33 and 16.67%, which was low as compared to obese and underweight women. Our study reveals that parameters such as GWG, type of family, intake of milk, fruits and junk food, haemoglobin concentration directly affects the pregnancy outcomes such as term of delivery, type of delivery and infant birth weight.

Keywords: preterm birth, prepregnancy, body mass index, weight gain, pregnant women

1. Introduction

The perinatal mortality rate, which is one of the important adverse pregnancy outcome and includes stillbirths and infant death within first week of life is estimated to be nearly 40 deaths per 1,000 pregnancies in Gujarat. Also the infant mortality rates have been estimated to be 50 deaths before age of one year per 1,000 pregnancies. It is stated that children whose mothers are illiterate or belong to low socio-economic class have two and half times more chances to die within 1 year of their birth compared to those whose mothers have completed atleast 10 years of education or belong to high socio-economic class. There are nearly 13% of women who does not receive proper antenatal care and facility during pregnancy [1].

In India, there are nearly half of the women (52%) who possess normal BMI range: rest are either underweight or overweight. Approximately 55% of the women of total population in India are anaemic. These maternal parameters directly affect the children causing 48% of the children to be malnourished and 43% to be underweight [2].

The impact of prepregnancy body mass index (BMI) on maternal as well as neonatal outcomes has attracted wide spread attention these days. Several of the recent studies had reported that the prepregnancy BMI is associated with the child birth weight and it is also reported that mothers' whose weight gain during pregnancy may be excessive or inadequate are more prone to poor maternal and child outcomes. The range of weight gain during pregnancy is constant since last 10 years, although it may differs from one to another according to the maternal BMI [3]. According to the recommendations for weight gain during pregnancy by Institute of Medicine (IOM), both prepregnancy BMI and GWG are associated with the outcomes of pregnancy, either in correlation to mother or neonate or in both. Maternal and neonatal complications associated with BMI and GWG are of public health importance because they add to the disease burden in women and children and also increase the medical costs. Prior to pregnancy, all women should strive for appropriate body weights [4]. Gestational weight gain is a modifiable factor which can be controlled through diet as well as nutritional counselling during pregnancy to modify the inadequate or excessive weight [5].

The antenatal care involves various actions such as prevention and health care promotion of mother as well as neonate, early diagnosis and appropriate treatment of any problem occurring during this period of time. For proper antenatal care, monitoring the nutritional intake and status of pregnant women is important along with examining the gestational weight gain, haemoglobin level which also possesses direct co-relation with maternal and foetal health [6].

Various studies have been conducted which suggests the correlation of different maternal parameters with adverse pregnancy outcomes. A study by Li et al. observed that maternal prepregnancy BMI was positively associated with risks of gestational diabetes mellitus (GDM), pregnancy-induced hypertension, caesarean delivery, preterm delivery, LGA, and macrosomia, and inversely associated with risks of SGA and LBW. They also found that maternal excessive GWG was associated with increased risks of pregnancy-induced hypertension, caesarean delivery, LGA, and macrosomia, and decreased risks of preterm delivery, SGA, and low birth weight [3]. Another study by Steer P.J observed that the minimum incidence of low birth weight (< 2.5 kg) and preterm labor (< 37 completed weeks) occurs in association with a haemoglobin concentration of 95–105 g/L. Thus associating the haemoglobin levels with infant birth weight and term of delivery [7]. Adverse pregnancy outcomes are more common in women who begin the gestation as undernourished or as obese in comparison to pregnant women whose weight is within normal ranges. Maternal malnutrition increases the risks of birth weight, premature birth, foetal growth retardation, SGA infants and is associated with perinatal morbidity and mortality; insufficient intake of certain nutrients is related to some foetal congenital anomalies and birth defects. Gestational underweight has also been linked to infant inclination to certain chronic illnesses (diabetes mellitus type 2, hypertension, coronary disease, and stroke) in adulthood [8].

Low prepregnancy BMI (<19.5) is associated with many adverse pregnancy outcomes. In a country like India, where maternal underweight remains more common than overweight, the influence of maternal underweight BMI can affect mother and neonate adversely in many ways. Low Prepregnancy BMI is said to be associated with pregnancy outcomes such as preterm birth, LBW (i.e. birth weight less than 2500grams) or small SGA [9]. Women with lower than normal maternal body weight are prone to elevated risk for adverse prenatal outcomes such as intrauterine growth restriction (IUGR) as well as increased risk of subsequent obesity and hypertension in the offspring [10]. Also the SGA neonates are at risk for low Apgar scores, meconium aspiration, seizures, respiratory complications, extended hospital stays, and long-term squeal, including metabolic syndrome and neurologic deficits [11].

The prevalence of overweight (BMI 25–29.9 kg/m^2) and obesity (BMI 30–34.9 kg/m^2) is increasing rapidly among obstetric population. Further studies report that complications due to obesity can cause excess health care service use, including increased hospital stay during or after pregnancy [12]. Women with higher BMI during pregnancy are at higher risk of antenatal, intrapartum, postpartum and neonatal complications. Antenatal complications include recurrent miscarriage, congenital malformations, pregnancy induced hypertension (PIH), pre-eclampsia, gestational diabetes mellitus (GDM) and venous thromboembolism. Overweight and obese women are more likely to be induced and require a caesarean. Infants of overweight and obese mothers are often macrosomic and require prolonged hospital admission [13].

The iron concentration is less in females compared to males because of blood loss due to menstruation. Moreover during pregnancy, the foetal demand of iron is increased so more iron intake is required. It is also observed that the absorption of iron from the food during pregnancy increases along with the increasing gestational week, but this occurs only if there if sufficient iron concentration in the diet. Although very rare, but incidences of anaemia causing low birth weight and pre-term birth have been reported [7].

It is very important to maintain maternal nutritional status during pregnancy since it directly affects the foetal growth prior and post-delivery. It is highly recommended to consume balanced diet during pregnancy which is described by Indian Council of Medical Research (ICMR). It is frequently observed that low or improper nutrition intake during pregnancy may lead to insufficient weight gain, pre-term delivery, still birth, IUGR, as well as increase the morbidity and mortality rates which directly affect the maternal and neonatal health [14].

In modern times, the stress is increasing day by day. Since antiquity, people have thought that the emotions and experiences of a pregnant woman impinge on her developing foetus. Maternal stress has been found to possess adverse effect on perinatal as well as future developmental outcomes. Various stressors may be responsible for causing stress in pregnant women such as various life events (death of a relative, divorce, serious illness etc.), any physical aggravations, financial, domestic or any such type of factor. Any of the stressors thus activates the hypothalamus–pituitary–adrenal cortex system (HPA axis) and the sympathetic nervous system–adrenal medulla system. Hormonal imbalance occurs within the system because of hormones like Corticotropin Releasing Hormone (CRH), Adrenocorticotropin-releasing Hormone (ACTH), cortisol, and noradrenaline release. Spontaneous abortions, structural malfunction, preeclampsia, preterm delivery and low birth weight are the general adverse outcomes of various types of stress during pregnancy [15, 16].

According to the recent estimates of third National Family Health Survey (NFHS-3, 2005–2006), more than one-third (33%) of ever-married women aged 15 ± 49 in India have a BMI below 18.5 indicating chronic nutritional deficiency (CED) or underweight, and 14.8% of women are overweight or obese. Out of 29 Indian states, in total 13 states, more than 35% of women are too thin, and the percentage of overweight are more than underweight women in the states of Delhi, Punjab, Sikkim, Kerala, that is, a significant proportion of underweight women coexisting with high rates of overweight or obese in these states. Thus, Indian women suffer from a dual burden of malnutrition, with nearly half (48%) being either too thin or overweight. On the other hand, the percentage of thinness and overweight or obese is somewhat lower for men aged 15 ± 49 (34 and 9%, respectively) than for women aged 15 ± 49 [17].

As such pregnancy and its complications can occur in any part of the world without any correlation with race or species. Various studies are conducted in India which correlate individually between various aspects of GWG and maternal pre-pregnancy BMI to preterm delivery, but no such studies are conducted in the state of Gujarat regarding the same. Hence a study was designed to investigate the correlation between GWG, pre-pregnancy BMI, haemoglobin concentrations, various stressors and diet during the period of pregnancy, with the preterm delivery. The main aim and objectives of the study were to study prevalence of underweight, overweight or obese pregnant women and GWG during pregnancy, to determine the risk of underweight, overweight or obese pre-pregnancy BMI, and other comorbidities in pregnant women, to study the correlation between Pre-pregnancy BMI as well as GWG during pregnancy and preterm birth.

2. Study methodology

2.1 Study design

This was a prospective, multi-centric study which involved pregnant women from various hospitals whose detailed information was filled in the case record form. The study involved pregnant women with gestation week ≤20 weeks.

Informed consent of the pregnant women and the permission from hospitals were study was conducted was taken. Study approval was obtained from Institutional Ethical Committee, in agreement with local legal prescriptions, for formal review and approval of the study conduct. CRF and ICF were also submitted along with this for ethics committee approval. The study proposal was approved by Institutional Ethical Committee, Nirma University (Approval No: IEC/NU/14/2).

A pre-designed case record form was used for data collection. Information on maternal and paternal demographic data, socio-economic status, education and habit was taken. Also details regarding type of family, physical or mental stress, dietary information, history regarding gravidity and parity, present data regarding last menstrual date, estimated delivery date, comorbid conditions, actual delivery date, type of delivery, infant weight and gender was noted. Details of laboratory investigations, vitals, GWG and current medications were recorded from the file of pregnant women given from respective hospitals. Weight and height were measured by standard protocol and calibrated instruments. BMI was calculated as weight (kg) divided by height (m^2).

Privacy and confidentiality of pregnant women was maintained at all levels and subject name, address or contacts was not revealed at any stage during the study.

2.2 Settings and location

Pregnant women were selected randomly from Gujarat Cancer Society Medical College, Hospital and Research Centre, Binal Maternity Nursing Home and Nanavati Maternity Hospital.

2.3 Sample size selection

Sample size calculated was 384. The sample size calculation was done based on the prevalence of pre-term delivery in pregnant women in India. Out of 384 women, study was done on 250 women due to limited time availability. Amongst them, 226 women appeared for delivery at the same hospital from which they were enrolled. So finally the data of 226 were used for the study purpose.

2.4 Sampling criteria

2.4.1 Inclusion criteria

- Women from age 19 years to 45 years.
- Women not suffering from diabetes mellitus at the time of enrolment.
- Women not suffering from hypertension at the time of enrolment
- Women who are of gestational age of not later than 20 weeks at the time of enrolment.

2.4.2 Exclusion criteria

- Women of age below 19 years and above 45 years.
- Women having previous history of epilepsy or other CNS disorders.
- Women having previous -history of any liver related disorders.

- Women with any type of cancer or previous history of any type of cancers.
- Women with pre-existing hypertension, diabetes
- Multiparous women were also not included.

2.5 Data collection tool

- Informed consent form (English and Gujarati) (Annexure IA and IB)
- Case record form (English and Gujarati) (Annexure IIA and IIB)
- Information for participants (English and Gujarati) (Annexure IIIA and IIIB)

2.6 Parameters

Following parameters were considered for occurrence of adverse pregnancy outcomes:

- Prepregnancy BMI
- GWG
- Previous obstetric history
- Diet
- Socioeconomic status
- Haemoglobin concentration

2.7 Data analysis method

After the collection of data, analysis was done by using various statistical parameters. Pearson Correlation was used to correlate the parameters with adverse pregnancy outcomes to find the significance. All continuous variables were presented as mean ± SD. Other variables were presented in the percentage of population having a specific value.

3. Results

A total of 226 pregnant women who met the inclusion and exclusion criteria's were enrolled and completed the study.

3.1 BMI distribution

It was observed during the study that out of 226 women enrolled, 44 women (19.47%) were underweight, 137 women (60.62%) were normal, 30 women (13.27%) were overweight and 15 women (6.64%) were obese. Thus maximum population was found to be normal according to BMI (**Figure 1**).

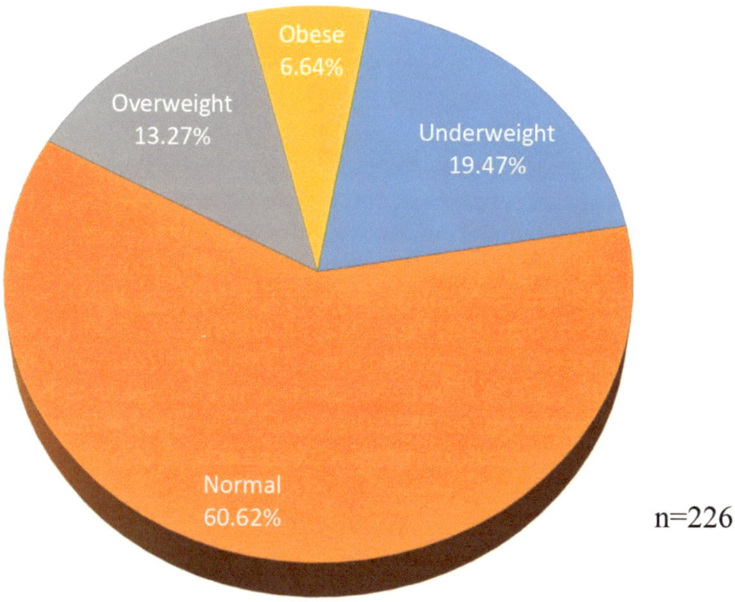

Figure 1.
Distribution of BMI ranges.

3.2 Maternal education

On grouping of maternal education with BMI, it was observed that in all the BMI ranges, there were very few subjects who were either illiterate or had just completed the primary education. Amongst underweight, 15.91% were illiterate or primarily educated, 50% had completed secondary education, and 34.09% had college or higher education completed. Within normal range, 12.41 were illiterate or primarily educated, 39.42% and 48.17% had their secondary and college or higher education completed. In overweight subjects, 23.33% were illiterate or primarily educated, 33.33% had secondary education and 43.33% had college or higher education completed respectively. In obese population, 13.33% were illiterate or primarily

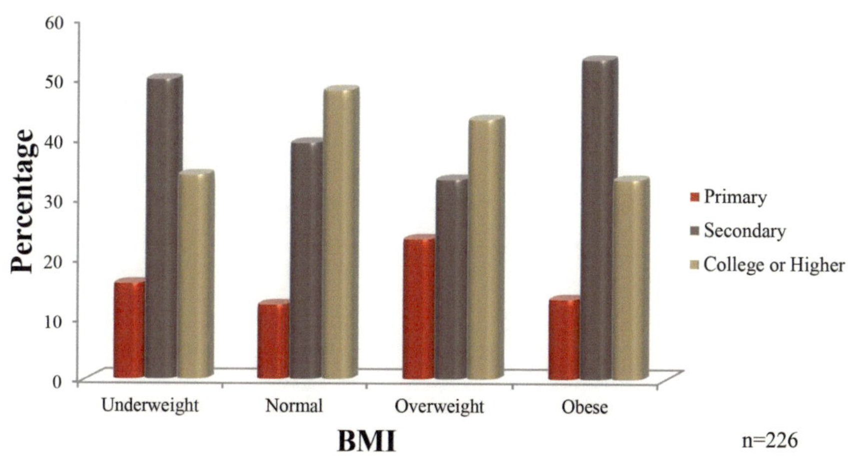

Figure 2.
Maternal education according to BMI.

educated, 53.33% had completed their secondary education and 33.33% had studied till college or higher education (**Figure 2**).

3.3 Paternal education

In paternal education also, there were more males who had their secondary or college or higher education finished compared to them who were just primary educated. In underweight population, 6.85% males were illiterate or had their primary education only. 61.36% and 31.82% had their secondary and college or higher education completed respectively. In normal BMI range, 8.03% were primarily educated, 35.77% had completed secondary education and 56.2% had completed college or higher education. In overweight class, 3.33% were illiterate or had their primary education, 40% and 56.67% had secondary and college or higher education completed. In obese population, 6.67% fathers were illiterate or primary educated, 53.33% had secondary education and 40% had college or higher education (**Figure 3**).

3.4 Total monthly income

An average subjects enrolled in all the BMI classes had their monthly income in range from 10,000-39,000. Very few had it below 5,000. In underweight population, 18.18% had monthly income below 4999, 31.82% had it between 5000–9999, 25% in 10,000-19,999, 15.91% in 20,000–39,999 and 9.09% had it above 40,000. In normal population, 11.68% had income below 4999, 19.71% between 5000–9999, 30.66% between 10,000-19,999, 27.01% between 20,000–39,999 and 10.95% above 40,000. In overweight population 13.33% were below 4999, 16.67% between 5000–9999, 30% between 10,000-19,999, 23.33% between 20–000-39,999 and 16.67% above 40,000. And in obese class, 13.33% were below 4999, 13.33% between 5000–9999, 26.67% between 10,000-19,999, 26.67% between 20,000–39,999 and 20% was above 40,000. It was found that in underweight, more subjects had income below 5,000 compared to other classes, whereas in obese, more subjects had income above 40,000 in comparison to other classes which indirectly reflected their nutritional status (**Figure 4**).

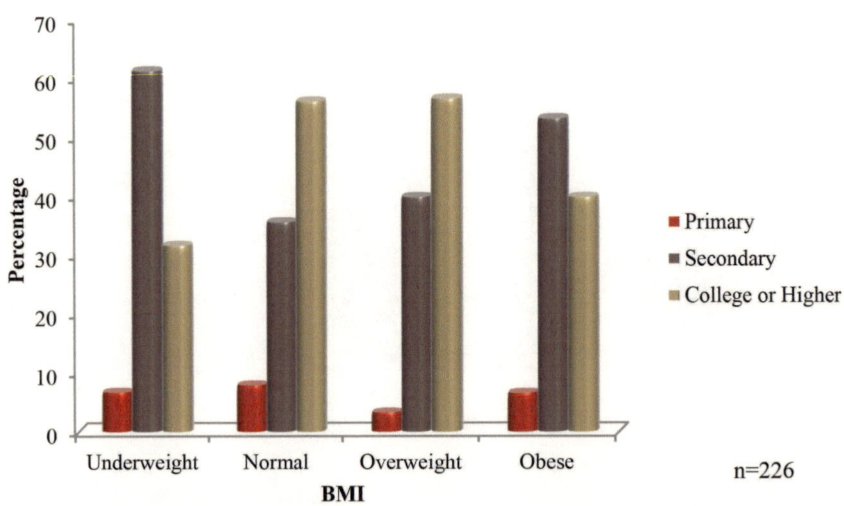

Figure 3.
Paternal education according to BMI.

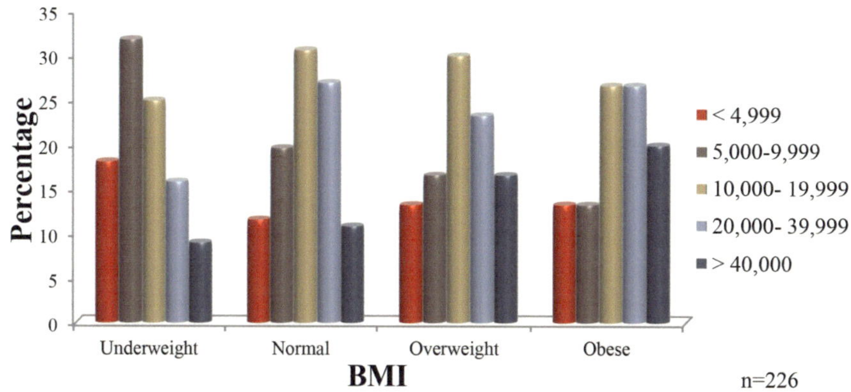

Figure 4.
Total monthly income of family according to BMI.

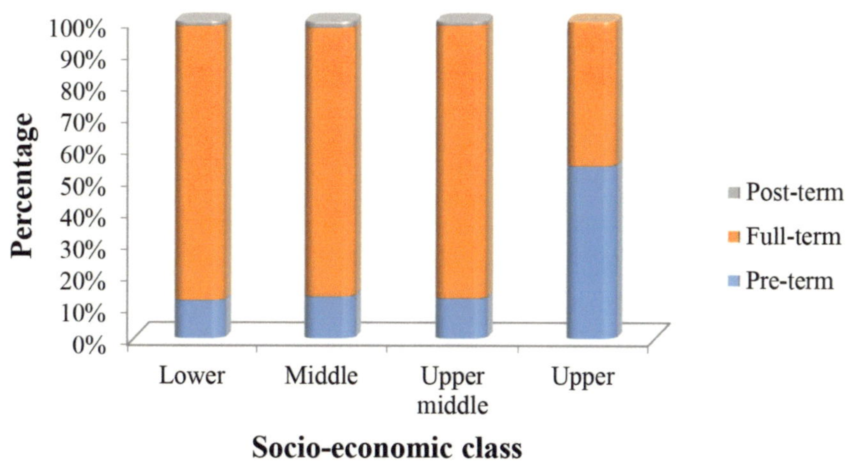

Figure 5.
Socio-economic status and term of delivery.

3.5 Socio-economic status

3.5.1 Socio-economic status and term of delivery

In present study, it was observed that in lower socio-economic class, incidence of pre-term birth (12%) was nearly equal to that observed in middle class (13.20%) and upper middle class (12.64%). But in upper socio-economic class, the incidence of pre-tem delivery was found 54.54%. In lower class, 86.67% had full-term and 1.33% had post-term delivery. In middle class, 84.90% and 1.89% had full-term and post-term delivery respectively. In upper middle class, 86.20% had full-term and 1.14% had post-term delivery. And in upper class, the rest of 45.54% had full-term delivery. A partial negative correlation (r = −0.116) was observed between socioeconomic status and term of delivery (**Figure 5**).

3.5.2 Socio-economic status and type of delivery

It was observed from the study that the frequency of normal delivery was lower in upper class compared to lower socio-economic class. In lower class, 58.67% had normal and 41.33% had caesarean section delivery. In middle class, 52.83% were having normal delivery, 43.39% were having caesarean section and 3.77 were having forcep delivery. In upper middle class, 48.27% were having normal, and 51.72% were having caesarean section delivery. And in upper class, 36.36%, 54.54% and 9.09% were having normal, caesarean section and forcep type of delivery respectively. A partial positive correlation (r = 0.177), thus is obtained between socio-economic class and type of delivery (**Figure 6**).

3.5.3 Socio-economic status and GWG

The study also showed, whether or not there is any correlation between socio-economic status and gestational weight gain. On an average, every class gained almost similar GWG. In lower class, underweight women gained 13.05 ± 2.01, normal gained 12.44 ± 1.61, overweight gained 9.88 ± 1.46 and obese gained 0.933 ± 0.58 of weight during gestational period. In middle class, underweight gained 12.5 ± 1.58, normal gained 12.1 ± 1.56, overweight gained 9.88 ± 1.55 and obese gained 9.6 ± 1.82 weight. In upper middle class women, underweight gained 13 ± 2.01, normal gained 12.48 ± 1.83, overweight gained 10.7 ± 1.06 and obese

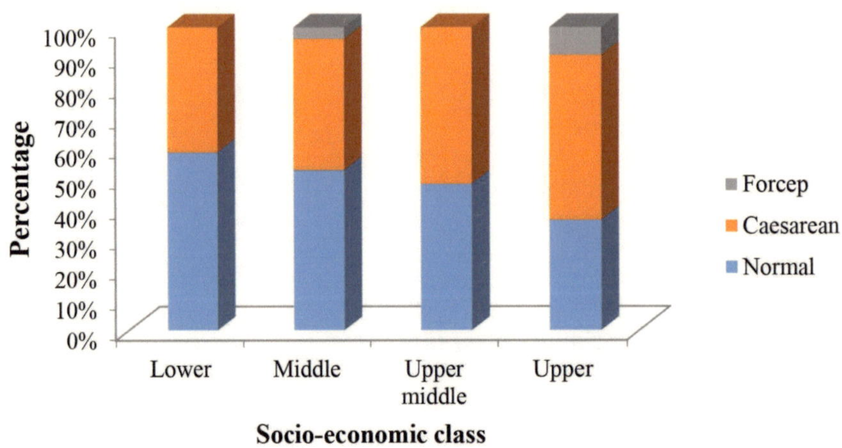

Figure 6.
Socio-economic status and type of delivery.

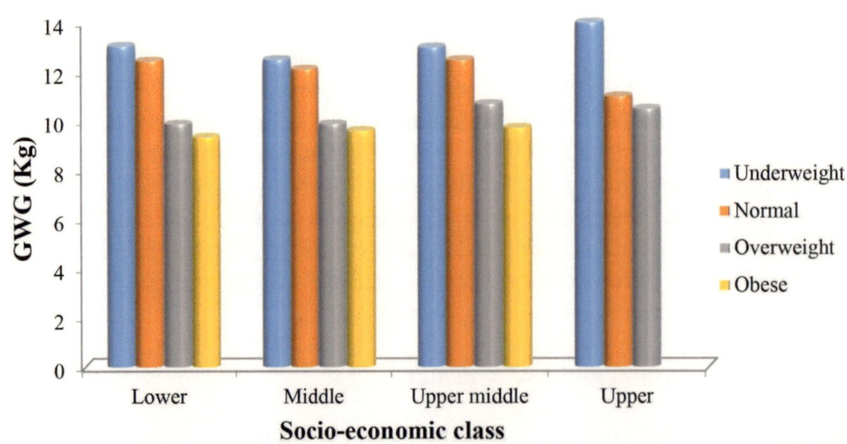

Figure 7.
Socio-economic status and GWG.

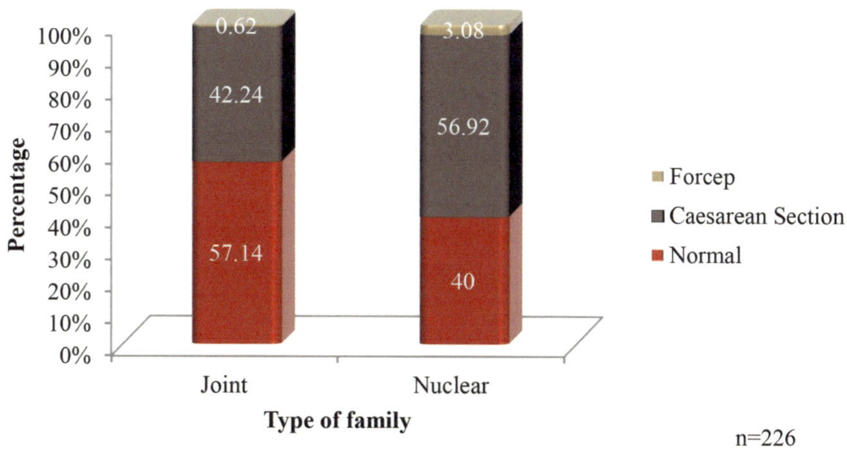

Figure 8.
Type of delivery according to type of family.

gained 9.71 ± 1.70. In obese women, underweight gained 14, overweight gained 11 ± 1.55 and overweight gained 10.5 ± 0.58 weight (**Figure 7**).

3.6 Type of family

In present study, 71.24% families were joint type and the rest 28.76% were nuclear. The incidence of caesarean delivery (56.92%) was more in nuclear family as compared to joint family (46.92%). 57.14% and 40% had normal delivery in joint and nuclear family respectively. Forcep delivery was observed in 0.62% in joint family and 3.08% in nuclear type of family. A fractional positive correlation ($r = 0.16$) is observed between type of family and type of delivery (**Figure 8**).

3.7 Past obstetric history

3.7.1 Previous delivery and present delivery

In present study we compared type of previous delivery(ies) to type of present delivery. It was observed that the risk of caesarean section delivery was more in women who had previous history of caesarean section. Rest 28.89% had previous caesarean section and 4.44% were such who had both type of deliveries. In women who presently had caesarean section delivery, 41.67% were having previous history of normal delivery and 58.33% were having previous history of caesarean section. In women who had previous normal delivery, 66.67% had normal delivery in present pregnancy also (**Figure 9**).

3.7.2 Number of abortions/miscarriage and term of delivery

It was observed during the study that not much of a significant correlation was observed between number of abortions/miscarriage and term of delivery. In women who had undergone no abortion/miscarriage, the incidences of pre-term, full-term and post-term delivery were 13.02%, 85.20% and 1.77% respectively. On the other hand, in females who had undergone 1 abortion/miscarriage, 20.45% had pre-term delivery and 79.54% had full-term delivery. In women who had more than 2 abortions/miscarriage, 15.38% and 84.61% had pre-term and full-term delivery respectively (**Figure 10**).

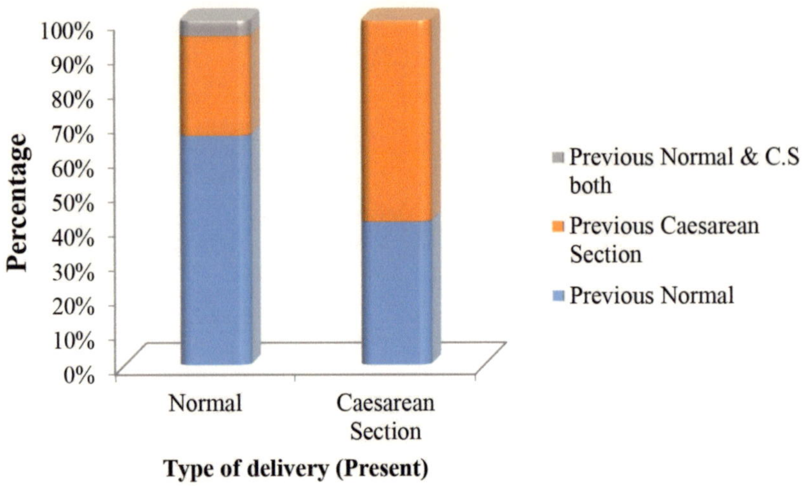

Figure 9.
Previous delivery and present delivery.

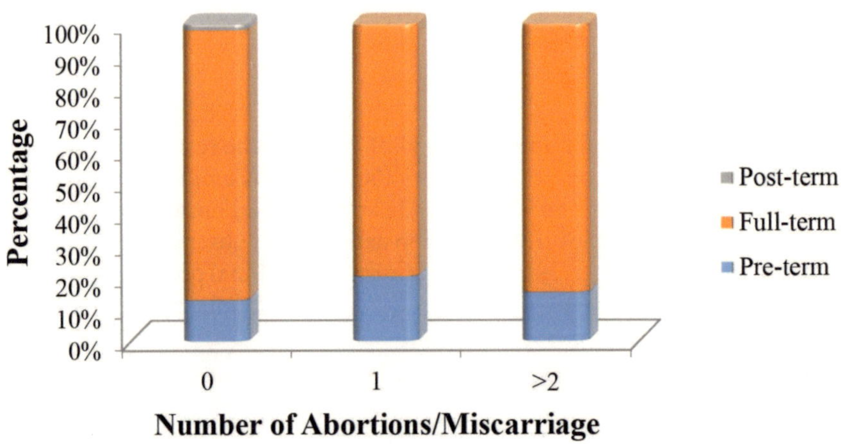

Figure 10.
Number of abortion/miscarriage and term of delivery.

3.7.3 Number of abortions/miscarriage and type of delivery

We also studied number of previous abortions/miscarriage and type of present delivery and tried to find out whether any correlation exists between the two or not. It was discovered that in women who had no history of abortion/miscarriage, 54.44% had normal delivery and 44.97% and 0.59% had caesarean section and forcep type of delivery respectively. In woman having 1 abortion/miscarriage, 47.73% had normal delivery, 47.7 had caesarean section and 4.4% had forcep delivery. And in women who had more than 2 abortions/miscarriage, 38.46% had normal delivery and 61.54% had caesarean section delivery (**Figure 11**).

3.8 Prevalance of stress

Current study showed that in underweight subjects, 50% had no stress at all. 34.09% had one type of stress. 13.64% had two types of stress and 2.27% had any 3 type of stress. In normal BMI women, 72.26% had no stress, 20.44%, 4.38% and

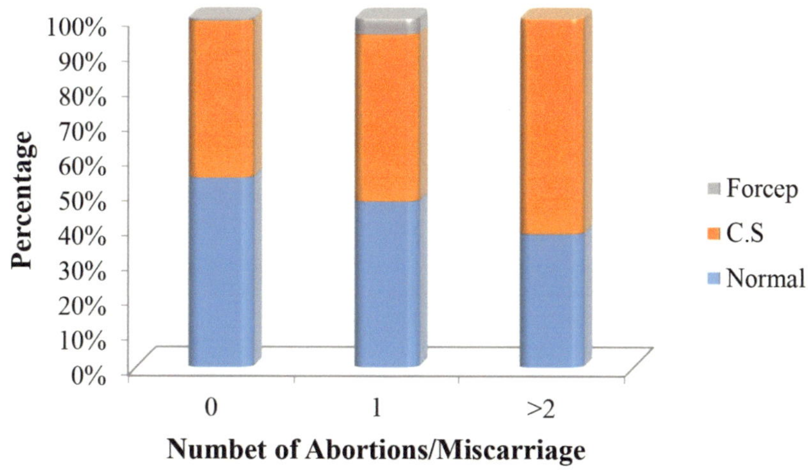

Figure 11.
Number of abortions/miscarriage and type of delivery.

2.92% had one type, two type and three type of stress respectively. In overweight women, 70% were stress free, 20% had one type and 10% had two types of stress. And in obese population, 33.33% had no stress, 40% had one type and 26.67% had two types of stress. The subjects having any 1 type of stress (physical, occupational, social, financial or pregnancy related) were more in underweight (34.09%) and obese (40%) class. The study revealed that in all BMI ranges, except obese, maximum subjects had no stress at all; whether physical or mental (**Figure 12**).

3.9 Dietary Information

3.9.1 Milk and infant birth weight

The study revealed that in women, who had consumed no milk during gestational period, 20.59% had LBW infant, 73.53% had normal and 5.88% had HBW infant. In subjects who occasionally had milk, 30.77% had LBW infant and 69.23% had normal infant birth weight. In women who had 1 glass milk daily, the incidence of LBW infant was 20.62%, normal birth weight was 75.26% and HBW was 4.12%. The mothers who drank 2 glass of milk, LBW, normal and HBW percentage was

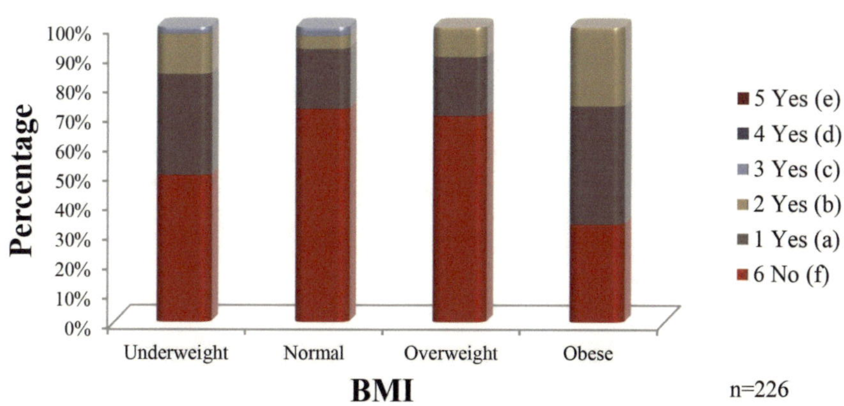

Figure 12.
Prevalence of stress according to BMI.

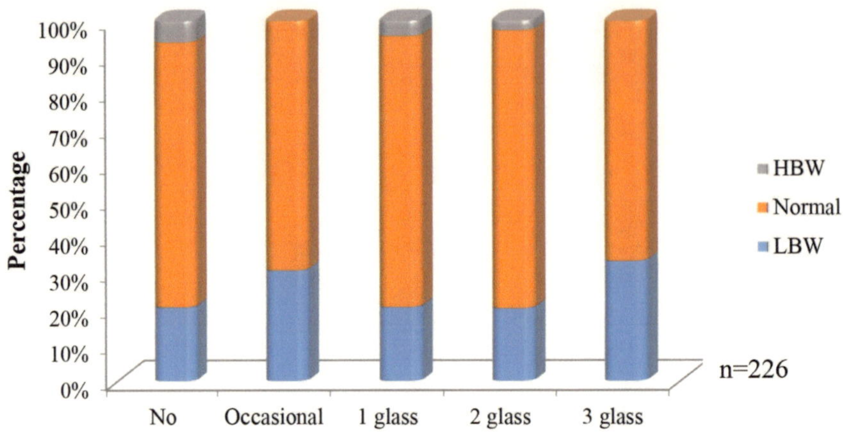

Figure 13.
Comparison of milk taken to infant birth weight.

found to be 20.25%, 77.22% and 2.53% respectively, while mothers who drank 3 glasses of milk, 33.33% were having LBW infant and 66.67% had normal infant weight. It was observed that the chances of LBW infant was less in women who had 1 or 2 glass of milk compared to them who had no milk or occasionally had milk (**Figure 13**).

3.9.2 Fruits and infant birth weight

It was observed in the study that 23.53% women who had no fruits during the gestational period were having LBW infant and 76.47% were having normal infant weight. In subjects who occasionally ate fruits, 23.29% were having LBW 76.71% normal birth weight infants. In women who had atleast 1 fruit the chances of LBW was 19.32%, normal birth weight was 74.62% and HBW was 6.15%. In women taking more than 1 fruit daily, 33.33% had LBW and 66.67% had normal birth weight infants. It is observed that the chances of LBW infant are comparatively less in women taking 1 fruit daily (**Figure 14**).

3.9.3 Junk food and infant birth weight

The frequency of junk food whether affects the infant birth weight was also determined in the study. It was found that in women taking no junk food at all, the chances of LBW were 16.39% and normal birth weight and HBW are 78.69% and 4.92% respectively. In women taking junk food once a month there were 22.33% LBW, 74.76% normal birth weight and 2.91% HBW infants. In women who took junk food every 15 days (fortnight), 25.58% were LBW, 72.09 were normal weight and 2.33% were HBW infants. Subjects who had junk food once or twice a week, 21.05%, 73.68% and 5.26% infants were LBW, normal weight and HBW respectively (**Figure 15**).

3.9.4 Diet and type of delivery

It was also observed that amongst women taking 1 glass milk daily (42.92%), about 55.67% of had normal type of delivery. Amongst women taking 1 fruit daily (57.52%), 53% women had normal delivery. No correlation was observed between junk food frequency and type of delivery.

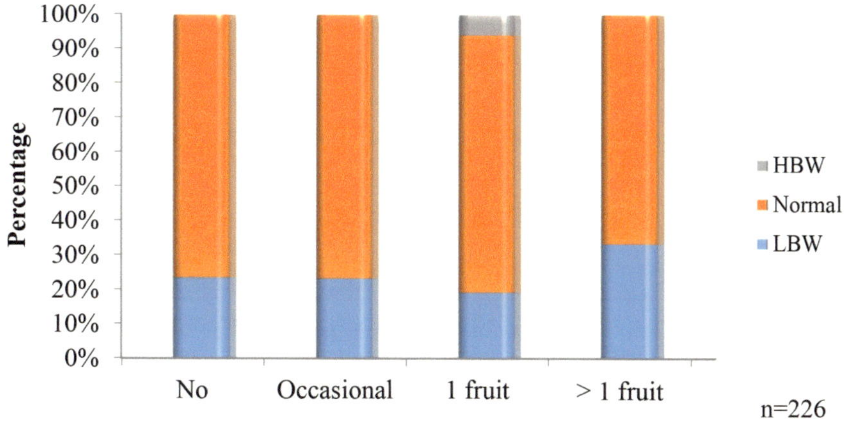

Figure 14.
Comparison of intake of fruits to infant birth weight.

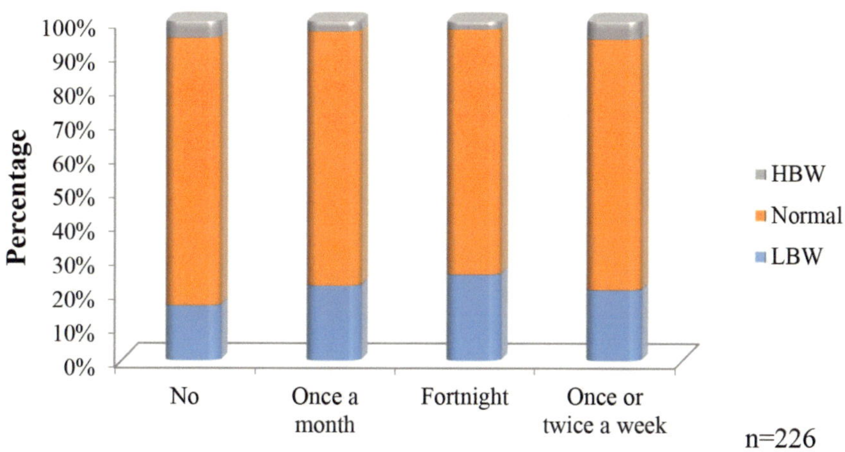

Figure 15.
Comparison of junk food to infant birth weight.

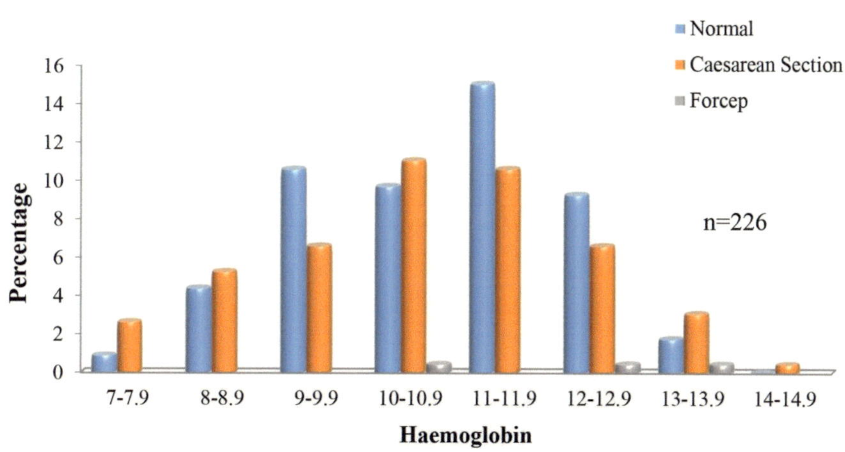

Figure 16.
Haemoglobin and type of delivery.

3.10 Haemoglobin

3.10.1 Haemoglobin and Type of delivery

From the present study it was spotted that an insignificant decrease in risk of caesarean delivery was observed with increase in maternal haemoglobin level from 9.0 gm/dl till 12.0 gm/dl (**Figure 16**).

3.10.2 Haemoglobin and GWG

No specific correlation was obtained between maternal haemoglobin concentration and GWG, as well as maternal haemoglobin concentration and term of delivery. It was observed that maximum weight gain is seen in the haemoglobin range 9.0–11.9 g/dl (**Figure 17**).

3.10.3 Haemoglobin and term of delivery

No exact correlation between haemoglobin level and term of delivery was observed within the current study. Maximum percentage of pre-term deliveries are observed within haemoglobin range 10–12.9 g/dl. As a fact it may be due to reason that this range contains maximum number of population (**Figure 18**).

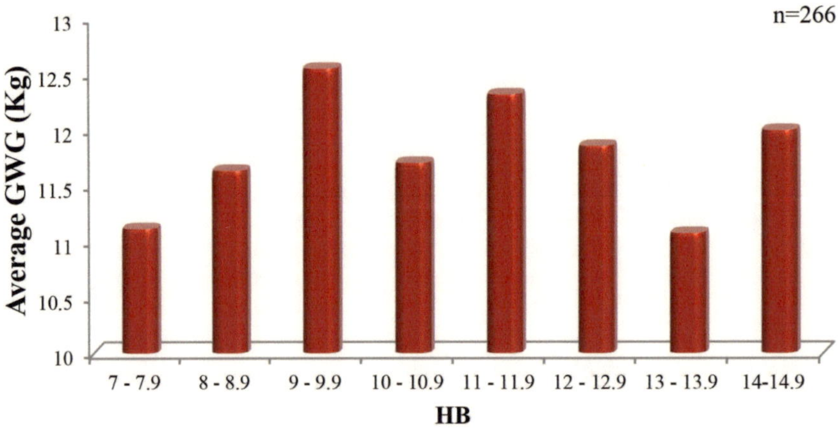

Figure 17.
Haemoglobin and average GWG.

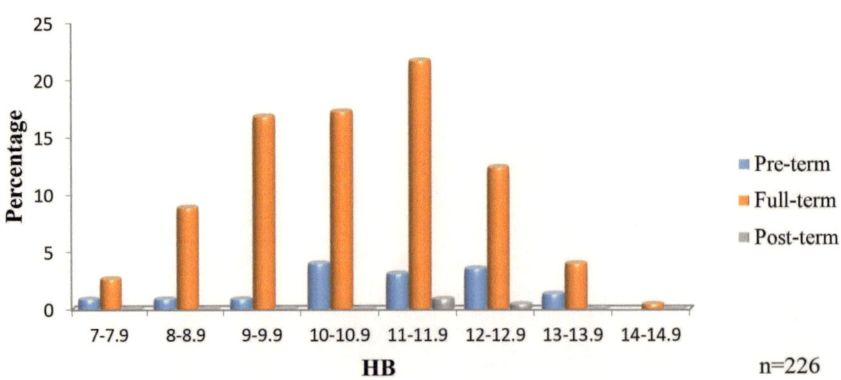

Figure 18.
Haemoglobin and term of delivery.

3.11 GWG

3.11.1 GWG according to BMI

The gestational weight gain observed in each BMI class was almost in accordance with that provided by IOM. Average weight gain observed in underweight was 12.93 ± 1.90, in normal 12.32 ± 1.71, in overweight 10.23 ± 1.28 and in obese 9.6 ± 1.50. A partial negative correlation ($r = -0.474$) was found between GWG and pre-pregnancy BMI, i.e. as pre-pregnancy BMI increases, the GWG decreases (**Figure 19**).

3.11.2 GWG and infant birth weight

It was observed that there is increase in infant birth weight as the GWG increases. But the increase is very minimal on observation. Thus as a fact, no correlation was obtained between GWG and infant birth weight.

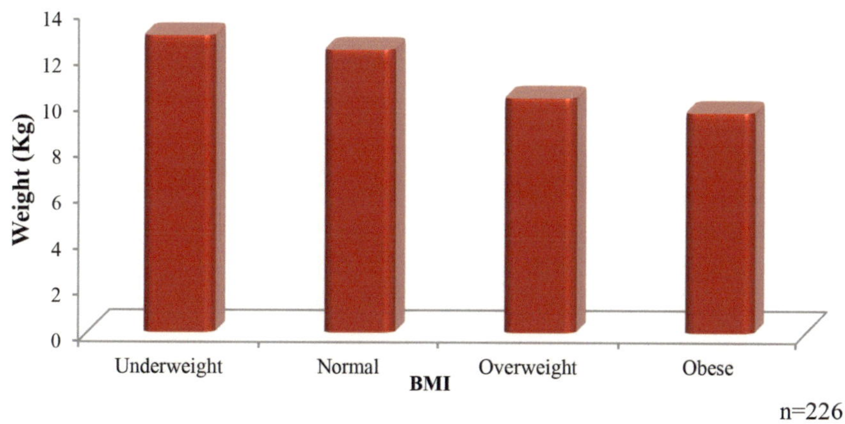

Figure 19.
Average GWG according to BMI.

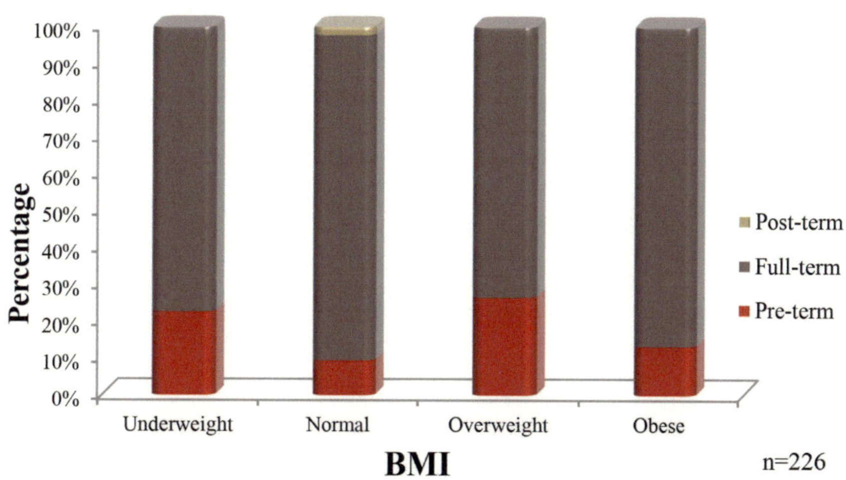

Figure 20.
Term of delivery according to BMI.

3.12 Term of delivery

The term of delivery is definitely affected by the pre-pregnancy BMI. In our study, in underweight women, 22.73% were pre-term and 77.28% were full-term deliveries. In normal BMI range, 9.49%, 88.32% and 2.19% were pre-term, full-term and post-term deliveries respectively. In overweight women, 26.67% were pre-term and 73.33 were full-term deliveries. In obese women, a total of 13.33% deliveries were pre-term and the rest of 86.67% were normal deliveries respectively. A partial positive correlation (r = 0.166) was found between term of delivery and pre-pregnancy BMI (**Figure 20**).

3.13 Infant weight

3.13.1 Maternal BMI and average infant birth weight

The association between maternal pre-pregnancy BMI and infant birth weight was clearly seen in the current study. The average weight in infant during birth is as shown in **Figure 21**. It is observed that highest birth weight is obtained in obese

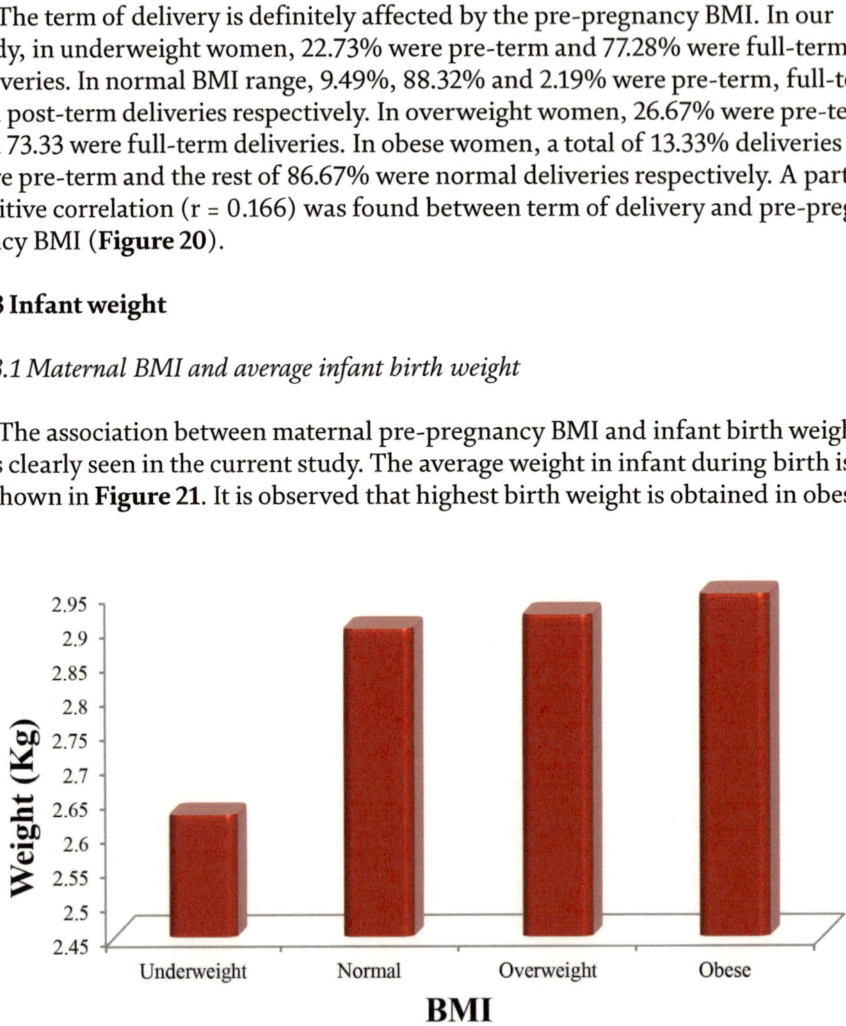

Figure 21.
Maternal BMI and average infant birth weight.

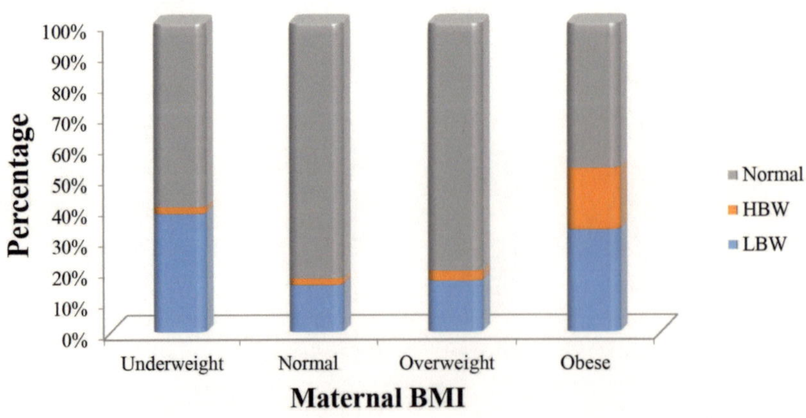

Figure 22.
Maternal BMI and average infant birth weight range.

women, which decreases as the maternal BMI range decreases. A partial positive correlation (r = 0.147) between pre-pregnancy BMI and infant birth weight.

3.13.2 Maternal BMI and infant birth weight range

An infant may have LBW, normal birth weight or HBW depending upon individual maternal gestational weight gain and other conditions. In our study, it was observed that in underweight women, 38.64% neonates are LBW, 2.27 with HBW and 59.09% with normal weight. In mothers with normal BMI, the infants born were 15.33%, 2.19% and 82.48% LBW, HBW and normal birth weight. In overweight women, 16.67% were LBW, 3.33% were normal birth weight and 80% were HBW infants. In obese population, 33.33%, 20% and 46.67% were LBW, normal birth weight and HBW infants respectively. A partial positive correlation (r = 0.16) is observed between maternal pre-pregnancy BMI and infant birth weight range (**Figure 22**).

4. Discussion

Different studies have been conducted in different parts of India, thus correlating pre-pregnancy BMI and GWG with the pregnancy outcomes. But very few or we can say no study have been conducted in Gujarat region which covers all such parameters affecting pregnancy. Thus we had conducted such as study which determines the prevalence and risk factors for BMI ranges like underweight, normal, overweight and obese. And also studies the GWG and correlation between GWG, pre-pregnancy BMI and different pregnancy outcomes. So we conducted a prospective, multicentric study including pregnant women in Ahmedabad for getting a better idea regarding GWG and pre-pregnancy BMI.

Our study possesses maximum population (62%) in normal BMI range followed by underweight, then overweight and finally least population was in obese BMI. A similar distribution of pre-pregnancy BMI was observed in a study conducted in Maharashtra in 2013, where amongst 400 pregnant women more than 50% had normal BMI and less than 10% population was found obese [18].

It was observed that in all the BMI ranges, there were more of women who had completed secondary or college or higher education compared to primary education. Same as that, there were nearly <10% males in all population range who either illiterate or were just primarily educated.

In present study, the upper socio-economic class showed higher incidences of pre-term delivery. A partial negative (r = −0.116) was observed between socio-economic status and term of delivery. In a similar study conducted by Wood et al., observed a modest increase in the risk of spontaneous preterm birth with low socio-economic status [19]. Regarding socio-economic status and type of delivery, decreasing incidence of normal delivery was observed from lower to upper socio-economic class. A partial positive correlation (r = 0.177), thus is obtained between socio-economic class and type of delivery.

Unlike this, a study by Gissler et al., concluded that women with the lowest socio-economic status were more likely to give birth by caesarean section delivery, indicating that increase in pregnancy complications increases the need for the same [20]. Socio-economic status showed no significant correlation to GWG. On an average, every BMI range belonging to every socio-economic class gained similar gestational weight during pregnancy. In contrast to this, a study by Andersson et al., observed that the mothers belonging to low socio-economic class gained only 5.5 kg weight during pregnancy while women from affluent societies gain about 12.5 kg.

They stated that the low gestational weight gain in low socio-economic family may be due to lack of food [21].

During our study, it was found that the incidence of caesarean type of delivery was more in nuclear family as compared to joint family. A fractional positive correlation (r = 0.16) was observed between type of family and type of delivery. Whereas in a study by Kilic, observed no correlation between type of family and type of delivery [22].

It was observed during the study that in women with previous caesarean section delivery, the risk of current delivery to be of caesarean section type increases. No significant correlation was observed between number of abortions/miscarriage and term of delivery. It was observed that as the number of abortions/miscarriage increases, the chances of caesarean section increases. Bhattacharya et al. [23], observed that the risk of preterm birth after abortion/miscarriage is lower than that after miscarriage but higher than that in a first pregnancy or after a previous live birth. This risk is not increased further in women who undergo two or more consecutive abortions [23]. Also in our study the incidence of increase in caesarean section and decrease in normal type of delivery is observed on increase in number of abortions.

Regarding stress, a partial positive correlation is observed in physical stress and GWG (r = 0.115) and type of delivery (r = 0.10). Thus as stress increase, there is increase in GWG. There is no correlation of physical stress with infant birth weight, whereas a negative partial correlation (r = −0.13) is observed with term of delivery. Any type of mental stress has no correlation with any of the outcomes such as GWG, type of delivery, term of delivery or infant birth weight. Study by Dole et al., stated that any psychosocial stress or anxiety is related to risk of pre-term delivery [24] another study by Zhu et al., observed that prenatal severe life events may increase the risk of pre-term birth or low birth weight infant [25].

The present study concluded that the risk of LBW infant in women who consumed 1 or 2 glass of milk daily was comparatively less than women who did not consumed milk at all. Also the risk of LBW infant decreases if minimum of 1 fruit is consumed everyday. No major deviation was observed in women who ate junk food as compared to them who did not have it. The occurrence of normal delivery is high in women consuming 1 glass of milk and 1 fruit daily.

Statistically no correlation was obtained between haemoglobin level and type of delivery. This is in contrast to the results obtained by Francis et al., who reported a significant relationship between maternal haemoglobin level and type of delivery [26]. It was observed during the study that no specific correlation occurs between haemoglobin level and term of delivery. A similar non-correlation was obtained between haemoglobin and term of delivery in a meta-analysis performed by Haider et al. [27] and Koura et al. [28]. Whereas a study by Bakhtiar et al. [29], observed that decrease in haemoglobin concentration can cause pre-term birth. No correlation was observed in present study between haemoglobin level and GWG [29]. Also no correlation has been found between haemoglobin level and GWG.

In our study a partial negative correlation (−0.474) was observed between GWG and pre-pregnancy BMI. As pre-pregnancy BMI increases, the gestational weight gain decreases. This is in contrast to study performed by Joshi et al. 2013, where they obtained significant association between prepregnancy BMI and GWG ($P < 0.001$). They suggested that the women with normal pre-pregnancy BMI gained adequate weight while women with low BMI gained inadequate weight and high BMI patients tend to move towards increased weight gain [18]. Another study by Montpetit et al., also observed a positive correlation (r = 0.35, P = 0.007) between pre-pregnancy BMI and GWG [30]. Unlike this, a study by Nohr et al. 2008, found high variation in weight gain, and it also increased across BMI groups. They observed that nearly 50% of underweight and normal weight women gained 10–15 kg, and that the low gain was more common among overweight and obese women than among underweight and normal weight women, and also that 40% of the obese women gained <10 kg [4].

The study shows a partial positive correlation (r = 0.421) between GWG and infant birth weight. However, a study by Chiba et al., observed no correlation between birth weight and GWG [31]. On contrary, a study by Mamun et al., found that mothers who gained excessive weight were more likely to have had higher birth weight infants [12]. A study by Rao et al., also found that with an increase in weight gain during pregnancy from 5 to 11 kg or more, there was a corresponding increase in mean birth weight. This increase was statistically significant ($P < 0.05$) [32].

Present study shows partial positive correlation (r = 0.166) between term of delivery and pre-pregnancy BMI. Various studies have been suggestive of effect of BMI on term of delivery. A study by Li et al. [3], suggested a positive association between maternal pre-pregnancy BMI and pre-term delivery ($P < 0.001$). Another study by Simas et al. also concluded the same association between BMI and term of delivery [11].

Present study found that the incidence of LBW (33.33%) and HBW (20%) was more in obese women compared to women with normal or underweight BMI. A study in Gorakhpur analysed maternal and foetal complications in overweight and obese women and observed that macrosomia and LBW were significantly (<0.05) more in overweight and obese women in contrast to normal BMI women [33]. Another study by Prabha et al. 2014, noted that LBW seemed to be more common with higher BMI groups; it was found to be non-significant after adjusting for confounders. However, macrosomia was more common and significant in the overweight and obese groups with ORs of 3.36 (95% CI: 1.51–7.49) and 8.30 (95% CI: 2.99–23.03) respectively, compared with the normal BMI group [34].

5. Conclusion

The percentage of pregnant women with normal BMI range is maximum followed by underweight, overweight and obese in Ahmedabad region. A partial negative co-relation was observed between socio-economic status and term of delivery. Moreover, there was a partial positive association of socio-economic class and type of family with type of delivery. In the women with previous caesarean section delivery, the risk of current delivery to be of caesarean section type increases. Additionally, it was observed that as the number of abortions/miscarriage increases, the chances of caesarean section increases. A negative partial correlation of physical stress is observed with term of delivery. Stress and dietary habits too modify the term of delivery, type of delivery and infant birth weight. As pre-pregnancy BMI increases, term of delivery decreases. As GWG decreases, the infant birth weight decreases. Present study found that the incidence of LBW and HBW was more in obese women compared to women with normal or underweight BMI.

Abbreviations

BMI	Body Mass Index
GWG	Gestational Weight Gain
HBW	high Birth Weight
LBW	Low Birth Weight
LGA	Large for Gestational Age
SGA	Small for Gestational Age

Author details

Bhavya Baxi[1] and Jigna Shah[2*]

1 IQVIA India, Ahmedabad, India

2 Institute of Pharmacy, Nirma University, Ahmedabad, Gujarat, India

*Address all correspondence to: jigna.shah@nirmauni.ac.in

References

[1] International Institute for Population Sciences (IIPS) and Macro International. 2008. National Family Health Survey (NFHS-3), India, 2005-06: Gujarat. Mumbai: IIPS.

[2] Arnold F, Parasuraman S, P. Arokiasamy, and Kothari M. 2009. *Nutrition in India*. National Family Health Survey (NFHS-3), India, 2005-06. Mumbai: International Institute for Population Sciences; Calverton, Maryland, USA: ICF Macro.

[3] Li N, Liu E, Guo J, Pan L, Li B, Wang P, et al. Maternal Prepregnancy Body Mass Index and Gestational Weight Gain on Pregnancy Outcomes. Jaddoe VWV, editor. PLoS ONE. 2013 Dec 20;8(12):e82310.

[4] Nohr EA, Vaeth M, Baker JL, Sørensen TI, Olsen J, Rasmussen KM. Combined associations of prepregnancy body mass index and gestational weight gain with the outcome of pregnancy. Am J Clin Nutr. 2008 Jun;87(6):1750-1759.

[5] Rozlan N, Mohd Abd M HA, Abas SS, Danis A, Anuar Md. K. The Association of Gestational Weight Gain and the Effect on Pregnancy Outcome Defined by BMI Group among Women Delivered in Hospital Kuala Lumpur (HKL), Malaysia: A Retrospective Study. Asian Journal of Clinical Nutrition. 2012 Apr 1; 4(4):160-167.

[6] Sato APS, Fujimori E. Nutritional status and weight gain in pregnant women. Rev Lat Am Enfermagem. 2012 Jun;20(3):462-468.

[7] Steer PJ. Maternal hemoglobin concentration and birth weight. Am J Clin Nutr. 2000 May;71(5 Suppl): 1285S– 1287S.

[8] Plecas D, Plesinac S, Kontic-Vucinic O. Nutrition in pregnancy: Basic principles and recommendations. Srpski arhiv za celokupno lekarstvo. 2014;142(1-2):125-130.

[9] Ronnenberg AG, Wang X, Xing H, Chen C, Chen D, Guang W, et al. Low preconception body mass index is associated with birth outcome in a prospective cohort of Chinese women. J Nutr. 2003 Nov;133(11):3449-3455.

[10] Yu Z, Han S, Zhu J, Sun X, Ji C, Guo X. Pre-Pregnancy Body Mass Index in Relation to Infant Birth Weight and Offspring Overweight/Obesity: A Systematic Review and Meta-Analysis. Baradaran HR, editor. PLoS ONE. 2013 Apr 16;8(4):e61627.

[11] Moore Simas TA, Waring ME, Liao X, Garrison A, Sullivan GMT, Howard AE, et al. Prepregnancy Weight, Gestational Weight Gain, and Risk of Growth Affected Neonates. Journal of Women's Health. 2012 Apr;21(4):410-417.

[12] Mamun AA, Callaway LK, O'CallaghanMJ,WilliamsGM,NajmanJM, Alati R, et al. Associations of maternal pre-pregnancy obesity and excess pregnancy weight gains with adverse pregnancy outcomes and length of hospital stay. BMC Pregnancy Childbirth. 2011;11:62.

[13] Athukorala C, Rumbold AR, Willson KJ, Crowther CA. The risk of adverse pregnancy outcomes in women who are overweight or obese. BMC Pregnancy Childbirth. 2010;10:56.

[14] Godhia M, Nigudkar M, Desai R. Associations Between Maternal Nutritional Characteristics and the Anthropometric Indices of Their Full-term and Pre-term Newborns. Pakistan Journal of Nutrition. 2012 Apr 1;11(4):343-349.

[15] Mulder EJH, Robles de Medina PG, Huizink AC, Van den Bergh BRH, Buitelaar JK, Visser GHA. Prenatal maternal stress: effects on pregnancy and the (unborn) child. Early Hum Dev. 2002 Dec;70(1-2):3-14.

[16] DiPietro JA. The Role of Prenatal Maternal Stress in Child Development. Current Directions in Psychological Science. 2004 Apr;13(2):71-74.

[17] Poluru R, and Mukherjee S. Concurrent prevalence of underweight and overweight among women in India: The case of Western States. Journal of Research and Practice in Social Sciences. 2010; 6(1): 22-42.

[18] Joshi S, Kulkarni A, Godbole G. Weight Gain, Correlation with Obstetric Outcome. Indian Journal Of Applied Research. 2013 May; 3(5): 467-469.

[19] Wood S, McNeil D, Yee W, Siever J, Rose S. Neighbourhood socio-economic status and spontaneous premature birth in Alberta. Can J Public Health. 2014 Oct;105(5):e383–e388.

[20] Räisänen S, Gissler M, Kramer MR, Heinonen S. Influence of delivery characteristics and socioeconomic status on giving birth by caesarean section – a cross sectional study during 2000-2010 in Finland. BMC Pregnancy and Childbirth. 2014;14(1):120.

[21] Andersson R, Bergström S. Maternal nutrition and socio-economic status as determinants of birthweight in chronically malnourished African women. Trop Med Int Health. 1997 Nov;2(11):1080-1087.

[22] Kilic M. The Delivery Methods and the Factors Affecting Among Giving Birth in Hospitals in Yozgat, Turkey. International Journal of Caring Sciences. 2012 May-August. 5(2): 157-161.

[23] Bhattacharya S, Lowit A, Bhattacharya S, Raja EA, Lee AJ, Mahmood T, et al. Reproductive outcomes following induced abortion: a national register-based cohort study in Scotland. BMJ Open. 2012 Aug 6;2(4):e000911–e000911.

[24] Dole N. Maternal Stress and Preterm Birth. American Journal of Epidemiology. 2003 Jan 1;157(1):14-24.

[25] Zhu P, Tao F, Hao J, Sun Y, Jiang X. Prenatal life events stress: implications for preterm birth and infant birthweight. American Journal of Obstetrics and Gynecology. 2010 Jul;203(1):34.e1-34.e8.

[26] Francis S and Nayak S. Maternal haemoglobin level and its association with pregnancy outcome among mothers. Nitte University Journal of Health Science. 2013 Sept; 3: 96-100.

[27] Haider BA, Olofin I, Wang M, Spiegelman D, Ezzati M, Fawzi WW, et al. Anaemia, prenatal iron use, and risk of adverse pregnancy outcomes: systematic review and meta-analysis. BMJ. 2013 Jun 21;346(jun21 3):f3443–f3443.

[28] Koura GK, Ouedraogo S, Le Port A, Watier L, Cottrell G, Guerra J, et al. Anaemia during pregnancy: impact on birth outcome and infant haemoglobin level during the first 18 months of life: Anaemia during pregnancy and its consequences. Tropical Medicine & International Health. 2011 Dec;no – no.

[29] Bakhtiar UJ, Khan Y, Nasar R. Relationship between maternal hemoglobin and Perinatal outcome. RMJ. 2007, [cited May 13, 2015]; 32(2): 102-104.

[30] Montpetit AE, Plourde H, Cohen TR, Koski KG. Modeling the impact of prepregnancy BMI, physical activity, and energy intake on gestational weight gain, infant birth weight, and postpartum weight retention. J Phys Act Health. 2012 Sep;9(7):1020-1029.

[31] Kashiwakura I. Influence of maternal body mass index on gestational weight gain and birth weight: A comparison of parity. Experimental and Therapeutic Medicine [Internet]. 2013 Jun 19 [cited 2015 May 14]; Available from: http://www.spandidos-publications.com/10.3892/etm.2013.1167.

[32] Rao P, KP P, Nair S. Influence of Pre-Pregnancy Weight, Maternal Height and Weight Gain During Pregnancy on Birth Weight. Bahrain Medical bulletin. *2001 March; 23(1):1-8.*

[33] Meenakshi, Srivastava R, Sharma NR, Kushwaha KP, Aditya V. Obstetric Behavior and Pregnancy Outcome in Overweight and Obese Women: Maternal and Fetal Complications and Risks in Relation to Maternal Overweight and Obesity. The Journal of Obstetrics and Gynecology of India. 2012 Jun;62(3):276-280.

[34] Kumari P, Malviya S, Gupta M, Kahlon P. Association between high maternal body mass index and feto-maternal outcome. Journal of Obesity and Metabolic Research. 2014;1(3):143.

Section 2

Caesarean Section Techniques

Chapter 8

Prevention of Cesarean Scar Defects: What Is Possible?

Christian Litzka, Annegret Schnabel,
Maria Emilia Solano and Angela Köninger

Abstract

Defect healing of the uterotomy at ceasarean section (CS) results in a morphological und probably functional disruption of the anterior uterine wall. Clinical sequelae concern subsequent pregnancies with a broad range of complications before and during pregnancy as well as at birth. In the following chapter, we provide an overview about the definition, diagnosis, symptoms and pathogenetical mechanisms of CS scar defects. Keeping in mind the pathogenesis allows to introduce preventative approaches.

Keywords: suture technique, peritoneum closure, contractions, immunology, tissue repair

1. Introduction

1.1 Definition of uterine scar defects

With the increasing rate of CS worldwide a meaningful long-term complication has been observed within the last two decades: the development of defects of the uterine scar. Previously, these defects were referred to as "pouch", "uterine/cesarean scar defect", "uterine diverticulum" or "sacculation" [1]. Nowadays, the terms "isthmocele" or "niche" are best established [2].

As niches occur almost exclusively after CS [3, 4], they are located within the uterine isthmus at the site of the former uterotomy [5]. There is still no international consensus about the exact definition of a niche or a standardized classification. Therefore, prevalence rates are of wide range [1]. Due to ongoing research, initial gaps in knowledge start to close [6]:

Most commonly, a niche is defined as any indentation of the myometrium at the location of the uterotomy with a depth of at least 2 mm [2]. The depth of a large niche either ranges between 50 and 80% of the myometrial thickness, or leaves a remaining myometrial thickness (RMT) thinner than 2.2 mm (measured by transvaginal ultrasound -TVUS-) or 2.5 mm (measured by contrast enhanced sonohysterography –SHG-), respectively [1]. Concerning the shape of the niche, the following subclassification was suggested: A simple niche (without any further branch), a simple niche with one branch, and a complex niche (with more than one branch) [2] (**Figures 1–3**). In most cases, the appearance of a niche is triangular in shape, but it can also be round [3]. A scar dehiscence is defined as a complete defect of the myometrium (**Figure 4**) [3].

IntechOpen

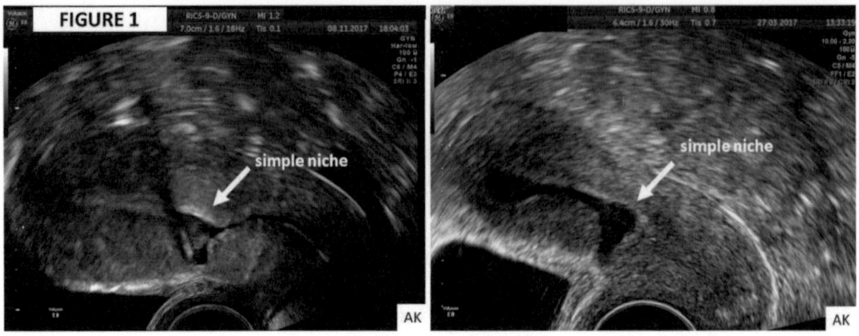

Figure 1.
Simple niches.

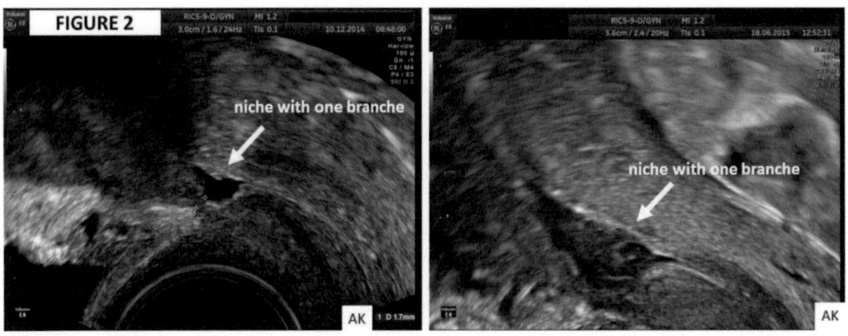

Figure 2.
Simple niches with branches.

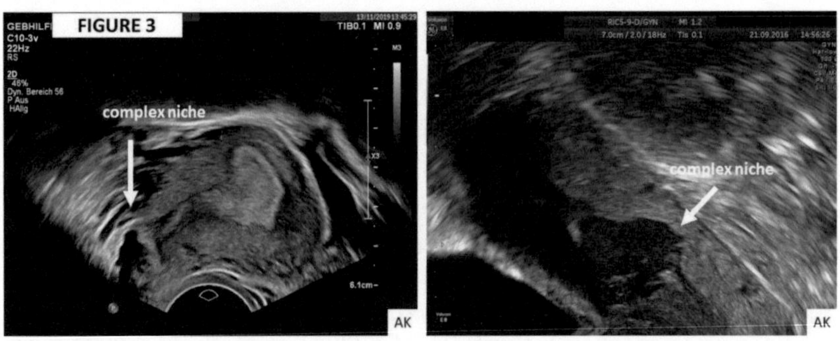

Figure 3.
Complex niches.

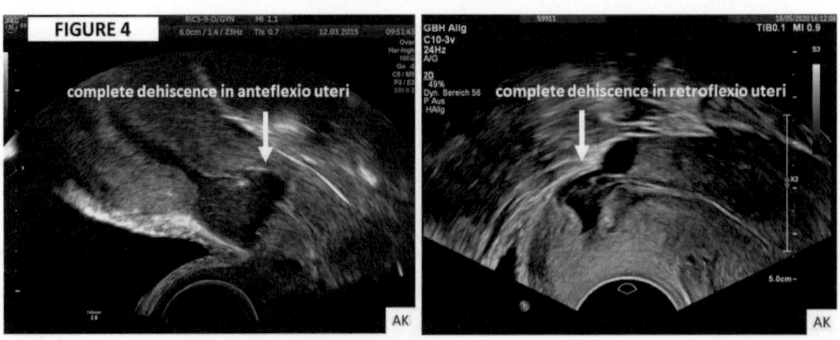

Figure 4.
Complete defect of the myometrium.

Several studies examined the prevalence of niches, resulting in a range from 22 to 84% of patients after CS [6, 7]. This rather wide range results from the different modes of assessment (TVUS or SHG) and the timing of the examination (several weeks up to 12 months after CS).

2. Niche diagnosis

2.1 Methods

Several methods exist to diagnose a niche: magnetic resonance imaging (MRI), hysteroscopy, two- or three-dimensional TVUS and SHG with the aid of saline or gel infusion.

By MRI, the thickness of the remaining myometrium can be measured quite exactly using T2 weighted views. As an advantage, the evaluation does not depend on the examiner's experience and consequently the measurements of RMT by MRI are more objective compared to those assessed by ultrasound [8]. On the other hand, MRI examinations are costly and not always available.

Hysteroscopy can simultaneously be used for diagnosis as well as for therapeutical interventions. As long as no mucus or residual blood obstruct the view, the potential defect can be visualized and treated in the same session. However, it is not possible to determine the RMT from inside the uterine cavity [9].

Ultrasound is widely available, harmless and rather unexpensive. However, diagnostic quality strongly depends on the examiner's experience. The exploration of a niche and the RMT can be facilitated by the use of saline or gel infusion enhancing the contrast. Several studies comparing ultrasound methods found that the use of contrast SHG is more sensitive and specific than simple TVUS for the identification of a niche [10]. In a prospective study of 371 patients, half of all myometrial defects remained undiagnosed with TVUS but could be seen with SHG, resulting in a higher prevalence of a niche using SHG (45,6% vs. 22,4%) [7] (**Figure 5**). A systematic review including 21 studies found a niche prevalence in up to 84% of women with a history of CS by using SHG for diagnosis [1]. SHG was considered as comparable to hysteroscopy in diagnosing defects of the myometrium with a sensitivity of 87%, specificity of 100%, a positive predictive value of 100%, a negative predictive value of 95% and an overall accuracy of 96% [1]. Because of the clear advantages of SHG, currently most authors consider it as a gold standard for diagnosing niches. If not available, simple TVUS with intrauterine fluid (e.g. blood during menstruation) to enhance the contrast [2, 7] constitutes a possible alternative.

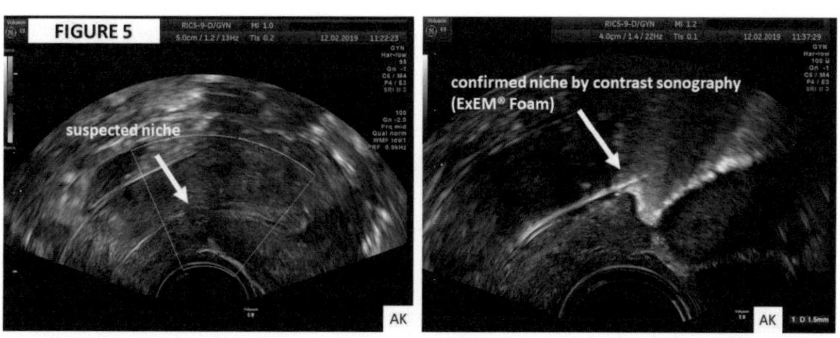

Figure 5.
Diagnosis of a niche without (left) and with (right) contrast enhanced sonohysterography.

2.2 Timing

For most exact results in measurement, optimal timing of the examination is necessary. This includes the day in the menstruation cycle as well as the interval to previous CS. Most authors agree that the best time for ultrasound is either during menstruation or in early follicular phase shortly after menstruation [2, 6]. The accumulation of blood in the isthmocele together with a thin endometrium facilitate the detection of the defect. Other authors prefer the time proximate to ovulation, when cervical mucus may distend a niche located within or near the cervix [11]. Using the follicular phase of menstrual cycle also is suitable to exclude the presence of an early pregnancy.

Unfortunately, data is limited concerning the best time interval to previous CS. The suggested time ranges from three to six months [2, 7]. Due to the fact that proper wound healing after CS takes up to six months [7], at least half a year interval before measuring the myometrial thickness is recommended.

2.3 Procedure

The assessment of the myometrium in search of a niche requires to follow a systematic workflow. A full bladder helps visualizing the lower uterine segment (LUS) but is not obligatory for the examination [2]. Variation in pressure with the probe is useful for an optimal image. Using doppler imaging, the differentiation between niche and myometrial vessels is possible. In 2019, Jordans et al. established a modified Delphi procedure for the sonographic examination of niches [2].

Briefly, the examination starts in the midsagittal plane including a proper visualization of the cervical canal. By panning the probe laterally left and right, the niche should become visible. Once the defect is identified measurements of length and depth are made. If the niche is complex with branches, both length and depth should be measured for every branch. Furthermore, the distance to the vesico-vaginal fold (VV) should be measured placing the caliper at the level where the residual myometrium is thinnest (**Figure 6**). Exactly at the same point measurement of the RMT is done. Next, adjacent myometrial thickness (AMT) is measured close to the niche. The last measurement in the midsagittal plane is the distance to the external os parallel to the cervical canal starting at the distal point of the niche (**Figure 7**).

Afterwards the niche is visualized in transverse plane by rotating the probe by 90 degree. Here, the niche's width can be measured. The transverse plane works best for detecting branches in case of complex niches.

Nevertheless, standardized cut off parameters for niche characterization, especially in the case of large niches, are not yet established. The following parameters

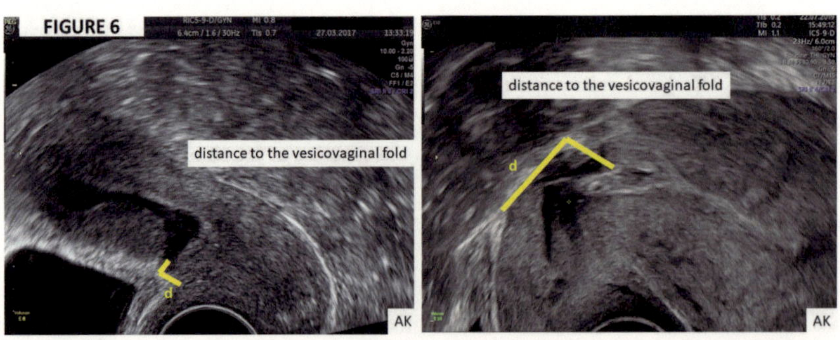

Figure 6.
Technique of niche measurement: distance between the niche and the vesicovaginal fold.

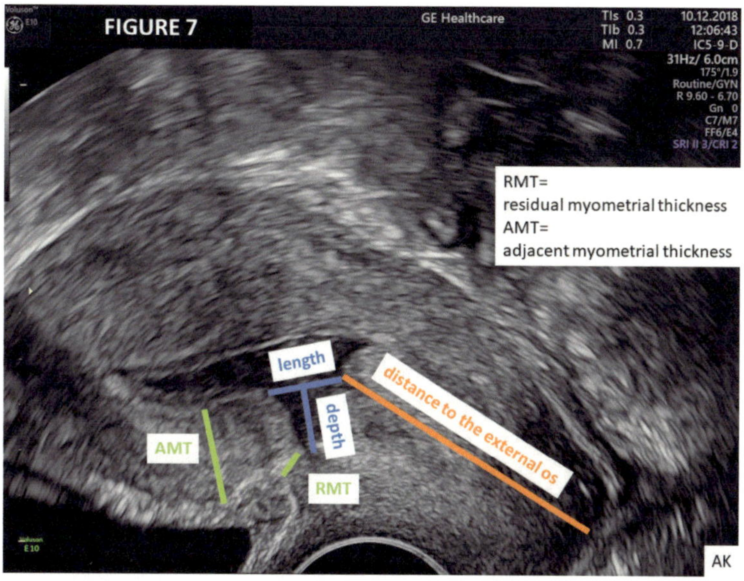

Figure 7.
Technique of niche measurement following the Delphi procedure [2].

seem to be suitable for clinical practice: the ratios RMT/AMT, depth/RMT, depth/AMT and RMT [1, 2, 7].

A further issue that needs to be considered in future studies is the clinical relevance of the size of the niche. To date, no study has clearly shown a direct correlation between the scar's thickness and the risk of e.g. uterine rupture [3, 5, 12, 13]. Therefore, further studies are needed to evaluate the association between a niche's size and clinical sequelae.

2.4 Niche symptoms

Although niches can also be asymptomatic [6], niche-associated problems differ between non-pregnant and pregnant women according to the symptoms and potential complications.

2.5 Non-pregnant women

Today there is international consensus that specific gynecological problems can be caused by a niche:

As the main symptom, abnormal uterine bleeding, e.g. postmenstrual spotting, results from a retention of menstruation blood in the indentation of the myometrium [14]. Nearly 30% of women with a niche report spotting compared to only 15% without a niche within 6–12 months after a CS [11]. An insufficient contractility of the myometrium seems to be the main reason [1]. Also the size of the niche is important since women with larger niches are reported to have more severe bleeding issues [2].

Several studies describe dysmenorrhea, dyspareunia or even chronic pelvic pain as further symptoms of a niche [6, 11]. The reason for pain during the menstruation bleeding might be found in the myometrium's distension caused by the accumulating blood.

Importantly, the presence of a niche may affect fertility: the accumulation of blood in the niche deteriorates the quality of cervical mucus, potentially inhibiting sperm transport or referring to an impaired implantation of the embryo [15]. It has been shown that the repair of scar defects is able to restore fertility [15].

Therefore, a symptomatic niche can mimic frequent gynecological issues like endometriosis or pelvic inflammatory disease and should be considered as a differential diagnosis.

Addionally, an elevanted risk for intervention-related complications during a curettage oder device placement should be considered in the presence of a niche.

2.6 Pregnant women

In contrast to non life-threatening problems in non-pregnant women, the presence of a niche may derive in major complications during pregnancy. There is an important risk of a CS scar ectopic pregnancy (CSP) at the site of the niche [16] (**Figure 8**). CSP occur with an overall incidence of 1: 1800–1: 2216 pregnancies [17]. Even in early-pregnancy, CSP treatment can be associated with severe hemorrhage [18].

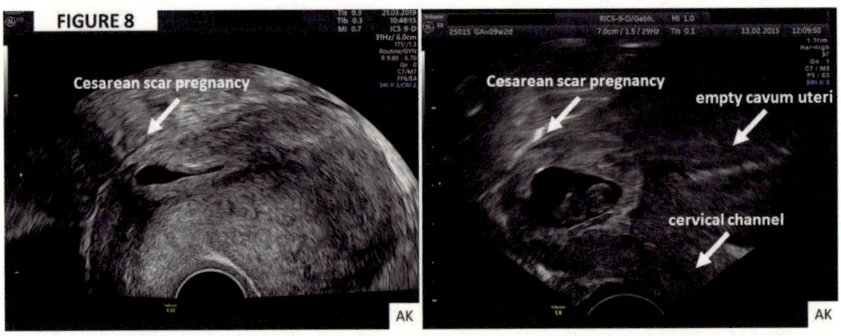

Figure 8.
Cesarean scar ectopic pregnancy.

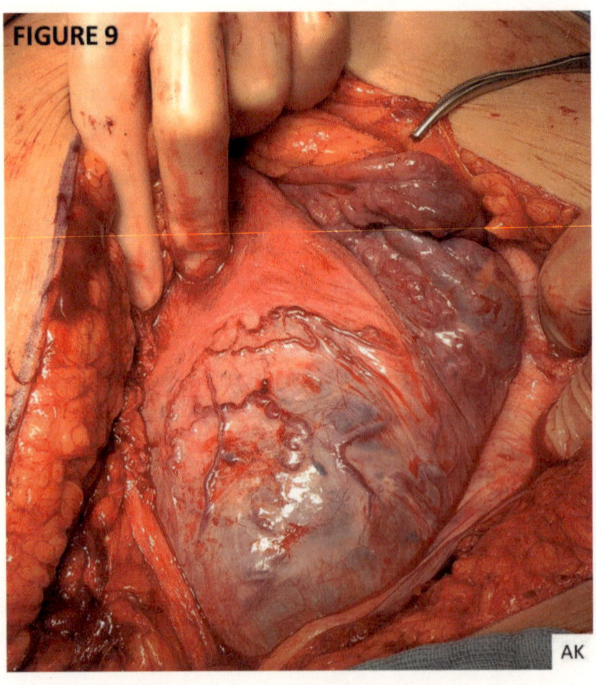

Figure 9.
Intraoperative demonstration of placenta percreta.

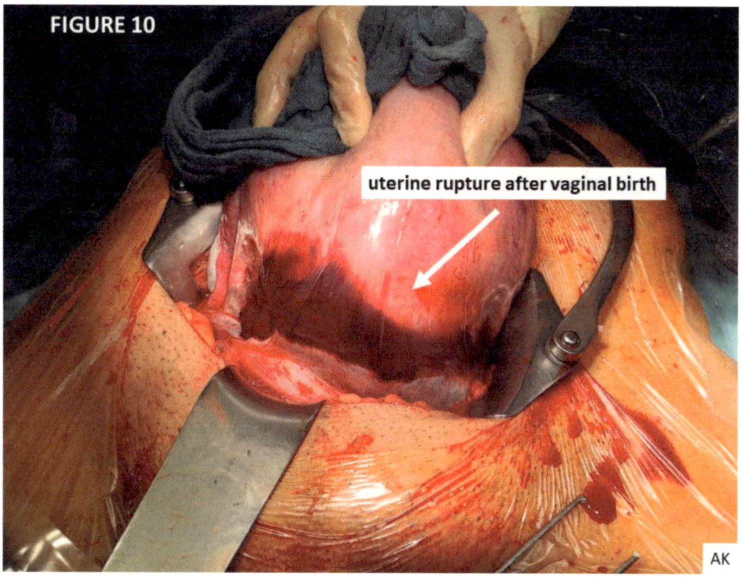

Figure 10.
Uterine rupture after vaginal delivery in a patient with a former Cesarean section.

In most cases, CSP results in morbidly-adhaerent placenta like placenta accreta, increta or percreta [19]. Short- and longterm complications can be detrimental [20] (**Figure 9**).

Uterine rupture during pregnancy and labour is a rare but life-threatening sequeleae both for the mother and the fetus [21] (**Figure 10**). It appears conclusive that a thinner myometrium increases the risk of a rupture. Unfortunately, no cut-off value of myometrial thickness was defined as a reliable predictor of uterine rupture. A RMT > 2.1–4.0 mm and LUS thickness between 3.1–5.1 mm were described as strong negative predictive values for uterine rupture. A RMT of 0.6–2.0 mm was considered as a positive predictive factor for uterine rupture [22].

Since the clinical consequences of niches can not be exactly predicted, the prevention of niches formation is crucial. Insights into the pathogenesis of niche development will allow the initiation of preventative approaches.

3. Pathogenesis of niches

Many studies focused on potential risk factors for developing niches after CS. The most promising considerations comprise problems in wound healing including a (reversible) retroflexio uteri, the number of previous CS and the location of the uterotomy. The latter is affected by the stage of labour and the dilation of the cervix when CS is done. For the surgeon the most important issue particularly might be the optimal technique for closure of the uterotomy.

3.1 (Reversible) Retroflexio uteri

In most women, the physiological direction of the uterus in the pelvic cavity is an anteflexion. A retroflexion is a non-pathologic alternative to the norm. In 2016, Ryo et al. reported that the uterus may change its flexion after delivery, shifting from ante- to retroflexion. Compared to vaginal delivery, a retroflexed uterus was observed significantly more frequently after CS, increasing with the number of previous CS [23]. Other findings demonstrated a higher prevalence of niches in retroflexed uteri and notably large defects in cases of retroflexion [12, 13, 24]. Nowadays, it is widely accepted that there is a strong coincidence of niches and a retroflexion of the uterus [11–13, 25].

However, an important question remains: Does a retroflexion of the uterus facilitate the development of a niche or does a niche cause a (reversible) retroflexion? There are explanations for both hypotheses:

On the one hand, after CS, adhesions might cause mechanical tension on the anterior uterine wall leading to a retraction of the scar tissue with poor blood perfusion and resulting in an impaired wound healing. The retraction might be intensified if the uterus is already retroflexed [11]. This hypothesis is supported by the finding that the risk of developing a niche is more than twice higher, when the uterus is retroflexed [1].

On the other hand, the consideration of a niche causing a (reversible) retroflexion also seems plausible. Ryo et al. did not only examine the changes in uterine flexion after delivery but also provided a fairly logic objection to the above-mentioned pathogenesis: If a niche developed due to mechanical tension and retraction of the scar, the defect would be found at the outside of the anterior uterine wall [23]. In contrast, niches are generally found at the cavitary side of the myometrium. The uterine incision and the developing niche may compromise the contractility of the myometrium, leading to an imbalance between the anterior and posterior wall, causing traction backwards and resulting in a retroflexion.

Therefore, it seems more plausible that first a niche develops and second the uterus becomes retroflexed. Further studies are needed to better understand the role of a retroflexion in the pathogenesis of niches.

3.2 Number of previous Cesarean sections

Niches are almost solely diagnosed in women after CS. No studies report myometrial defects after vaginal birth. Osser et al. described a median myometrial thickness at the isthmus of 11.6 mm after vaginal delivery, compared to 8.3 mm/6.7 mm/4.7 mm after one/two/three or more CS [3]. Largely all studies report a positive correlation between the number of previous CS and increasing rates of niches [1, 3, 6, 23, 25]. The niche prevalence was found to be up to 63,1% after one, 76–81% after two and 88–100% after three CS, respectively [3, 7]. Not only the number of niches increase, but also the scar defect itself becomes larger the more CS found in the patient's history [3]. Total defects with no remaining RMT were more frequently found in women with multiple CS: 6%, 7% and 18% after one, two and $\geq$ three or more CS, respectively [1].

The possible explanation seems to be impaired wound healing: trauma to the uterine wall disrupts the physiological healing process due to a reduction of vascular perfusion [25].

Addionally, increasing CS rates correlate with higher prevalence of retroflexed uteri, underscoring the hypothesis about the association of retroflexed uteri with niches development [23].

Therefore, the careful evaluation of each CS in terms of its necessity seems to be the most promising step to reduce myometrial defects.

3.3 Position of the uterotomy and timing of the CS

The most common technique of uterotomy performance is a transversal incision of the isthmo-cervical region. During labour, the isthmo-cervical region undergoes continuous changes. First, the thinning and elongation, recognizable by a lifted

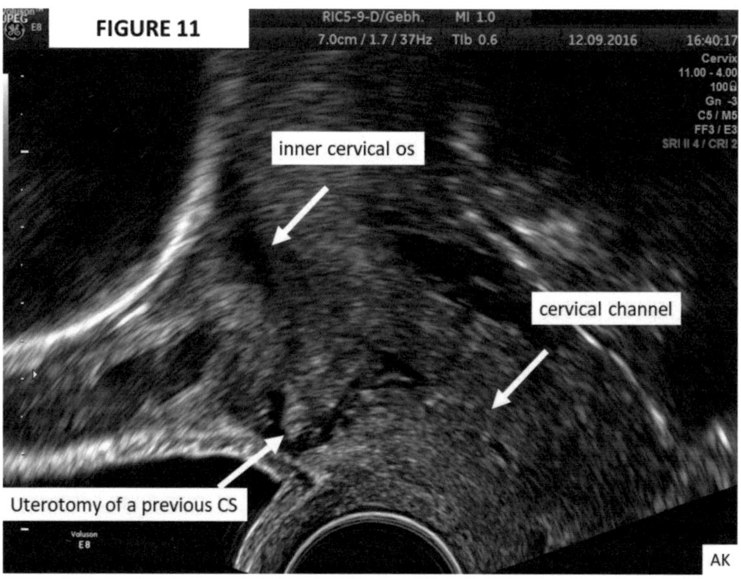

Figure 11.
Uterine incision of a former CS within the cervical channel.

urinary bladder or plica vesicouterina. Consecutively, also the inner cervical os with its mucous glands and only few muscular tissue moves upwards. Hence, if the surgeon incides the uterus at the same height in late labour as in an earlier stage of labour, the incision is placed either lower or even beneath the inner cervical os (**Figure 11**). The most likely explanation for distinct wound healing effects is found in the morphological difference between the region around the inner cervical os and the myometrium above. The mucus may dilate the sutured rims of the uterotomy or cause retention cysts, both leading to impaired wound healing [11, 26]. Furthermore, as a result of poor contraction in this area, wound edge adaptation may be insufficiently.

Therefore, CS at advanced stage of labor may provoke a lower incision including cervical tissue and resulting in more scar defects. On the other hand, contractions or rupture of membranes have already occurred in advanced stage of labor with a crucial and beneficial influence on the postoperative healing process of the uterine scar.

The following chapters discusses the effects of both of these opposite forces on scar healing:

On the one hand, CS performed before the onset of labour resulted in a thinner uterine wall in subsequent pregnancies than CS performed during labour [27, 28]. Jastrow et al. [29] showed significantly decreased LUS measurements depending on stage of labour prior to the CS (full LUS after CS in latent phase: 2.8 mm, in active phase: 3.1 mm and in CS prior to labour 2.4 mm, $p < 0.01$). Importantly, Park et al., were able to demonstrate no increased risk to develop a niche when CS was performed in situations with >8 cm dilated cervix [6].

A CS performed intrapartum reduces the probability to develop a placenta praevia in a following pregnancy [30] as well as the risk of uterine rupture in cases of vaginal birth after a CS [31], underlining the importance of contractions on wound healing. A case control study of 307 women showed a threefold increased risk to develop a morbidly adherent placenta after an elective CS compared to an emergency CS. In this study, the increasing severity of a morbidly adherent placenta (placenta accreta versus increta versus percreta) was associated with a higher probability of a prior elective CS, respectively [32]. Hence, we hypothesize that uterine contractions and their immonological triggers may contribute to the postpartum tissue repair. To elucidate possible mechanisms, we shortly discuss this topic on the end of this chapter.

On the other hand, several studies demonstrated, that the incidence of defect wound healing increased significantly when CS was performed in advanced labour [1, 6, 33].

It was shown that a prolonged labour beyond 5 hours or a CS performed during active labour with the cervix is dilated >5 cm, is associated with an increased risk to develop a niche (5–9 hours OR 13.0 (2.2–76.6), > 10 hours OR 33.1 (6.6–166.9); $p < 0.001$) [21].

Also, a higher percentage of RMT < 3 mm was observed in cases with advanced cervical dilatation at CS [7]. Park et al. showed a higher risk of niches in cases with a CS at a cervical dilatation of 5–7 cm compared to cases with CS at closed cervix [6].

But how can these conflicting results be explained?

The hypothesis to answer this question is that in cases of CS at advanced stage of labor, the uterotomy position is closer to the internal cervical os and wound healing is compromised in this area. This hypothesis can be confirmed by the following observations:

As shown by Vikhareva Osser, the uterotomy position was exactly positioned at the internal os in 97% of cases with a cervical dilatation >5 cm compared to 55% in cervical dilatation <5 cm [21].

Hanacek et al. demonstrated that if the CS is performed at full cervical dilatation, the resulting scars were closer to the external os and the RMT was markedly thinner [34]. These findings might be explained by the localization of the uterine incision, which is often overly caudal, due to cervical incorporation into the lower uterine part.

A very recently published prospective cohort study showed a higher prevalence of scar defects when the uterotomy was placed cranially of the internal os compared to a uterotomy placed caudally of the internal os in patients with a first CS [35]. Subgroup analysis, however, showed that in cases of a CS before the onset of labor, the uterotomy position was mostly cranial of the internal os whereas in cases with advanced labor, the position was rather caudal. Therefore, the beneficial effect of advanced labor was undermined by the more caudally position of the uterotomy.

In order to confirm the negative effects of a low uterine incision, a prospective randomized study published in 2019 compared the incidence of niches in patients with low and high incision (2 cm below vs. 2 cm above the plica vesicouterina) 6–9 months after an elective CS. Large scar defects occurred significantly more often in the low-incision group (41% vs. 7%) [33]. This leads to the conclusion, that the position of the uterotomy is one of the most important factors in the pathogenesis of niches.

In summary, CS performed under contractions in active stages of labour may elicit mechanisms that improve scar healing subsequently resulting in thicker RMT and in reduced development of niches. However, this benefit inverts when labour or cervical dilatation is too advanced and the uterotomy is localized overly caudal. In consequence, every obstetrician needs to consider the stage of labour and the cervical dilation for choosing the optimal position of uterine incision.

3.4 Closure of the uterotomy

Closure of the uterotomy is a crucial and very controversially discussed topic. Several studies addressed this important step in order to optimise scar integrity, endometrium rehabilitation, postoperative recovery and the reduction of risks in subsequent pregnancies. The following section illustrates partially contrary strategies to close a uterotomy in order to prevent a niche.

3.5 Single versus double layer

Single vs. double layer sutures of the myometrium were discussed in a large number of studies and reviews. It is currently postulated that double layer is superior to single layer as it is associated with a thicker RMT (4.6 vs. 5.2 mm) [34, 36–38] and lower niche prevalence (4.2% vs. 1.3%, $p < 0.001$, RR 0.32, [28]).

These observations were confirmed in a large review including 20 randomised controlled trials or prospective cohort studies and more than 15000 women. Here, a double layer suture resulted in a thicker RMT (+ 1.26 mm double layer vs. single layer), a better healing ratio (=anterior wall thickness/anterior wall thickness + height of the wedge-shaped defect) and less dysmenorrhoea than single layer suture [39]. A 50% reduced risk of uterine rupture during subsequent pregnancy was also assumed following a double layer suture compared to a single layer [40]. Finally, Vachon-Marceau et al. demonstrated a significantly higher rate on scar dehiscence in the single- compared to double-layer group [28].

Of note, a number of studies pointed out that a proper single layer (unlocked) suture might not be inferior to double layer [36]. The RMT is commonly lower compared to double-layer suture, but interestingly the risk of uterine rupture in a subsequent pregnancy is influenced only marginally [38, 41, 42]. However, since the frequency of uterine rupture is very low in general, the sample size of most studies was too small to reach reliable data.

One large review including 9 randomised controlled trials (3969 patients) demonstrated a thinner RMT in the single layer suture group (mean difference – 2.19 mm), but no statistically significant differences regarding uterine scar defects, uterine dehiscence or uterine rupture. The authors acknowledged that even if uterine scar defects are associated with lower RMT, it remains questionable whether RMT alone is a proper marker for prospective uterine ruptures [38]. Jastrow et al. calculated that a cut-off value for myometrial layer tickness in third trimester below 1.4–2 mm and complete lower LUS of less than 2–3.5 mm correlates with a higher risk of niche incidence and therefore uterine rupture. Unfortunatly, the retrospective study design and small sample size limit the scope of these results [29].

A proper single layer suture was suggested to be helpful when the CS is performed during advanced labour and myometrial layers cannot be correctly identified [28]. One trial demonstrated that double layer suture results in a higher RMT than single layer suture only in elective CS but not in CS at advanced labor [43].

In summary, although there is no evidence for a higher uterine rupture rate following a single layer suture compared to a double-layer suture, RMT and therefore probably the integrity of the lower uterine segment is improved by the double-layer suture of the uterus, at least in cases with an elective CS.

3.6 Locked versus unlocked suture

Locking a suture was used for long time to reduce bleeding. However, there is some evidence that a locked suture may provoke defect scar healing.

One trial showed that only unlocked double-layer, but not locked double-layer suture was superior to locked single-layer in either RMT (3.8 $\pm$ 1.6 mm vs. 6.1 $\pm$ 2.2 mm) and healing ratio [36]. Higher rates of scar separation were described when a continuous suture was locked (OR 5.4, 95% CI 3.17–9.20, $p < 0.001$, [41]).

Stegwee et al. reviewed data from three randomized controlled trials and two prospective cohort studies to compare locked and unlocked suture. RMT decreased significantly and niche prevalence was non-significantly higher when a locked suture was performed (RR 1.23, 95% CI 0.93–1.61, $p = 0.14$). Also one study including 48 women reported the healing ratio, which was lower in locked vs. unlocked sutures [39].

In summary: Locking a suture decreases healing due to the reduction in blood flow and consequently in oxygen supply to the scar, which is required for the healing process [44].

3.7 Single stitches versus continuous suture

A small number of studies is available comparing continuous suture with single stitches to close the uterine incision.

One case–control study (n = 98) analysed the effect of prior uterine closure on placenta location and placentation disorders. Half of the double-layer group had continuous suture of the inner layer, the others had interrupted sutures of the inner layer. Continuous suture of the inner layer of the myometrium was an independent risk factor for subsequent placenta accreta, total placenta praevia and anterior location. The risk for morbidly adherent placenta was 6-fold higher after continuous suture compared to interrupted stitches [45]. An additional prospective randomized study in primiparae with an elective CS demonstrated larger and more numerous niches in patients after locked continuous sutures compared to interrupted sutures (95% niches and 77% niches after 12 months, respectively). In this study, the decidua was excluded and a single layer suture without closure of the visceral peritoneum was performed [46].

Overall, conclusive evidence in this topic is limited by the small size of the studies. Currently, interrupted stitches of the inner layer of myometrial closure might favour the healing process.

3.8 Inclusion versus exclusion of the decidua in the suture

Including the decidua (endometrium) in the suture might lead directly to a worsened scar integrity and niche development. Roberge et al. observed, as mentioned before, that excluding the decidua in double-layer suture supports better scar healing than including it [36].

A recently published double-blind, randomised controlled study (2Close Trial) examined the presence of postmenstrual spotting after a single- versus a double- layer suture. In the double-layer group, the decidua was integrated in the scar, however, in the single-layer group, this integration was optional. Surprisingly, a significantly increased niche prevalence was found after double- compared to single-layer suture (73.6 versus 68.9%). The authors draw the conclusion that rather by the number of sutured layers this result was provoked by the integration of the decidua in the suture. In line with this, subgroup analysis of the single-layer group revealed a significantly lower niche incidence in cases of exclusion of the decidua (59.3 versus 71.8%) [47].

A retrospective cohort study showed no morbidly adherent placenta in a cohort of 109 patients with previous CS, although in 44% an anterior wall placentation was present. The authors concluded that the exclusion of the endometrium from the suture, which was a standard practice in the study center, chiefly contributed to the results. However, there was no control group and the study group was compared with historical cohorts [48].

A critical view on this approach raises the concern that less myometrium might be adapted if the endometrium is not included in the scar, probably contributing to a defect healing. Yazicioglu et al. observed a higher incomplete healing ratio in sutures that excluded the endometrium compared to those including all layers [49]. However, the examination was performed 6 weeks after the CS, which is known to be rather early for a final assessment of wound healing. Furthermore, cervical dilatation was performed at a lower percentage in patients with incomplete healing, probably explaining the results. This study also was part of a meta-analysis pooling two studies recording niches after sutures including or excluding the decidua [39]. The second study, which was included in this meta-analysis, showed contrary results [50]: Three study groups were compared (group A: inclusion of all layers; group B: double-layer suture with inclusion of the decidua, group C: double-layer suture with a separate suture of the decidua and a separate suture of the myometrial layer). The group with the separate suture of the endometrium showed significantly lower niche rates (34%, 16% and 5.6% niches in group A, B and C, respectively).

In summary, the exclusion of the decidua from the suture seems favourable in preventing niches.

3.9 Closure of the peritoneum viscerale/parietale

The closure of the peritoneum reveals no advantages with regards to operation time, pain and bleeding amounts, as currently recommended the German Guideline Cesarean Section [51]. But does the closure of the peritoneum help to prevent a niche?

Verwoort et al. discussed several hypotheses on niche development. During laparoscopic scar repair surgery dense fibrotic adhesions attached on top of the niches were found [11]. One hypothesis is that adhesions pull the uterine scar towards the abdominal wall and induce scar development due to traction. One explanation for this adhesion between the anterior uterine and the abdominal wall might be the incision of the utero-vesical fold and subsequent dissection of the urinary bladder with the aim to keep the bladder out of the surgical area. This may create adhesions and provoke niche formation as well as a fixed retroflexio uteri [52].

Moreover, a systematic review including 249 patients evaluated whether the parietal peritoneum should be closed. This study showed that closure of the peritoneum prevents adhesions from abdominal to uterine wall [53].

In conclusion, further investigation is needed to be able to answer the question about the contribution of closure of the visceral and parietal peritoneum to niche prevention.

3.10 Dilatation of the cervix uteri

The rationale of dilating the cervix uteri during elective CS is to facilitate the proper drain of blood and "products of conception" postpartum. On the one hand, retained blood after CS is ought to impair scar healing and results in scar defects [54]. On the other hand, a risk of infection by a possible transmission and contamination from vaginal microorganisms to uterine or abdominal wounds is discussed [55]. A randomised trial analysed the different outcomes of CS after cervical dilatation (CD) was performed with Hegar dilator or not. 400 women with a singleton pregnancy were included and planned for elective CS at term. All patients received vaginal disinfection preoperatively with povidone iodine. No difference was observed regarding wound infection or endometritis between the groups. In the cervical dilatation group, indicators of better healing of the scar were found: Significantly higher scar width and depth, thicker RMT, and fewer scar defects were found together with better blood supply to the scar. In comparison, women without cervical dilatation were at higher risk for subinvolution of the uterus [54].

In another recently published trial (DONDI-Trial, prospective, open-label, randomized controlled trial), 447 women randomly received cervical dilation or not during CS. Women with current antibiotic therapy, chorioamnionitis, onset of labour with dilatation of the cervix and gestational age below 24 weeks were excluded. Dilatation of the cervix had no effect on infectious morbidity (puerperal fever, endometritis, wound infection and urinary tract infection), blood loss or even operating time. The only benefit observed in the dilatation group was a lower prevalence of patients that had retained products in the uterus cavity compared to the no-dilation group (0 vs. 6.2%, $p < 0.001$) [56]. Although scar healing was not examined in this study, retention of products may potentially disturb wound healing.

A recently published review underlined the following findings, too: performing or not CD at elective CS at term either with double gloved index or Hegar dilator caused no differences regarding postpartum haemorrhage, postoperative fever, endometritis or subinvolution. Cervical dilatation led to a slightly higher mean blood loss, thicker endometrial cavity, less retained products of conception, less distortion of uterine incision and better healing ratio. Operating time, wound infection, urinary tract infection and integrity of scar (defined as scar thickness less than 2.3 mm) were not affected [57].

In conclusion, dilatation of the cervix has positive effects on scar integrity, wound healing and RMT due to less retention of products in utero. It is safe regarding infections; however, vaginal disinfection should be considered before CS.

4. Add on: role of labor on post partum tissue repair

Since scar defects represent a kind of defect wound healing, we here focus on possible mechanisms which are involved in postpartum tissue repair. As shown in the section "Timing of the CS", there is evidence that an unplanned CS after the onset of labor has advantages concerning niche incidence and further pregnancy complications like uterine rupture and morbidly adherent placenta. Probably, immunological changes which only occur at the time of contractions, may have the potential to contribute to the clinical benefits of a CS after the onset of labor.

The human endometrial tissue holds the capacity to achieve complete regeneration after injures [58]. Particularly, childbirth and the detachment of the deeply invading placenta is generally followed by the restoration of the endometrial layer at the former implantation site. This regeneration is essential for successive pregnancies, as incomplete healing and repair results in endometrium fibrosis or scarring, with potential consequences on the uterine cavity shape or on the adhesiveness and invasiveness of the embryo [59–61]. Despite their relevance, the precise mechanisms of post partum tissue repair and the factors contributing to an impaired endometrial re-epithelialization e.g. after caesarean section remain still poorly described.

To date it is well known that labour entails a series of drastic changes that provoke uterine contractions and birth. This process is characterized by rapid fluctuations in maternal hormones, including the upregulation of glucocorticoids and oxytocin as well as the reduction in progesterone signalling [62, 63]. Simultaneously, there is a shift in the immune responses at the feto-maternal interface from the predominantly anti-inflammatory phenotype throughout pregnancy to a sterile inflammation-like response during labour [64]. This includes inflammasome activation, the release of cytokines and chemokines, and the further recruitment of leukocytes to the feto-maternal interface [65], as studied in detail in relevant animal models.

In line with this, it is tempting to hypothesize that the effects of labour and uterine contractions may surpass the birth and detachment of the placenta, conveying a central role to the labor-triggered recruitment of immune cells in the machinery of postpartum tissue regeneration. Indeed, the immune system critically orchestrates repair processes in multiple organisms and tissues. Danger signals prompted by tissue injure activate pattern recognition receptors to initiate an immune response [66, 67]. This dynamic response is characterized by the stepwise recruitment of granulocytes, monocytes/macrophages, and T cells [68]. Both recruited and tissue resident leukocytes play scavenger functions and secrete cytokines and growth factors that promote lympho- and angiogenesis, proliferation of tissue cells, and consequently repair [66, 69]. Recently, regulatory T cells have also emerged as important players that ensure regeneration of multiple tissues [70]. Particularly in the case of macrophages and T cells, the balance between inflammatory and anti-inflammatory responses may hold the capacity to tilt the repair process towards scarring or regeneration respectively [68].

Noteworthy, the specific features of the repair process are contingent on the particularities of the tissue affected and little is known about uterine wound healing and prevention of scarring in the postpartum period. In the rodent postpartum uterus, macrophages with an anti-inflammatory M2-like phenotype have been observed in the former implantation sites together with abundant expression of VEGF and its receptors in the uterine stroma and blood vessels that may jointly favour angiogenesis and healing [71, 72]. In contrast, accumulation of M1-like macrophages, neutrophils, and T cells was detected in the uterus of mice exhibiting dysfunctional postpartum uterine repair due to impaired Notch signalling [73]. These findings support that in the uterus, such as in other tissues, an anti-inflammatory milieu is required to prevent the formation of fibrosis upon wound healing. Despite this emerging evidence on the role of immune responses in postpartum tissue healing, further mechanisms and players remain still to be elucidated. In particular, it is still unknown whether labour-induced recruitment of immune cells under the regulatory influence of high levels of steroid hormones contribute to tissue healing, and whether the failure of such a recruitment, e.g. in caesarean deliveries without induction of labour, may hinder endometrial regeneration and result in scar formation.

5. Conclusion: how to perform a CS in 2021

Taken together all aspects which influence the risk of a defect scar healing, we advise to perform a CS as following:

1. CS after the onset of labour seems to be superior than an elective CS. Childbaering women should be encouraged to undergo vaginal birth whenever possible.

2. Uterotomy should be placed not overly caudal, avoiding an incorporation of the cervix or the region around the internal cervical os into the scar.

3. After delivery of the placenta, performing cervical dilatation is recommended in cases without cervical dilatation due to the absence of contractions.

4. The decidua should be excluded from the suture.

5. Double-layer-suture is recommended.

6. Single stitches (of the first layer) are superior to a continous suture.

7. Locked sutures (of the first layer) should be avoided.

   Personal opinion of the authors: We recommend to perform a double layer suture with single stitches of the first layer and a continuous unlocked second layer including the superficial muscle layer and the peritoneum viscerale.

8. Closure of the peritoneum parietale may be advantageous.

Author details

Christian Litzka[1†], Annegret Schnabel[1†], Maria Emilia Solano[2] and Angela Köninger[1*]

1 University Department of Obstetrics and Gynecology at the Hospital St. Hedwig of The Order of St. John, University of Regensburg, Regensburg, Germany

2 Laboratory for Translational Perinatology, University Department of Obstetrics and Gynecology at the Hospital St. Hedwig of the Order of St. John, University of Regensburg, Regensburg, Germany

*Address all correspondence to: angela.koeninger@ukr.de

† These authors contributed equally.

References

[1] Bij de Vaate AJM, van der Voet LF, Naji O, Witmer M, Veersema S, Brolmann HAM, Bourne T, Huirne JAF. **Prevalence, potential risk factors for development and symptoms related to the presence of uterine niches following Cesarean section: systematic review.** Ultrasound Obstet Gynecol 2014; 43: 372-382.

[2] Jordans IPM, de Leeuw RA, Stegwee SI, Amso NN, Barri-Soldevila PN, van den Bosch T, Bourne T, Brölmann HAM, Donnez O, Dueholm M, Hehenkamp WJK, Jastrow N, Jurkovic D, Mashiach R, Naji O, Streuli I, Timmerman D, van der Voet LF, Huirne JAF. **Sonographic examination of uterine niche in non-pregnant women: a modified Delphi procedure.** Ultrasound Obstet Gynecol. 2019 Jan;53(1):107-115.

[3] Osser OV, Jokubkiene L, Valentin L. **High prevalence of defects in Cesarean section scars at transvaginal ultrasound examination.** Ultrasound Obstet Gynecol. 2009 Jul;34(1):90-97.

[4] Pan H, Zeng M, Xu T, Li D, Mol BWJ, Sun J, Zhang J. **The prevalence and risk predictors of cesarean scar defect at 6 weeks postpartum in Shanghai, China: A prospective cohort study.** Acta Obstet Gynecol Scand. 2019 Apr;98(4):413-422.

[5] Woźniak A, Pyra K, Tinto HR, Woźniak S. **Ultrasonographic criteria of cesarean scar defect evaluation.** J Ultrason. 2018;18(73):162-165.

[6] Park IY, Kim MR, Lee HN, Gen Y, Kim MJ. **Risk factors for Korean women to develop an isthmocele after a cesarean section.** BMC Pregnancy Childbirth. 2018 May 15;18(1):162.

[7] Antila-Långsjö R, Mäenpää JU, Huhtala H, Tomás E, Staff S. **Comparison of transvaginal ultrasound and saline contrast sonohysterography in evaluation of cesarean scar defect: a prospective cohort study.** Acta Obstet Gynecol Scand. 2018 Sep;97(9):1130-1136. doi: 10.1111/aogs.13367. Epub 2018 May 29.

[8] Tang X, Wang J, Du Y, Xie M, Zhang H, Xu H, Hua K. Caesarean scar defect: Risk factors and comparison of evaluation efficacy between transvaginal sonography and magnetic resonance imaging. Eur J Obstet Gynecol Reprod Biol. 2019 Nov;242:1-6.

[9] Abacjew-Chmylko A, Wydra DG, Olszewska H. **Hysteroscopy in the treatment of uterine cesarean section scar diverticulum: A systematic review.** Adv Med Sci. 2017 Sep;62(2):230-239.

[10] Roberge S, Boutin A, Chaillet N, Moore L, Jastrow N, Demers S, Bujold E. **Systematic review of cesarean scar assessment in the nonpregnant state: imaging techniques and uterine scar defect.** Am J Perinatol. 2012 Jun;29(6):465-471.

[11] Vervoort AJ, Uittenbogaard LB, Hehenkamp WJ, Brölmann HA, Mol BW, Huirne JA. **Why do niches develop in Caesarean uterine scars? Hypotheses on the aetiology of niche development.** Hum Reprod. 2015 Dec;30(12):2695-2702.

[12] Osser OV, Jokubkiene L, Valentin L. Cesarean section scar defects: agreement between transvaginal sonographic findings with and without saline contrast enhancement. Ultrasound Obstet Gynecol. 2010a Jan;35(1):75-83.

[13] Osser OV, Jokubkiene L, Valentin L. **Cesarean section scar defects: agreement between transvaginal sonographic findings with and without saline contrast enhancement.**

Ultrasound Obstet Gynecol. 2010b Jan;35(1):75-83.

[14] Bij de Vaate AJ, Brölmann HA, van der Voet LF, van der Slikke JW, Veersema S, Huirne JA. **Ultrasound evaluation of the Cesarean scar: relation between a niche and postmenstrual spotting**. Ultrasound Obstet Gynecol. 2011 Jan;37(1):93-99.

[15] Gubbini G, Centini G, Nascetti D, Marra E, Moncini I, Bruni L, Petraglia F, Florio P. **Surgical hysteroscopic treatment of cesarean-induced isthmocele in restoring fertility: prospective study.** J Minim Invasive Gynecol. 2011 Mar-Apr;18(2):234-237.

[16] Timor-Tritsch IE, Monteagudo A, Cali G, Vintzileos A, Viscarello R, Al-Khan A, Zamudio S, Mayberry P, Cordoba MM, Dar P. Cesarean scar pregnancy is a precursor of morbidly adherent placenta. Ultrasound Obstet Gynecol. 2014 Sep;44(3):346-353.

[17] Rotas MA, Haberman S, Levgur M. Cesarean scar ectopic pregnancies: etiology, diagnosis, and management. Obstet Gynecol. 2006 Jun;107(6): 1373-1381.

[18] Timor-Tritsch I, Buca D, Di Mascio D, Cali G, D'Amico A, Monteagudo A, Tinari S, Morlando M, Nappi L, Greco P, Rizzo G, Liberati M, Jose-Palacios-Jaraquemada, D'Antonio F. Outcome of cesarean scar pregnancy according to gestational age at diagnosis: A systematic review and meta-analysis. Eur J Obstet Gynecol Reprod Biol. 2021 Mar;258:53-59.

[19] Calì G, Timor-Tritsch IE, Palacios-Jaraquemada J, Monteaugudo A, Buca D, Forlani F, Familiari A, Scambia G, Acharya G, D'Antonio F. **Outcome of Caesarean scar pregnancy managed expectantly: systematic review and meta-analysis.** Ultrasound Obstet Gynecol 2018;51(2):169-175.

[20] Maheux-Lacroix S, Li F, Bujold E, Nesbitt-Hawes E, Deans R, Abbott J. Caesarean Scar Pregnancies: A Systematic Review of Treatment Options. Minim Invasive Gynecol 2017;24(6):915-925.

[21] Vikhareva Osser O, Valentin L. **Risk factors for incomplete healing of the uterine incision after caesarean section.** BJOG. 2010 Aug;117(9):1119-1126.

[22] Kok N, Wiersma IC, Opmeer BC, de Graaf IM, Mol BW, Pajkrt E. **Sonographic measurement of lower uterine segment thickness to predict uterine rupture during a trial of labor in women with previous Cesarean section: a meta-analysis.** Ultrasound Obstet Gynecol. 2013 Aug;42(2):132-139.

[23] Ryo E, Sakurai R, Kamata H, Seto M, Morita M, Ayabe T. **Changes in uterine flexion caused by cesarean section: correlation between post-flexion and deficient cesarean section scars.** J Med Ultrason (2001). 2016 Apr;43(2):237-242.

[24] Chen Y, Han P, Wang YJ, Li YX. **Risk factors for incomplete healing of the uterine incision after cesarean section.** Arch Gynecol Obstet. 2017 Aug;296(2):355-361. doi: 10.1007/s00404-017-4417-6. Epub 2017 Jun 6.

[25] Antila- Långsjö RM, Mäenpää JU, Huhtala HS, et al. **Cesarean scar defect: a prospective study on risk factors**. Am J Obstet Gynecol 2018; 219:458.e1-458.e8.

[26] Kremer TG, Ghiorzi IB, Dibi RP. **Isthmocele: an overview of diagnosis and treatment.** Rev Assoc Med Bras (1992). 2019 Jun 3;65(5):714-721.

[27] Bérubé L, Arial M, Gagnon G, Brassard N, Boutin A, Bujold E. **Factors associated with lower uterine segment thickness near term in women with**

previous caesarean section. J Obstet Gynaecol Can. 2011 Jun;33(6):581-587.

[28] Vachon-Marceau C, Demers S, Bujold E, Roberge S, Gauthier RJ, Pasquier JC, Girard M, Chaillet N, Boulvain M, Jastrow N. **Single versus double-layer uterine closure at cesarean: impact on lower uterine segment thickness at next pregnancy.** Am J Obstet Gynecol. 2017 Jul;217(1):65.e1-65.e5.

[29] Jastrow N, Gauthier RJ, Gagnon G, Leroux N, Beaudoin F, Bujold E. **Impact of labor at prior cesarean on lower uterine segment thickness in subsequent pregnancy.** Am J Obstet Gynecol. 2010 Jun;202(6):563.e1-563.e7.

[30] Downes KL, Hinkle SN, Sjaarda LA, Albert PS, Grantz KL. **Previous prelabor or intrapartum cesarean delivery and risk of placenta previa.** Am J Obstet Gynecol. 2015 May;212(5):669.e1-669.e6. doi: 10.1016/j.ajog.2015.01.004.

[31] Algert CS, Morris JM, Simpson JM, Ford JB, Roberts CL. **Labor before a primary cesarean delivery: reduced risk of uterine rupture in a subsequent trial of labor for vaginal birth after cesarean.** Obstet Gynecol. 2008 Nov;112(5):1061-1066.

[32] Shi XM, Wang Y, Zhang Y, Wei Y, Chen L, Zhao YY. Effect of Primary Elective Cesarean Delivery on Placenta Accreta: A Case-Control Study. Chin Med J (Engl) 2018 Mar 20;131(6):672-676.

[33] Vikhareva O, Rickle GS, Lavesson T, Nedopekina E, Brandell K, Salvesen KÅ. **Hysterotomy level at Cesarean section and occurrence of large scar defects: a randomized single-blind trial.** Ultrasound Obstet Gynecol. 2019 Apr;53(4):438-442.

[34] Hanacek J, Vojtech J, Urbankova I, Krcmar M, Křepelka P, Feyereisl J, Krofta L. Ultrasound cesarean scar assessment one year postpartum in relation to one- or two-layer uterine suture closure. Acta Obstet Gynecol Scand. 2020

[35] Kamel R, Kaelin Agten A, Noel L, Eissa T, Sharaf M, Negm S, Thilaganathan B. **Position and integrity of the uterine scar is determined by cervical dilation at the time of Caesarean section.** Ultrasound Obstet Gynecol. 2021 Mar;57(3):466-470.

[36] Roberge S, Demers S, Girard M, Vikhareva O, Markey S, Chaillet N, Moore L, Paris G, Bujold E. **Impact of uterine closure on residual myometrial thickness after cesarean: a randomized controlled trial.** Am J Obstet Gynecol. 2016 Apr;214(4):507.e1-507.e6.

[37] Di Spiezio Sardo A, Saccone G, McCurdy R, Bujold E, Bifulco G, Berghella V. Risk of Cesarean scar defect following single- vs double-layer uterine closure: systematic review and meta-analysis of randomized controlled trials. Ultrasound Obstet Gynecol. 2017

[38] Bamberg C, Hinkson L, Dudenhausen JW, Bujak V, Kalache KD, Henrich W. **Longitudinal transvaginal ultrasound evaluation of cesarean scar niche incidence and depth in the first two years after single- or double-layer uterotomy closure: a randomized controlled trial.** Acta Obstet Gynecol Scand. 2017 Dec;96(12):1484-1489.

[39] Stegwee SI, Jordans I, van der Voet LF, van de Ven PM, Ket J, Lambalk CB, de Groot C, Hehenkamp W, Huirne J. **Uterine caesarean closure techniques affect ultrasound findings and maternal outcomes: a systematic review and meta-analysis.** BJOG. 2018 Aug;125(9):1097-1108.

[40] Bujold E, Goyet M, Marcoux S, Brassard N, Cormier B, Hamilton E,

Abdous B, Sidi EAL, Kinch R, Miner L, Masse A, Fortin C, Gagné GP, Fortier A, Bastien G, Sabbah R, Guimond P, Roberge S, Gauthier RJ. **The role of uterine closure in the risk of uterine rupture.** Obstet Gynecol. 2010 Jul;116(1):43-50.

[41] Roberge S, Chaillet N, Boutin A, Moore L, Jastrow N, Brassard N, Gauthier RJ, Hudic I, Shipp TD, Weimar CH, Fatusic Z, Demers S, Bujold E. **Single- versus double-layer closure of the hysterotomy incision during cesarean delivery and risk of uterine rupture.** Int J Gynaecol Obstet. 2011 Oct;115(1):5-10.

[42] Hesselman S, Högberg U, Ekholm-Selling K, Råssjö EB, Jonsson M. **The risk of uterine rupture is not increased with single- compared with double-layer closure: a Swedish cohort study.** BJOG. 2015 Oct;122(11):1535-1541.

[43] Bamberg C, Dudenhausen JW, Bujak V, Rodekamp E, Brauer M, Hinkson L, Kalache K, Henrich W. **A Prospective Randomized Clinical Trial of Single vs. Double Layer Closure of Hysterotomy at the Time of Cesarean Delivery: The Effect on Uterine Scar Thickness.** Ultraschall Med. 2018 Jun;39(3):343-351.

[44] Roberge S, Demers S, Berghella V, Chaillet N, Moore L, Bujold E. **Impact of single- vs double-layer closure on adverse outcomes and uterine scar defect: a systematic review and metaanalysis.** Am J Obstet Gynecol. 2014 Nov;211(5):453-460.

[45] Sumigama S, Sugiyama C, Kotani T, Hayakawa H, Inoue A, Mano Y, Tsuda H, Furuhashi M, Yamamuro O, Kinoshita Y, Okamoto T, Nakamura H, Matsusawa K, Sakakibara K, Oguchi H, Kawai M, Shimoyama Y, Tamakoshi K, Kikkawa F. **Uterine sutures at prior caesarean section and placenta accreta in subsequent pregnancy: a case-control study.** BJOG. 2014 Jun;121(7):866-874; discussion 875.

[46] Ceci O, Cantatore C, Scioscia M, Nardelli C, Ravi M, Vimercati A, Bettocchi S. **Ultrasonographic and hysteroscopic outcomes of uterine scar healing after cesarean section: comparison of two types of single-layer suture.** J Obstet Gynaecol Res. 2012 Nov;38(11):1302-1307.

[47] Stegwee SI, van der Voet LF, Ben AJ, de Leeuw RA, van de Ven PM, Duijnhoven RG, Bongers MY, Lambalk CB, de Groot C, Huirne J; 2Close study group. **Effect of single- versus double-layer uterine closure during caesarean section on postmenstrual spotting (2Close): multicentre, double-blind, randomised controlled superiority trial.** BJOG. 2021 Apr;128(5):866-878.

[48] Antoine C, Pimentel RN, Reece EA, Oh C. **Endometrium-free uterine closure technique and abnormal placental implantation in subsequent pregnancies.** J Matern Fetal Neonatal Med. 2019 Oct 3:1-9.

[49] Yazicioglu F, Gokdogan A, Kelekci S, Aygun M, Savan K. **Incomplete healing of the uterine incision after caesarean section: Is it preventable?** Eur J Obstet Gynecol Reprod Biol. 2006 Jan 1;124(1):32-36.

[50] Hayakawa H, Itakura A, Mitsui T, Okada M, Suzuki M, Tamakoshi K, Kikkawa F. **Methods for myometrium closure and other factors impacting effects on cesarean section scars of the uterine segment detected by the ultrasonography.** Acta Obstet Gynecol Scand. 2006;85(4):429-434.

[51] https://www.awmf.org/leitlinien/detail/ll/015-084.html (Feb 16th, 2021)

[52] Vervoort A, van der Voet LF, Hehenkamp W, Thurkow AL, van Kesteren P, Quartero H,

Kuchenbecker W, Bongers M, Geomini P, de Vleeschouwer L, van Hooff M, van Vliet H, Veersema S, Renes WB, Oude Rengerink K, Zwolsman SE, Brölmann H, Mol B, Huirne J. Hysteroscopic resection of a uterine caesarean scar defect (niche) in women with postmenstrual spotting: a randomised controlled trial. BJOG. 2018 Feb;125(3):326-334.

[53] Cheong YC, Premkumar G, Metwally M, Peacock JL, Li TC. **To close or not to close? A systematic review and a meta-analysis of peritoneal non-closure and adhesion formation after caesarean section.** Eur J Obstet Gynecol Reprod Biol. 2009 Nov;147(1):3-8.

[54] Dawood AS, Elgergawy A, Elhalwagy A, Ataallah WM, Elbohoty SB, Elshwaikh SL, Elsokary AA, Elkhyat AM, Elbadry AT, Abbas AM. **The impact of mechanical cervical dilatation during elective cesarean section on postpartum scar integrity: a randomized double-blind clinical trial. Int J Womens Health.** Int J Womens Health. 2019 Jan 10;11:23-29.

[55] Sherman D, Lurie S, Betzer M, Pinhasi Y, Arieli S, Boldur I. **Uterine flora at cesarean and its relationship to postpartum endometritis.** Obstet Gynecol. 1999 Nov;94(5 Pt 1):787-791.

[56] Kirscht J, Weiss C, Nickol J, Berlit S, Tuschy B, Hoch B, Trebin AV, Große-Steffen T, Sütterlin M, Kehl S. **Dilatation or no dilatation of the cervix during cesarean section (Dondi Trial): a randomized controlled trial.** Arch Gynecol Obstet. 2017 Jan;295(1):39-43.

[57] Liabsuetrakul T, Peeyananjarassri K. **Mechanical dilatation of the cervix during elective caeserean section before the onset of labour for reducing postoperative morbidity.** Cochrane Database Syst Rev. 2018 Aug 10;8(8):CD008019.

[58] Evans J, Salamonsen LA, Winship A, Menkhorst E, Nie G, Gargett CE, Dimitriadis E. Fertile ground: human endometrial programming and lessons in health and disease. Nat Rev Endocrinol. 2016 Nov; PMID: 27448058

[59] Köninger A, Rusch P, Kimmig R. Successful myometrial closure over protruding Cesarean scar pregnancy. Ultrasound Obstet Gynecol. 2020 Jun 30.

[60] Stanley R, Ohashi T, Mowa C. Postpartum cervical repair in mice: a morphological characterization and potential role for angiogenic factors. Cell Tissue Res. 2015 Oct;362(1):253-63.

[61] Jauniaux E, Grønbeck L, Bunce C, Langhoff-Roos J, Collins SL. Epidemiology of placenta previa accreta: a systematic review and meta-analysis. BMJ Open. 2019; Nov

[62] Carr BR, Parker CR Jr, Madden JD, MacDonald PC, Porter JC. Maternal plasma adrenocorticotropin and cortisol relationships throughout human pregnancy. Am J Obstet Gynecol. 1981 Feb 15;139(4):416-22.

[63] Solano ME, Arck PC. Steroids, Pregnancy and Fetal Development. Front Immunol. 2020 Jan 22;10:3017.

[64] Green ES, Arck PC. Pathogenesis of preterm birth: bidirectional inflammation in mother and fetus. Semin Immunopathol. 2020 Aug;42(4):413-429.

[65] Romero R, Dey SK, Fisher SJ. Preterm labor: one syndrome, many causes. Science. 2014 Aug 15;345(6198):760-5.

[66] Murphy K, Travers P, Walport M & Janeway C. Janeway's immunobiology. 2008. New York: Garland Science.

[67] Kono H, Onda A, Yanagida T. Molecular determinants of sterile

inflammation. Curr Opin Immunol. 2014 Feb;26:147-56.

[68] Julier Z, Park AJ, Briquez PS, Martino MM. Promoting tissue regeneration by modulating the immune system. Acta Biomater. 2017 Apr 15;53:13-28.

[69] Horst AK, Najjar SM, Wagener C, Tiegs G. CEACAM1 in Liver Injury, Metabolic and Immune Regulation. Int J Mol Sci. 2018 Oct 11;19(10):3110.

[70] Delacher M, Imbusch CD, Hotz-Wagenblatt A, Mallm JP, Bauer K, Simon M, Riegel D, Rendeiro AF, Bittner S, Sanderink L, Pant A, Schmidleithner L, Braband KL, Echtenachter B, Fischer A, Giunchiglia V, Hoffmann P, Edinger M, Bock C, Rehli M, Brors B, Schmidl C, Feuerer M. Precursors for Nonlymphoid-Tissue Treg Cells Reside in Secondary Lymphoid Organs and Are Programmed by the Transcription Factor BATF. Immunity. 2020 Feb 18;52(2):295-312.e11.

[71] Sağsöz H, Liman N, Alan E. Expression of vascular endothelial growth factor receptors and their ligands in rat uterus during the postpartum involution period. Biotech Histochem. 2015 Jul;90(5):361-74. Solano ME, Arck PC. Front Immunol. 2020 Jan 22;10:3017.

[72] Yoshii A, Kitahara S, Ueta H, Matsuno K, Ezaki T. Role of uterine contraction in regeneration of the murine postpartum endometrium. Biol Reprod. 2014 Aug;91(2):32.

[73] Strug MR, Su RW, Kim TH, Mauriello A, Ticconi C, Lessey BA, Young SL, Lim JM, Jeong JW, Fazleabas AT. RBPJ mediates uterine repair in the mouse and is reduced in women with recurrent pregnancy loss. FASEB J. 2018 May;32(5):2452-2466.

Chapter 9

Optimizing Techniques and Suture Materials for Caesarean Section

Padmasri Ramalingappa, Raksha Shivaramegowda and Shruthi Holavanahalli SrinivasaMurthy

Abstract

Cesarean section is an important part of comprehensive emergency obstetric and neonatal care and their numbers are increasing worldwide in the recent times. Proper healing of the scar after cesarean section is of paramount importance to avoid various obstetrical complications in future pregnancies. There is no standard technique on the method of closure following cesarean delivery. It is unclear as which technique and suture material should be used for closure of cesarean section in order to get the best results with minimal complications. The objective of this chapter is to review the literature, analyze the available resources and evaluate the evidence for closure of each layer post cesarean section. The following discussion will review closure of each step post cesarean section and provide evidence-based recommendations for closure technique.

Keywords: Cesarean section, closure technique, suture material

1. Introduction

Cesarean is a commonly performed obstetric surgery and in the recent times its number is constantly increasing. Standard technique for abdominal wall closure should be practiced considering the need to provide good support, prevent infections, sinus formation, and incision pain and scar dehiscence. There are multiple sutures and suturing techniques practiced worldwide for the closure of abdominal layers following cesarean section.

The history of sutures begins more than 2,000 years ago. Surgical and suture techniques evolved in the late 1800s with the development of sterilization procedures. It has been said that the scar is the "autograph of a surgeon". Every surgeon wants cosmetically acceptable scars along with optimal healing.

An ideal suture material should be cheap, sterile, non-electrolytic, non-allergenic, with adequate tensile strength, good handling characteristics, should not induce tissue reaction or cut through tissue.

A good suturing technique should ideally eliminate the dead space and minimize tension that causes wound separation. It involves correct wound placement with respect to relaxed tension lines. Consideration should focus on factors, such as systemic diseases and selection of ideal suture material that influence the outcome. The surgical technique used to close a given wound depends on the force and direction of tensions on the wound, the thickness of the tissues to be opposed and anatomic considerations.

1.1 Wound healing and inflammatory response

The physiology of wound healing has 3 phases: inflammation, proliferation, and remodeling. Various factors like cytokines, cellular mediators are involved in the healing process.

Phase I: Inflammation (Onset of injury to day 4–6): The first phase of wound healing is characterized by hypoxic, ischemic environment with macrophages, neutrophils and platelet. Collagen, platelet, thrombin, fibronectin and fibrin with complements form a blood clot which has 3 major functions

- Expresses cellular mediators
- Serves as reservoir to amplify cellular signaling
- Provides support and communication matrix for arriving inflammatory cells

Phase II: Proliferation (Days 4–14): It is marked by rapid construction of new tissue. Macrophages emit nitrous oxide thus dilating the vessels to accommodate influx of new cells. Granulation begins to form at this phase. Fibroblast which are recruited from the surrounding normal tissue starts synthesizing and depositing collagen.

Phase III: Maturation and remodeling (1 week- 1 year): The final stage of wound healing is characterized by evolution of matrix into ordered collagen complex. At one week, the wound has about 3 percent of its final strength, 30 percent of final strength at 3 weeks and ultimately achieves 80 percent of its final strength at 3 months and beyond. However wound will never regain the strength of an uninjured tissue.

2. Closure following Cesarean section

2.1 Uterine closure

A scarred uterus carries long term consequences. Thus, the technique and the suture material used are crucial for the uterine scar healing. But strong evidence regarding optimal techniques is scarce [1]. There are multiple techniques and suture materials used for closure of uterus during cesarean section.

Usually intraperitoneal repair of the uterus is undertaken. RCOG [2] and Cochrane review [3] on exteriorization of the uterus for repair of the uterine incision does not recommend routine exteriorization of the uterus as it is associated with more pain and does not improve operative outcomes such as hemorrhage and infection. However, a RCT conducted by Isabela Cristina et al., showed that number of sutures required is lower and the surgical time is shorter with extra-abdominal repair, although moderate and severe pain at 6 hours is less frequent with in situ uterine repair [4]. A meta-analysis in 2015 also showed that uterine repair by exteriorization may reduce blood loss and the associated decrease in hemoglobin, but did not find any difference between the two techniques with respect to intraoperative nausea, vomiting, or pain [5].

Uterine closure can be done either in a single layer or by double layer and both interlocking and unlocked suturing techniques have been used. Methods concerning closure of the uterine incision need to be considered with regards to benefit and potential harm in order to offer the best available surgical care to women undergoing cesarean section.

Blumenfeld in a study with 127 women opines that single layer closure is associated with 7 fold increase in the risk of developing bladder adhesions compared to double layer closure but there was no difference in the outcome of other pelvic or abdominal adhesions thus favoring double layer closure [6].

Glavind in a similar study, using 2D TVS (Transvaginal sonography), assessed for the residual myometrial thickness, scar defect, depth, width and length in 68 women with single layer and 81 women with double layer closure. Study concluded that double layer closure improves the quality of the scar with significantly higher myometrial thickness and shorter scar defect. He also favors double layer closure for better long term outcomes [7].

A Cochrane review based on 19 studies on single versus double layer closure of the uterus, found that there was no statistically significant differences for the primary outcome, febrile morbidity, although the meta-analysis suggested single layer closure was associated with a reduction in mean blood loss [8]. RCOG recommends that, except within research content, the uterine incision should be sutured within two layers [2]. A meta-analysis of 9 RCTs including 3969 women, showed that single layer closure and double layer closure are associated with similar incidence of cesarean scar defects, uterine dehiscence, uterine rupture in subsequent pregnancies [9].

2.1.1 Locking vs. non locking sutures

Single layer closure and double layer closure carry the same risk of uterine rupture in subsequent pregnancy. However a LOCKED single layer closure is associated with an increase of uterine rupture compared to double layer closure. They demonstrated that the double-layer uterine closure with a first unlocked layer that excludes the decidua, compared with locked single-layer closure that includes the decidua, is associated with a greater residual myometrial thickness (RMT) and healing ratio, which suggests that this technique is associated with better healing of the uterine scar (**Figure 1**) [10].

However Jun Woo Han in his study on impact of uterine closure on residual myometrial thickness after cesarean section disagrees with the Roberge study. He believes the main causative factor of the RMT is the coaptation ratio of incised myometrium (BX/A_0B; **Figure 2A**). When a single layer with a locking suture is used to penetrate the full thickness of myometrium and the decidua, the 2 points of A_0 and A_0' barely join each other, even after the absorption of suture materials (**Figure 2B–D**), because the uterus that delivered the baby is a dynamically contracting, globular, and muscular organ. Moreover, the presence and length of the uncoaptated portion (X-A_0) are the predominant factors that influence the different degree of RMT. Therefore, the surgeon should aim to minimize the length of the line "D_0-D_1" and not exclude the decidua itself. This would minimize the potential adverse effect that is associated with the inversion of the decidua (such as adenomyosis) or influence RMT and prevent the postoperative endometrial defect of exposure of the myometrium to the endometrial cavity [11].

2.1.2 Decidua exclusion

Including full thickness of the uterine wall may bring decidua into the scar. Decidual inclusion results in defective uterine healing in 78% of cases. When deciduas was excluded from the suture, all cases resulted in perfect healing [12].

Isthmocele is a uterine scar defect as a result of poor healing of uterine incision. It results in menstrual spotting, dysmenorrhea, dyspareunia, chronic pelvic pain, with an increased risk of scar pregnancy, placentation abnormalities and development of uterine rupture in future pregnancies. Uterine closure technique is

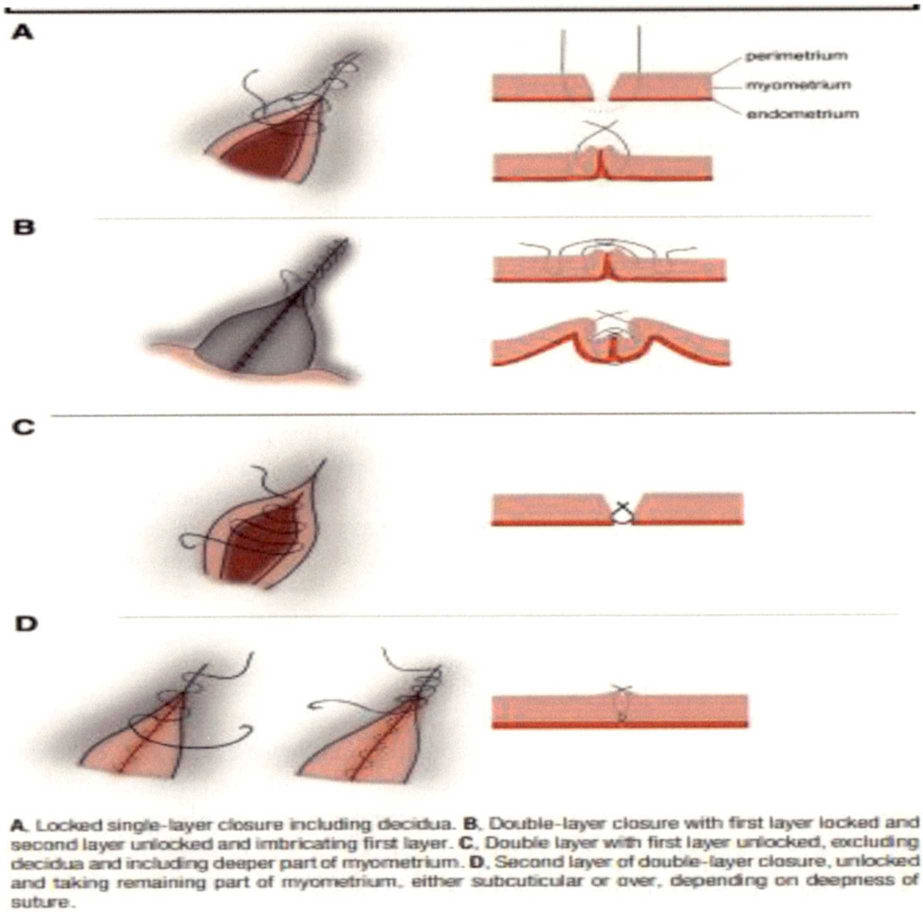

Figure 1.
Locked versus unlocked suturing techniques.

considered to be the most important factor associated with isthmocele formation. A study to demonstrate the factors associated with isthmocele concluded that uterine closure using the FFNN (Far far near near technique) continuous unlocked double layer technique is beneficial in terms of providing protection from isthmocele formation and ensuring sufficient RMT [13].

2.1.3 Types of suture material

The uterine incision is closed using an absorbable suture of number 0 or number 1. The commonly used suture materials are chromic catgut and polyglactin. Chromic catgut, being a natural suture material, has comparatively marked tissue reactivity, inconsistent tensile strength retention and reabsorption.

2.1.3.1 Catgut

Plain catgut is a natural suture material derived from the submucosa of sheep intestine or the serosa of cattle intestine. Chromic catgut is a modification of plain catgut that is tanned with chromic salts to improve strength and delay dissolution. Catgut is absorbed by phagocytosis, and is associated with a marked tissue inflammation that can be detrimental to healing. Conversely, tissue inflammation may lead to a more rapid breakdown of catgut. Plain gut has a median survival time of

DOI: http://dx.doi.org/10.5772/intechopen.97930

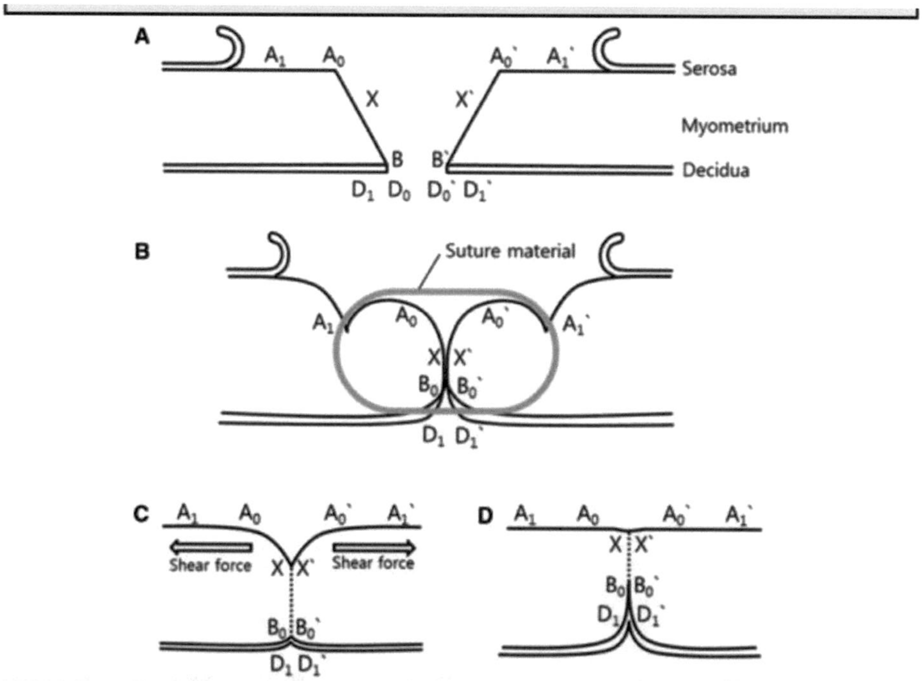

Initial state of myometrium **A,** before suturing, **B,** when sutured, **C,** at the moment of suture material absorption, and **D,** in the final state of incised, sutured, and healed myometrium.

A_0 and A_0', outer edge of incised myometrium; A^1, point of needle entry; A_1', point of needle exit; B_0 and B_0', inner edge of incised myometrium; D_0 and D_0', each edge of incised decidua; D_1, the point of needle exit; D_1', the point of needle entry; X and X', the end point of coaptated myometrium from B_0 and B_0'.

Figure 2.
Cut plane of uterine incision site when closing with single layer locking suture that penetrates the full thickness of myometrium and includes the decidua.

4 days in the oral cavity, whereas chromic gut retains its strength for 2 to 3 weeks. In moist environments such as the oral cavity, the strength of gut is reduced by 20–30%.Gut is a stiff material that must be moistened in alcohol, and forms knots that can be irritating to the oral tissues. Infection rates may increase with the use of gut. The advent of synthetic materials preferable to gut, with less tissue reactivity and more predictable resorption, has almost made catgut obsolete [14].

2.1.3.2 Polyglactin 910

Polyglactin 910 is a absorbable, braided, multifilament, coated synthetic suture. It is a heteropolymer consisting of 90% of glycolideand 10% of lactide and is degraded by hydrolysis. It is available with an antibiotic impregnation with triclosan. The residual tensile strength of a polyglactin 910 suture is consistently greater than that of polyglycolic acid suture and is absorbed more rapidly. Absorption starts at 40 days, and completes by day 70 with no remains by day 90. It retains 75% of its tensile strength at 2 weeks and 50% at 3 weeks. It elicits less tissue reactions and promote faster wound healing with good strength [15].

But, chromic gut has an excellent historical record in obstetrics and the knotted tensile strength of 0 chromic gut is adequate to withstand the disruptive forces on the repaired hysterotomy [16].

2.1.3.3 Polyglycolic acid (PGA) (Dexon, Dexon II)

PGA is a synthetic, braided polymer. When compared with chromic catgut, PGA is less reactive and is experimentally better able to resist infection from contaminating bacteria. PGA has excellent knot security and maintains at least 50% of its tensile strength for 25 days. The main drawback of PGA is that it has a high friction coefficient and "binds and snags" when wet. It is for the same reason that some experience is required to pass this material properly through tissues and to "seat" the throws during knotting. There is a modified PGA (dexon plus) which is coated with poloxamer 188, an agent that significantly reduces the friction and drag through the tissues. Although handling has become easier with this modification, more throws (four to six) are required to prevent knot slippage than for plain PGA (three to four). The main uses of PGA are for closures of superficial fascia (subcutaneous tissue) in wounds and ligature of small blood vessels for effective hemostasis [17].

A study to assess different suturing techniques and different materials (catgut plain, Dexon and Vicryl) on healing of uterine incision in Cesarean section (CS) concluded that the best uterine scar was seen after using one layer interrupted Vicryl and Dexon suture and the worst healing results were obtained after two-row interrupted and continuous sutures using catgut [18]. As compared to catgut, use of synthetic sutures were associated with thicker myometrium in subsequent delivery. Increased inflammation in natural absorbable suture may lead to increase in fibrosis and impaired healing rendering difficulty in subsequent pregnancies and delivery [19].

The CORONIS trial on the cesarean section surgical techniques compared the chromic catgut and polyglactin-910 for uterine closure. There were no statistically significant differences noted in the primary outcome, which was the composite of death, maternal infectious morbidity, further operative procedures, or blood transfusion (>1 unit) up to the 6 weeks follow up visit [20]. A 3 year follow up study was done to the CORONIS trial and there was no evidence of a difference in the main comparisons for adverse pregnancy outcomes in subsequent pregnancy, such as uterine rupture [21].

Thus, it can be concluded that both chromic catgut and polyglactin-910 of number 0 or 1 can be safely used for the uterine repair during cesarean section, though polyglactin has been used more often in the recent times.

2.1.4 Uterine compression sutures

The B-Lynch surgical technique is used for the management of massive postpartum hemorrhage (PPH) secondary to uterine atony with failed conservative management. Long term study demonstrated, the B-Lynch surgical technique is safe, effective and free of short- and long-term complication [22].

2.1.4.1 B Lynch sutures

A large Mayo needle with absorbable suture is used to enter the uterine cavity from below the uterine incision and exit just above the incision. The suture is looped over the fundus, then enters and exits the uterine cavity posteriorly, forms a second loop over the fundus and finally enters just above and exits just below the uterine incision The suture should be pulled very tight at this point and tied anteriorly (**Figure 3**).

2.1.4.2 Hayman sutures

It is performed to control bleeding in atonic postpartum hemorrhage post vaginal delivery and rarely after uterine incision closure in cesarean delivery. Two loops are formed over the fundus and tied after applying compression (**Figure 4**).

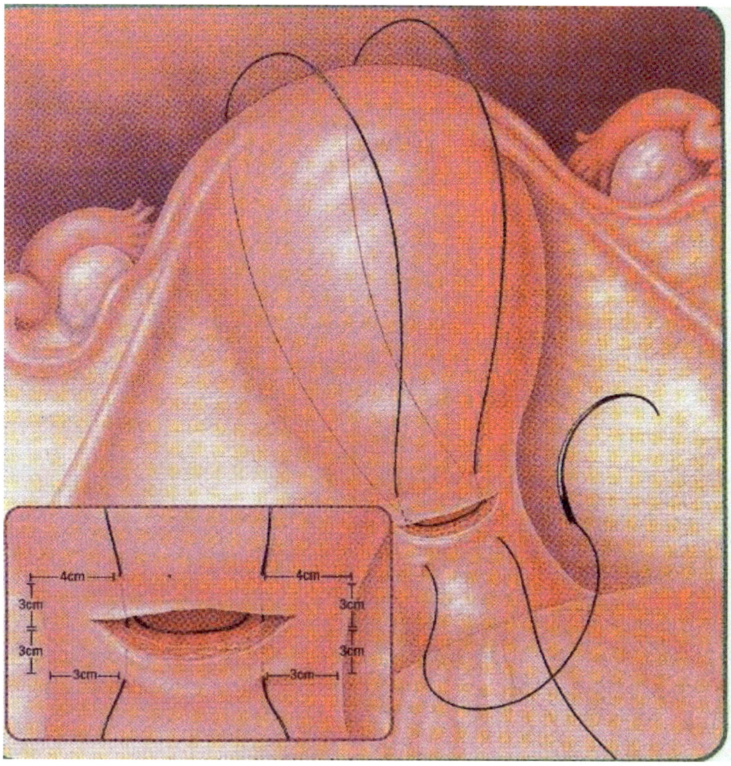

Figure 3.
B lynch suture.

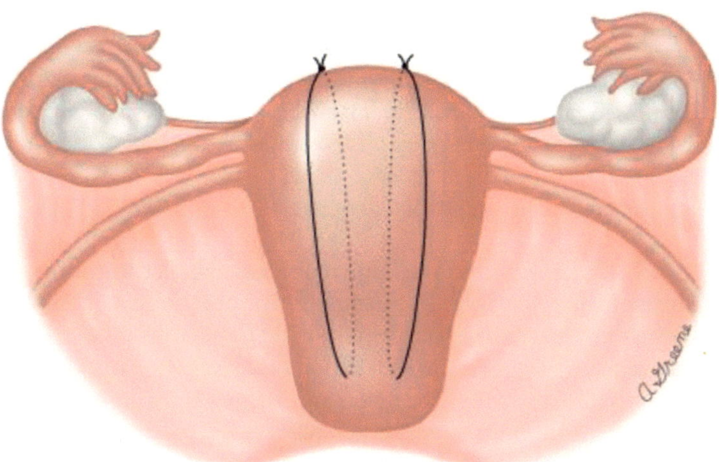

Figure 4.
Hayman suture.

2.1.4.3 Cho square sutures

A needle transfixes the uterus from anterior to posterior(point 1) and then from posterior to anterior (point 2), the same is done again at points 3 and 4 to approximate the uterine walls in a square manner. Usually 4 to 5 sutures are required **Figure 5a** and **b**.

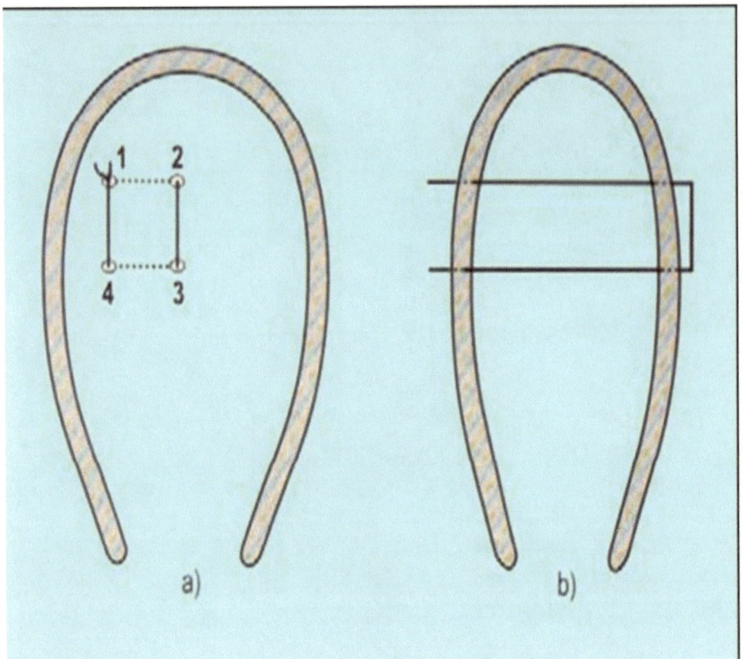

Figure 5.
Cho square suture.

Several studies are conducted to assess the ideal suture and size for uterine compression sutures but they have concluded no variations in outcome with type of suture used but it was observed that uterine preservation rate was significantly higher in cases with size 2 suture than in those with size 1 suture [23].

Placement of compression sutures that transverse the uterine cavity postpartum for PPH may be associated with a significant risk of uterine synechiae. Risk of synechiae following uterine compression sutures in the management of major postpartum hemorrhage [24].

2.2 Peritoneal and rectus muscle closure

The closure of peritoneum and the approximation the rectus muscle at cesarean section has always been debatable. The promoters of practicing peritoneal closure argue that this leads to less adhesion formation and comparative ease during a repeat cesarean section, but it also has an added disadvantage of prolonging the operative time and increased need for maternal analgesia. As far as peritoneal closure is concerned, visceral peritoneum is generally not closed as bladder adhesion is increased [25]. A review of 21 trials comparing closure versus non closure of the peritoneum showed that there was a reduction in operative time and the evidence on adhesion formation was limited and inconsistent [26]. RCOG too recommends that neither the visceral nor the parietal peritoneum should be sutured at cesarean section because this reduces operating time and the need for postoperative analgesia and improves maternal satisfaction [2]. Rectus muscle reapproximation increases immediate postoperative pain without difference in operative time, surgical complications, or maternal satisfaction but, closure of the rectus muscles at cesarean delivery was found to reduce adhesions.

If peritoneal closure and rectus muscle approximation is done in cases with diastasis recti abdominis, use absorbable sutures such as chromic catgut and polyglactin-910. A new modified undermined suture technique for rectus muscle, which gives increased post-operative satisfaction, has been tried, using Z suture method with absorbable 1/0 suture material [27].

2.3 Rectus sheath closure

Different techniques and suture materials are used in cesarean section for closure of the rectus sheath. Few general principles are to be followed while closing the abdominal wall to achieve good healing and reduce complications. All sutures used to close the musculofascial wall must be tied with enough tension to approximate the edges of the incision. If greater tension is applied, the tissue will become ischemic and necrosis will develop. The sutures should be placed at least 1 to 1.5 cm from the wound edge. In patients at increased risk of wound disruption, sutures should be placed 2 cm from the edge [28].

The commonly used technique is to put continuous sutures without any locking. Continuous suture when used in one layer avoids high tension on suture and does not compress the wound edges. This prevents devascularization of the sheath and formation of a good quality collagen, i.e., type I [29]. Running sutures have the advantage of speed, since knots need only be tied at two or three points. Interrupted and figure-of-eight sutures can be used for reinforcing in thin rectus sheath and has an advantage, of not coming apart if insecurely tied.

Rectus sheath closure is routinely performed with non-absorbable or delayed absorbable sutures. It is generally accepted that non-absorbable sutures cause less tissue reaction and are more resistant to infection than the absorbable sutures. However, these sutures are associated with higher incidence of buttonhole hernias and sinus formation leading to increased wound pain. Care should be taken while tying the knots to avoid slippage. The commonly used suture materials for rectus sheath closure are polyglactin-910 number 1 and polypropylene number 1. Cochrane review found no studies examining different suture techniques or material for rectus sheath closure.

2.4 Subcutaneous tissue and skin closure

Suturing of the subcutaneous tissue has always been debated. Level one evidence says that suture closure of the subcutaneous fat at the time of CS reduces the risk of wound disruption in women with a subcutaneous tissue larger than two centimeters. Doing so will not only reduce collection in this space but also decrease wound tension. Though studies do show that it does not affect long-term cosmetic outcome [30].

A basic need of skin closure is good approximation. Apart from cosmetically good scars it is also necessary that the skin closure technique should be technically easy, acceptable, speedy and economical. Good tissue union and cosmetically acceptable scars are vital for ideal surgical practice.

Technique of skin closure in a cesarean section can be continuous subcuticular stitch, interrupted mattress stitch, staples or adhesive compounds.

With a plethora of skin closure materials currently available, choosing a solution that combines excellent and rapid cosmetic results with practicality and cost-effectiveness can be difficult, if not tricky. Suture materials currently available are natural, synthetic, absorbable, or non-absorbable, single filament or braided.

Mattress sutures have an advantage of occluding dead space and keeping the skin edges everted without tension. This is useful especially in older women where skin tends to get inverted.

The disadvantage with this type of suture is that there can be difficulty in approximation and prominent suture marks as sutures tend to be removed later.

To overcome the disadvantage of traditional interrupted mattress suture, Hohenleutner et al., described the intradermal buried vertical mattress suture [31]. This suture technique is safe, easy and fast to perform, everts skin edges and achieves good cosmetic results without leaving suture marks.

Subcuticular suture was first described by Halsted [32]. It is a cosmetic stitch, more difficult, but a good choice especially in younger women whose skin is soft and supple, hence making approximation easy. It is preferable to use absorbable suture for this stitch as the ends are also buried and suture removal is not required.

Though subcuticular stitch has better patient compliance than mattress stitch, the post-operative scar assessment at 6 weeks have yielded similar results in both.

Staples are attractive because of the speed of application.

An RCT study of staples with subcuticular stitch by Figueroa D showed that surgical staples were significantly associated with a higher incidence wound disruptions among those randomized to staples. This observation persisted when the outcome is restricted to disruptions >1 cm in length or > 0.5 cm in depth and typically led to additional scheduled clinic follow-up visits [33].

Another RCT by Madsen AM, comparing absorbable subcuticular staples with suture showed that wound complications, and cosmesis were similar [34]. So if one wants to use staples for closure then the absorbable one would be preferred, as metal staples though faster, has more wound morbidity.

There are many advantages of tissue adhesives over suturing and other methods of wound closure, such as a lower infection rate, less operating room time, good cosmetic results, lower costs, ease of use, immediate wound sealing, faster return to work, elimination of needle-stick injuries and eliminating the need for post-operative suture removal [35]. An RCT by Daykan Y, says that skin closure with glue or synthetic subcuticular suture have similar outcomes with respect to surgical site infection and wound disruptions [36]. The commonly used adhesive is octyl-2-cyanoacrylat.

3. Conclusion

Various techniques and suture materials for closure of uterus and the abdominal wall following cesarean section have been described. Many studies and meta-analysis have been done to compare different methods with varying results. It is best left to the decision of the operating surgeon and the institutional protocols to decide about the technique of closure and the suture material to be used.

Conflict of interest

Authors declare no conflict of interest.

DOI: http://dx.doi.org/10.5772/intechopen.97930

Author details

Padmasri Ramalingappa*, Raksha Shivaramegowda
and Shruthi Holavanahalli SrinivasaMurthy
Department of Obstetrics and Gynaecology, Sapthagiri Institute of Medical Sciences and Research Centre, Bangalore, India

*Address all correspondence to: drpadmasuraj@gmail.com

References

[1] Emmanuel B. The optimal uterine closure technique during cesarean. N Am J Med Sci. 2012 Aug; 4(8): 362-363.

[2] National Institute for Health and Care Excellence; Clinical guideline; Caesarean section; Nov 2011, Updated Sept 2019.

[3] Wilkinson C, Enkin MW. Uterine exteriorization versus intraperitoneal repair at caesarean section. Cochrane Database Syst Rev. 2000;

[4] Coutinho IC, Ramos de Amorim MM, Katz L, Bandeira de Ferraz AA. Uterine exteriorization compared with in situ repair at cesarean delivery: a randomized controlled trial. Obstet Gynecol. 2008 Mar;111(3):639-647

[5] Zaphiratos V, George RB, Boyd JC, Habib AS. Uterine exteriorization compared with in situ repair for Cesarean delivery: a systematic review and meta-analysis. Can J Anaesth. 2015 Nov;62(11):1209-1220.

[6] Blumenfeld YJ et al, BJOG. 2010 May;117 (6); 690-694.

[7] Glavind J et al., Ultrasound Obstet Gynecol. 2013 Aug; 42(2):201-212.

[8] Dodd JM, Anderson ER, Gates S, Grivell RM. Surgical techniques for uterine incision and uterine closure at the time of caesarean section. Cochrane Database of Systematic Reviews 2014, Issue 7. Art. No.: CD004732

[9] Di SpiezioSardo A, Saccone G, McCurdy R, Bujold E, Bifulco G, Berghella V. Risk of Cesarean scar defect following single- vs double-layer uterine closure: systematic review and meta-analysis of randomized controlled trials. Ultrasound Obstet Gynecol. 2017 Nov;50(5):578-583

[10] Roberge et al. International Journal of Gynaecology and Obstetrics. 115 (2011) 5-10

[11] Jelsema et al. J Reprod Med. 1993 May; 38(5):393-6.

[12] Poidevin L. ObstetGynaecol Br Emp 1961 Dec;68;1025-1029.

[13] ZiyaKalem, AskiEllibes Kaya, BatuhanBakırarar, AlperBasbug&MüberraNamlıKalem (2019): An Optimal Uterine Closure Technique for Better Scar Healing and Avoiding Isthmocele in Cesarean Section: A Randomized Controlled Study, Journal of Investigative Surgery

[14] Suture materials and biomaterials, Anson J. Tsugawa, Frank J.M. Verstraete, in Oral and Maxillofacial Surgery in Dogs and Cats, 2012.

[15] Barham RE, Butz GW, Ansell JS. Comparison of wound strength in normal, radiated and infected tissues closed with polyglycolic acid and chromic catgut sutures. Surg Gynecol Obstet. 1978;146:901-907

[16] James AG, Rachel MC. Advances in suture material for obstetric and gynecologic surgery. Rev Obstet Gynecol. 2009 Summer; 2(3): 146-158.

[17] Instruments, suture materials, and closure choices. Alexander T. Trott MD. In wounds and Lacerations(Fourth Edition), 2012.

[18] Sestanović, Zeljan& Mimica, Marko &Vulić, Marko &Roje, Damir &Tomic, Snjezana. (2003). [Does the suture material and technique have an effect on healing of the uterotomy in cesarean section?]. Liječničkivjesnik. 125. 245-51.

[19] (Berube et al. J ObstetGynaecol Can. 2011 Jun; 33(6); 581-7.

[20] CORONIS Collaborative Group, Abalos E, Addo V, Brocklehurst P, El Sheikh M, Farrell B, Gray S et al. Caesarean section surgical techniques (CORONIS): a fractional, factorial, unmasked, randomized controlled trial. Lancet. 2013 Jul 20; 382(9888): 234-248.

[21] CORONIS collaborative group, Abalos E, Addo V, Brocklehyrst P, El Sheikh M, Farrell B, Gray S et al. Caesarean section surgical techniques: 3 year follow up of the CORONIS fractional, factorial, unmasked, randomized controlled trial. Lancet. 2016 Jul 2;388(10039) : 62-72.

[22] Tsitlakidis C, Alalade A, Danso D, B-Lynch C. Ten year follow-up of the effect of the B-Lynch uterine compression suture for massive postpartum hemorrhage. Int J Fertil Womens Med. 2006 Nov-Dec;51(6):262-265.

[23] Matsuzaki, S., Jitsumori, M., Hara, T. *et al.* Systematic review on the needle and suture types for uterine compression sutures: a literature review. BMC Surg **19,** 196 (2019).

[24] Poujade O, Grossetti A, Mougel L, Ceccaldi P, Ducarme G, Luton D. Risk of synechiae following uterine compression sutures in the management of major postpartum haemorrhage. BJOG 2011;118:433-439.

[25] Lyell DJ, Caughey AB, Hu E, Blumenfeld Y, El-Sayed YY, Daniels K. Rectus muscle and visceral peritoneum closure at cesarean delivery and intraabdominal adhesions. Am J Obstet Gynecol. 2012 Jun;206(6):515.e1-5.

[26] Bamigboye AA, Hofmeyr GJ. Closure versus non-closure of the peritoneum at caesarean section: short- and long-term outcomes. Cochrane Database Syst Rev. 2014 Aug 11;(8):CD000163. doi: 10.1002/14651858.CD000163.

[27] Yek Song Quek, Michelle Jia Ni Ling, Jamiyah Binti Hassan. New modified undermined suture technique for rectus muscle re-approximation at cesarean delivery—Case report, International Journal of Surgery Case Reports, Volume 73, 202, 235-238.

[28] DeLancey, J, Hartman, R, Operations on abdominal wall, *Glob. libr. women's med.,(ISSN: 1756-2228)* 2008; DOI 10.3843/GLOWM.10038

[29] Hintamani Editorial: Ten Commandments of Safe and Optimum Abdominal Wall Closure. Indian J Surg **80,** 105-108 (2018). https://doi.org/10.1007/s12262-018-1776-6

[30] Husslein H, Gutschi M, Leipold H, Herbst C, Franz M, Worda C (2014) Suture Closure versus Non-Closure of Subcutaneous Fat and Cosmetic Outcome after Cesarean Section: A Randomized Controlled Trial. PLoS ONE 9(12): e114730

[31] Hohenleutner U, Egner N, Hohenleutner S, Landthaler M. Acta DermVenereol. 2000 Sep-Oct; 80(5):344-347.

[32] Fisher GT, Fisher JB, Stark RB. Origin of the use of subcuticular sutures. Ann Plast Surg. 1980 Feb;4(2):144-148

[33] Figueroa D, Jauk VC, Szychowski JM, et al. Surgical staples compared with subcuticular suture for skin closure after cesarean delivery: a randomized controlled trial [published correction appears in Obstet Gynecol. 2013 May;121(5):1113.

[34] Madsen AM, Dow ML, Lohse CM, Tessmer-Tuck JA. Absorbable subcuticular staples versus suture for caesarean section closure: a randomised clinical trial. BJOG. 2019 Mar;126(4):502-510.

[35] Daykan Y, Sharon-Weiner M, Pasternak Y, Tzadikevitch-Geffen K, Markovitch O, Sukenik-Halevy R, Biron-Shental T. Skin closure at cesarean delivery, glue vs subcuticular sutures: a randomized controlled trial. Am J Obstet Gynecol. 2017 Apr;216(4):406.e1-406.e5

[36] Toriumi DM, O'Grady K, Desai D, Bagal A. Use of octyl-2-cyanoacrylate for skin closure in facial plastic surgery. PlastReconstr Surg. 1998;102:2209-2219

Section 3

Caesaren Section Preterm Birth

Chapter 10

Characteristics of Catch-Up Growth in Very Low Birth Weight Infants (<1500 g)

Teodoro Durá-Travé, Isabel San Martín-García, Fidel Gallinas-Victoriano, María Malumbres-Chacón, Paula Moreno-González and María Urretavizcaya-Martinez

Abstract

Features of catch-up growth are not well established in very low birth weight infants (VLBW). The aim of this study is to analyze the catch-up growth in height and some factors associated in a cohort of VLBW (<1500 g) from birth to age 14 years. Retrospective registration of weight and height at birth and ages 0.5, 1, 2, 3, 4, 6, 8, 10, 12 and 14 years in a cohort of 170 VLBW have been recorded Anthropometric variables were compared with those from a control group. Sixty-nine (40.6%) were small for gestational age (SGA subgroup) and 101 (59.4%) were appropriate for gestational age (AGA subgroup). Thirty-seven (21.8%) were extremely low birth weight (ELBW), and 32 (18.8%) extremely preterm (EPT). At age 2, 4 and 10 years, 49.4%, 78.9% and 87.1% VLBW, respectively, did reach normal height. Between 4 and 10 years of age, only 8.2% of VLBW reached normal height. At 10 years of age, 7% of VLBW (1000–1500 g) and 35% of ELBW (<1500 g) showed short stature (p = 0.001). Almost the entire sample of VLBW with normal height at age 2, 4 and 10 have reached an adequate catch-up growth in weight in the previous evaluations. ELBW, SGA and EPT were found to be independent predictors for inadequate catch-up growth in height at 2, 4, and 10 years of age. The growth pattern of children born preterm has particular features: they have a lower rate and/or slowness in the catch-up growth in height with respect to that described in full-term small-for-gestational-age infants. Catch-up in weight appears to be a decisive factor for catch-up in height, and, on this basis, we recommend a rigorous nutritional follow-up in these individuals. If these measures do not help improve catch-up in height, they may be eligible for the establishment of rhGH therapy.

Keywords: Catch-up growth, Extremely low birth weight, Growth pattern, Intrauterine growth retardation, Preterm infant, Very low birth weight infant

1. Introduction

Full-term infants who present with intrauterine growth restriction constitute a varied group with multifactorial conditions. These infants, along with high rates of perinatal morbidity and mortality, undergo an increased risk of cardiovascular and/or metabolic disease in adult life [1]. They subsequently experience an accelerated compensating growth, known as catch-up growth, which usually ceases at age 2 [2–4]. As a matter of fact, those children whose catch-up is inadequate have low chance to reach a normal size in adult life; that is one of the approved indications for the treatment with recombinant growth hormone [5–8].

Nevertheless, the features of catch-up growth are not well characterized in very preterm infants (<32 weeks of gestation) or very low birth weight infants (<1.500 g). In accordance with current knowledge, there is evidence that supports the need to experience adequate extrauterine growth in order to acquire optimal development of all their organic capacities. The increased survival rate of very low birth weight infants (<1500 g) at present time, as a consequence of the recent advances in obstetric and perinatal care, entails a higher risk of sensorineural morbidity and/or disability [5, 9, 10]. In any case, the follow-up of these patients, even though there is no actual consensus, suggests that this catch-up could extend to a later stage, and so condition the prognosis of adult size [11–18].

Catch-up is defined as a fast paced growth after a period of growth failure whose aim is to approach to the measurements of normal term-born infants [2–4]. When this event fails to develop during the initial stages of life, neurological deficits like behavioral difficulties and neurocognitive deficits in very preterm infants are likely to be found [19–21]. In addition, correlations between rapid and early growth (especially of weight) in preterm-born infants and the progression to metabolic syndrome in adulthood have been reported [19, 22, 23]. There is still poor understanding on the factors that determine when catch-up growth occurs in very preterm infants or very low birth weight infants, but it is well-known that low birth weight, early gestational age and medical complications have a particularly negative effect on postnatal growth [16]. In addition, the catch-up growth in weight in these children, which presents simultaneously to catch-up growth in length, has been less frequently studied, even though it has been proved that caloric intake has a positive impact on postnatal growth in preterm infants [24–27].

The main aim of the work is to perform a longitudinal descriptive study of anthropometric measurements in a group of very low birth weight (VLBW) infants, aged from birth to 14 years of age, and to analyze the features of catch-up growth in height and some of the factors associated in these children.

2. Methods

There is a specific program in our region (Comunidad Foral de Navarra), fostered by the Regional Health Service, that intends to promote healthy lifestyle and monitors child growth and development. By means of periodic consultation (usually at birth and during the first year, and ages 0.5, 1, 2, 3, 4, 6, 8, 10, 12 and 14 years), the program accomplish the registration of anthropometric measurements (weight and height) and saves different data in the clinical records.

These children, who represent a cohort of VLBW infants (<1500 g), have been evaluated by a pediatrician and/or pediatric nurse by the use of the different facilities available (our public Health Service guarantees universal accessibility in distance and personal assistance). The different consultations were programmed at birth and ages 0.5, 1, 2, 3, 4, 6, 8, 10, 12 and 14 years. A brief medical history, basic physical exam and the anthropometric measurements (weight and height) were recorded. The only requirements to be included were a Caucasian origin from Spanish parents, and the birth place (the Neonatal Unit of the Navarra Hospital Complex in Pamplona, Spain, which is the reference Hospital) in the period January, 2001-December, 2005.

Body measurements (weight and height) were taken during physical exam in underwear and barefoot. We used an Año-Sayol scale (reading interval 0 to 120 kg and a precision of 100 g) for the measurement of weight and a Holtain wall stadiometer (reading interval 60 to 210 cm, precision 0.1 cm) for the measurement of height.

We collected a sample of 217 births of babies who met the criteria of VLBW, 47 of whom were excluded due to different reasons: perinatal mortality in 20 (9.2%), the finding of severe malformations or chromosomopathies in 6 (2.8%), severe neurosensory disability and motor sequelae in 5 (2.3%), ethnic origin in 8 (3.7%) and other reasons (geographical distance to hospital and difficulties for transportation, absence of continuity in the evaluations of the pediatric health screening, etc.) in 8 cases (3.7%).

The children (VLBW) in this cohort were divided in two subgroups: newborn infants who were appropriate for gestational age (AGA subgroup) and newborn infants who were small for gestational age (SGA subgroup). The difference between both groups was that birth weight and/or length were higher or equal/lower than two standard deviations below the average of a reference population for gestational age and sex, respectively. We used the growth reference charts for newborns from the anthropometric growth patterns of preterm from Carrascosa et al. [28]. In addition, when birth weight was lower than 1.000 g they were defined as extremely low birth weight (ELBW). Another way to classify newborns was based on gestational age: extremely preterm (EPT) when gestational age was lower than 28 weeks, very preterm (VPT) when gestational age was between 28–32 weeks, and late preterm (LPT) when gestational age was between 32–37 weeks.

A control group was established by recruiting children from a different observational epidemiological study made of an infant population (healthy full-term infants, Caucasian and children from Caucasian parents); the periodic evaluations followed the same patterns as those for VLBW infants (482 boys and 448 girls) [29].

An adequate catch-up growth in height or weight was defined when height or weight in VLBW infants, respectively, surpassed the value of 2 standard deviations below the mean in the growth charts of the control group [2–4].

3. Statistical analysis

Results are presented in the successive tables as percentages (%) and means (M) with corresponding standard deviations (s.d.) and confidence intervals (95% CI). The statistical analysis (descriptive statistics, Student's t-test, analysis of variance, Chi-square and multiple logistic regression analysis) was executed with the program *Statistical Packages for the Social Sciences* version 20.0 (Chicago, IL, USA). The statistical significance was reached with a P-value of 0.05.

This study was submitted and subsequently approved by the Ethics Committee for Human Investigation of the Navarra Hospital Complex, Pamplona, Spain (in compliance with the ethical standards of the 1964 Declaration of Hensinki and later amendments). Parents and/or legal guardians were aware of the characteristics and requirements of the study and provided acceptance for the participation in all cases.

4. Results

The sample of VLBW infants who have been recruited for this study consists of 170 children (82 boys and 88 girls). In the aggregate, 40.6% (n = 69) of the infants were included as small for gestational age (SGA subgroup) and the remaining 59.4%

(n = 101) as appropriate for gestational age (AGA subgroup). In the SGA subgroup, 59.4% (n = 41) of children had a history of weight and height alterations at birth, while specific alterations of height (23.2%, n = 16) or weight (17.4%, n = 12) were less frequent (**Figure 1**).

Multiple pregnancies amount to 42.4% (n = 72), being twin pregnancies predominant, (**Figure 2**).

On the basis of gestational age, they have been subdivided into extremely preterm (n = 32, 18.8%), very preterm (n = 72, 42.4%) and late preterm (n = 66, 38.8%) (**Figure 3**). Thirty-seven (21.8%) infants were included as ELBW.

Table 1 exposes and compares the values of the anthropometric measurements at birth of VLBW infants in the AGA and SGA subgroups and classified by sex. We do not appreciate statistically significant differences in the mean weight and height values at birth between the two groups. The values of gestational age were significantly higher in the SGA subgroup than in the AGA subgroup.

Table 2 displays and compares the mean values for height, weight and growth rate in VLBW infants and the control group from birth to 10 years of age. Figures for height and weight were significantly lower in VLBW than in the control group. In contrast, growth rate in the first two years of life in was significantly higher in VLBW infants than in the individuals of the control group.

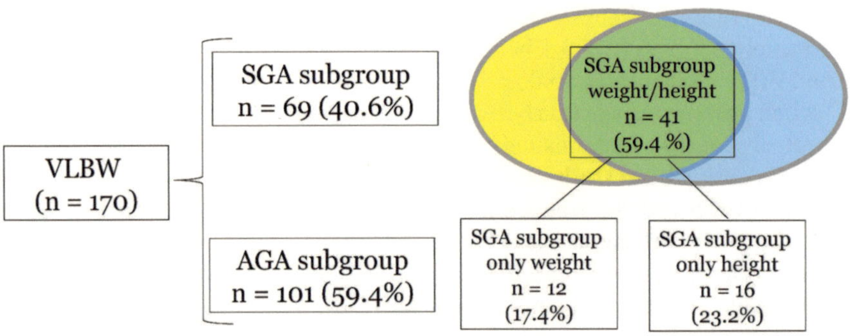

Figure 1.
Classification of VLBW according to weight and/or height at birth.

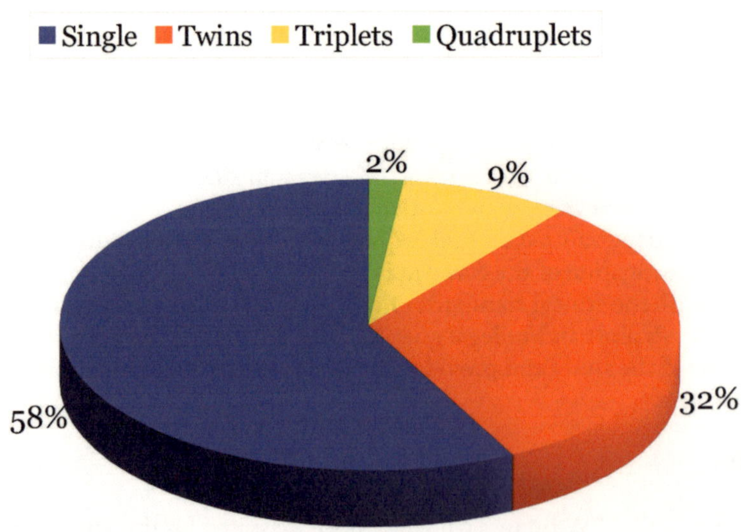

Figure 2.
Distribution of VLBW according to the type of pregnancy.

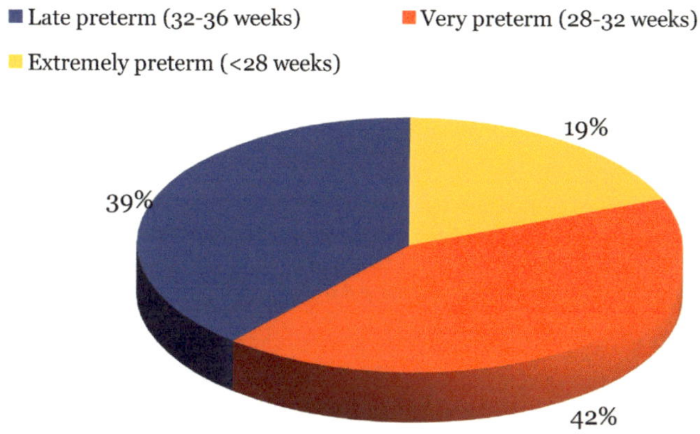

Figure 3.
Distribution of VLBW according to the degree of prematurity.

	Boys		Girls	
	AGA subgroup (n = 52)	**SGA subgroup (n = 30)**	**AGA subgroup (n = 49)**	**SGA subgroup (n = 39)**
Gestational age* (weeks)	28.7 ± 1.9	33.3 ± 1.9	28.9 ± 2.1	32.6 ± 3.1
Weight (g)	1204.3 ± 222.8	1257.4 ± 179.9	1145.8 ± 229.7	1134.0 ± 256.5
Height (cm)	38.3 ± 3.1	39.0 ± 2.4	38.2 ± 2.6	37.4 ± 3.5

**Student's t-test, p < 0.05 among AGA and SGA.*
AGA: appropriate for gestational age. SGA: small weight for gestational age.

Table 1.
Gestational age, weight and height data from VLBW infants at birth in both sexes (M ± SD).

Figure 4 shows the percentage of VLBW infants who reached normal height at the different stages that were evaluated in the study. At age 2, 4 and 10 years, 49.4%, 78.9% and 87.1%of infants, respectively, had gained normal height. In this sense, 8.2% of VLBW infants presented with normal height between ages 4 and 10 years.

The analysis reveals that 86% of VLBW infants that had gained normal weight after the first year of life reached normal height ($P < 0.001$) by age 2 years. Additionally, 98.6% of VLBW infants with normal weight at age 2 had reached normal height ($P < 0.001$) by age 4. In the same way, 97.2% of VLBW infants with normal weight at age 4 appear with normal values for height ($P < 0.001$) by age 10, 99.2% of VLBW infants with normal weight at age 6 showed normal values for height by age 8 ($P < 0.001$), and finally, all VLBW infants that presented with normal weight at age 10 had also normal height at this age ($P < 0.001$).

Table 3 states the comparison of mean values for height, weight and growth rate between AGA y SGA subgroups from birth to 10 years of age. The AGA subgroup features significantly higher values for height with respect to SGA subgroup at age 1, 2, 3, 4 and 6, as well as higher values for weight at age 1, 2, 3 and 6. There were no statistically significant differences in growth rate between both groups in every stage evaluated.

Figure 5 shows the figures of the percentages of infants in the AGA and SGA subgroups that gained normal size at the different stages under assessment. There were no statistically significant differences between the groups, except at age 10:

Height (cm)			
Age (years)	**VLBW group**	**Control group**	**p-value**
0	38.2 ± 3.3	50.0 ± 2.0	<0.001
6 mo	60.2 ± 3.5	67.2 ± 2.2	<0.001
1	70.9 ± 3.4	75.9 ± 2.7	<0.001
2	83.8 ± 4.0	88.1 ± 3.1	<0.001
3	92.5 ± 4.2	96.5 ± 3.4	<0.001
4	100.2 ± 4.9	104.0 ± 4.2	<0.001
6	113.8 ± 5.6	117.3 ± 4.8	<0.001
8	125.6 ± 6.0	129.6 ± 5.4	<0.001
10	136.2 ± 6.9	140.7 ± 6.2	<0.001
Weight (kg)			
Age (years)	**VLBW group**	**Control group**	**p-value**
0	1.2 ± 0.2	3.3 ± 0.4	<0.001
6 mo	5.7 ± 1.0	7.7 ± 0.8	<0.001
1	8.0 ± 1.2	10.0 ± 1.2	<0.001
2	10.5 ± 1.5	12.7 ± 1.4	<0.001
3	12.7 ± 2.0	15.2 ± 1.8	<0.001
4	14.8 ± 2.5	17.6 ± 2.4	<0.001
6	19.5 ± 3.5	22.7 ± 3.6	<0.001
8	25.0 ± 5.4	29.6 ± 5.6	<0.001
10	31.5 ± 8.1	37.2 ± 7.4	<0.001
Velocity height (cm/y)			
Age (years)	**VLBW group**	**Control group**	**p-value**
0–6 mo	44.1 ± 4.9	34.0 ± 6.5	<0.001
0–12 mo	32.6 ± 3.1	26.0 ± 2.6	<0.001
1–2	12.9 ± 1.8	11.9 ± 2.4	<0.001
2–3	8.8 ± 2.2	8.4 ± 1.9	0.060
3–4	7.5 ± 1.9	7.7 ± 1.8	0.190
4–6	6.6 ± 1.4	6.7 ± 1.0	0.895
6–8	6.1 ± 1.1	6.1 ± 1.1	0.453
8–10	5.5 ± 1.3	5.6 ± 1.3	0.558

VLBW: very low birth weight.

Table 2.
Changes in the values of height, weight and growth rate of VLBW and control group (M ± SD).

17% of children in the SGA subgroup (n = 12) and 10% of children in the AGA subgroup (n = 10) presented with low height values (P = 0.018).

Table 4 describes the mean values for height, weight and growth rate in ELBW (<1000 g) and VLBW (1001–1500 g) infants from birth to 10 years. Mean values for weight and height were significantly lower in ELBW than in VLBW in every age considered except for 10 years. There were no significant differences in growth rate between both groups in any period of age.

Figure 6 presents the percentages of VLBW (1000–1500 g; n = 133) and ELBW (<1000 g; n = 37) infants that reached normal height at the different ages under assessment. There were significant differences between groups at every age evaluated. In this way, 7% of VLBW infants (n = 9) and 35% of ELBW infants (n = 13) showed short stature (P = 0.001) at age 10.

In the SGA subgroup, 7 out of the 12 children that presented with short stature at age 10 (7 of whom were ELBW) had reached normal values in height by age 14 (6 of them had taken treatment with recombinant human growth hormone [rhGH]); the remaining 5 (3 of whom were ELBW) maintained short stature (3 of them had treatment with rhGH). Treatment with rhGH was started between ages 6.5

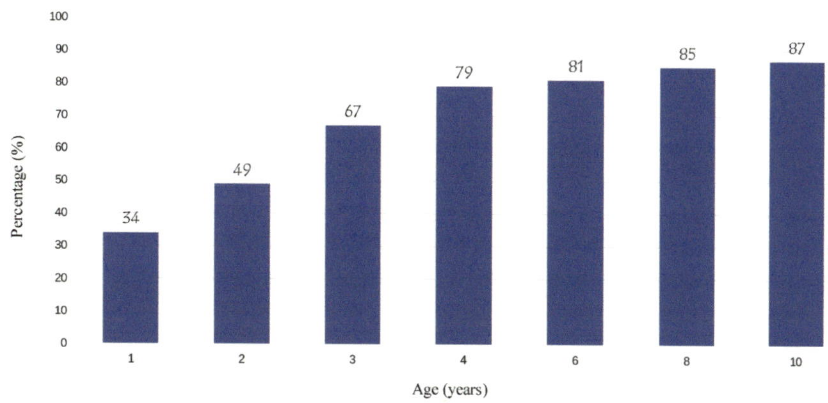

Figure 4.
Percentages of adequate catch-up growth in height in VLBW infants.

Height (cm)			
Age (years)	**SGA subgroup**	**AGA subgroup**	**p-value**
0	38.1 ± 3.8	38.2 ± 2.8	0.786
6 mo	60.1 ± 4.0	60.4 ± 3.4	0.702
1	70.2 ± 3.6	71.4 ± 3.4	0.008
2	82.9 ± 3.9	84.5 ± 3.9	0.027
3	91.6 ± 3.8	93.1 ± 4.4	0.030
4	99.1 ± 4.8	100.9 ± 5.0	0.035
6	112.4 ± 6.0	114.6 ± 5.7	0.025
8	124.6 ± 5.7	126.4 ± 6.2	0.109
10	135.5 ± 6.6	137.0 ± 7.2	0.409
Weight (kg)			
Age (years)	**SGA subgroup**	**AGA subgroup**	**p-value**
0	1.2 ± 0.2	1.2 ± 0.2	0.730
6 mo	5.5 ± 1.0	5.9 ± 0.9	0.081
1	7.6 ± 1.2	8.3 ± 1.1	0.002
2	10.0 ± 1.6	10.8 ± 1.5	0.002
3	12.1 ± 1.6	13.2 ± 2.1	0.001
4	14.4 ± 2.3	14.8 ± 3.4	0.355
6	18.7 ± 3.3	19.9 ± 3.6	0.032
8	24.4 ± 5.2	25.5 ± 5.4	0.258
10	31.5 ± 8.1	31.7 ± 8.3	0.902
Velocity height (cm/y)			
Age (years)	**SGA subgroup**	**AGA subgroup**	**p-value**
0–6 mo	44.5 ± 5.4	43.9 ± 4.4	0.511
6–12 mo	20.3 ± 4.0	21.9 ± 4.6	0.068
0–12 mo	32.2 ± 3.4	33.0 ± 2.8	0.170
1–2	12.8 ± 1.5	13.1 ± 2.1	0.423
2–3	8.6 ± 2.1	8.9 ± 2.2	0.553
3–4	7.4 ± 2.0	7.6 ± 1.7	0.650
4–6	6.4 ± 1.3	6.7 ± 1.4	0.225
6–8	6.1 ± 1.3	6.2 ± 1.0	0.678
8–10	5.4 ± 1.2	5.5 ± 1.5	0.750

AGA: appropriate for gestational age. SGA: small weight for gestational age.

Table 3.
Changes in the values of height, weight and growth rate of VLBW (AGA and SGA subgroups. (M ± SD).

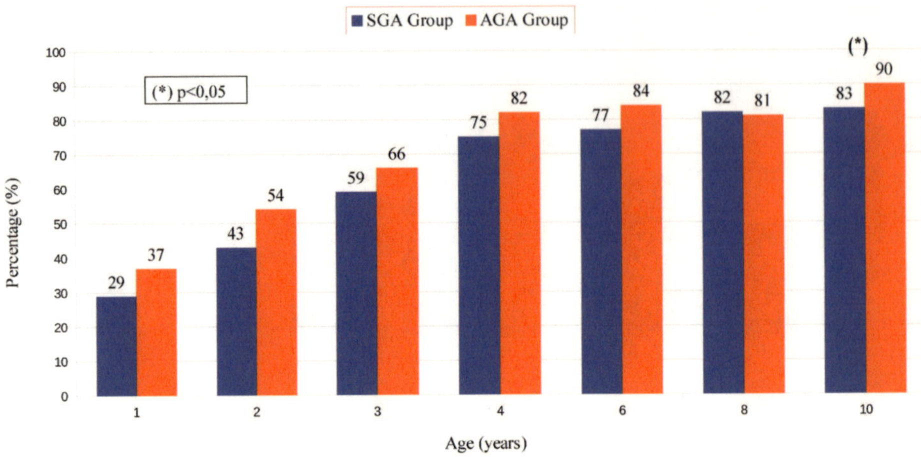

Figure 5.
Percentages of adequate catch-up growth in height in AGA and SGA groups (chi-square).

Height (cm)			
Age (years)	**ELBW group (<1000 g)**	**VLBW group (1000–1500 g)**	**p-value**
0	33.6 ± 2.7	39.4 ± 2.1	<0.001
6 mo	55.8 ± 2.8	61.4 ± 2.7	<0.001
1	67.0 ± 2.8	71.8 ± 2.8	<0.001
2	75.9 ± 3.9	84.8 ± 3.2	<0.001
3	79,7 ± 4.2	93.5 ± 3.5	<0.001
4	96.4 ± 5.9	101.1 ± 4.1	<0.001
6	110.5 ± 6.1	114.5 ± 5.2	<0.001
8	121.1 ± 6.8	126.8 ± 5.3	<0.001
10	133.8 ± 7.3	136.8 ± 6.7	0.179
Weight (kg)			
Age (years)	**ELBW group (<1000 g)**	**VLBW group (1000–1500 g)**	**p-value**
0	0.8 ± 0.1	1.3 ± 0.2	<0.001
6 mo	4.7 ± 0.8	6.0 ± 0.8	<0.001
1	6.8 ± 1.1	8.3 ± 1.0	<0.001
2	9.2 ± 1.3	10.9 ± 1.3	<0.001
3	11.2 ± 1.5	13.1 ± 1.8	<0.001
4	13.0 ± 2.0	15.3 ± 2.3	<0.001
6	17.1 ± 2.7	20.0 ± 3.4	<0.001
8	21.5 ± 4.1	26.1 ± 5.2	<0.00
10	32.6 ± 8.3	32.7 ± 8.3	0.048
Velocity height (cm/y)			
Age (years)	**ELBW group (<1000 g)**	**VLBW group (1000–1500 g)**	**p-value**
0–6 mo	44.9 ± 6.3	43.9 ± 4.4	0.409
6–12 mo	22.8 ± 4.5	20.8 ± 4.3	0.039
0–12 mo	33.9 ± 3.7	32.3 ± 2.9	0.065
1–2	12.7 ± 2.3	13.0 ± 1.7	0.492
2–3	9.0 ± 2.5	8.7 ± 2.1	0.621
3–4	7.4 ± 2.1	7.5 ± 1.7	0.698
4–6	6.5 ± 1.2	6.7 ± 1.3	0.595
6–8	5.8 ± 1.1	6.2 ± 1.1	0.171
8–10	5.7 ± 1.1	5.5 ± 1.3	0.530

ELBW: extremely low birth weight. VLBW: very low birth weight.

Table 4.
Changes in the values of height, weight and growth rate of VLBW (1000–1500 g) and ELBW (< 1000 g). (M ± SD).

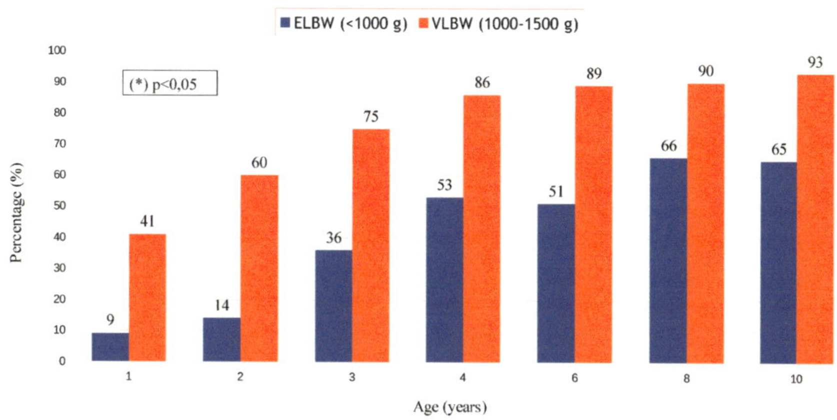

Figure 6.
Percentages of adequate catch-up growth in height in ELBW and VLBW infants (chi-square).

Items	Inadequate catch-up growth in height		
	At 2 years OR (95% CI) P-value	At 4 years OR (95% CI) P-value	At 10 years OR (95% CI) P-value
Birth weight VLBW (1000–1500 g), n = 133 ELBW (<1000 g), n = 37	Referent 8,9 (3.3–24.5) 0.001	Referent 5,9 (3.6–13.6) 0.001	Referent 5.3 (2.1–13.4) 0.001
AGA group, n = 69 SGA group (weight/height), n = 41	Referent 1,6 (0,8–2.9) 0,150	Referent 1,5 (0.7–3.1) 0,300	Referent 2.6 (1.1–6.4) 0.038
AGA group, n = 69 SGA group (only weight), n = 12	Referent 1.4 (0.7–2.7) 0.291	Referent 1.3 (0.6–2.9) 0.457	Referent 2.3 (0.9–5.5) 0.069
AGA group, n = 69 SGA group (only height), n = 16	Referent 2.0 (1.3–1.7) 0.048	Referent 1.9 (1.2–4.0) 0.033	Referent 2.8 (1.1–6.8) 0.024
Gestation type Single, n = 98 Multiple, n = 72	Referent 0,9 (0.5–1.5) 0.620	Referent 0.9 (0.4–1.9) 0.862	Referent 1.4 (0.6–3.6) 0.431
Gestational age 32–37 weeks (LPT), n = 66 <28 weeks (VPT), n = 72 28–32 weeks (EPT), n = 32	Referent 2.5(1.1–5.9) 0.035 2.6 (1.1.6.4) 0.033	Referent 7.2(2.6–19.8) 0.001 4.2 (1.6–10.8) 0.003	Referent 4.5(1.3–14.9) 0.015 1.9 (0.7–5.3) 0.242

VLBW: very low birth weight. ELBW: extremely low birth weight. AGA: appropriate for gestational age. SGA: small weight for gestational age. LPT: late preterm. VPT: very preterm. EPT: extremely preterm.

Table 5.
Logistic regression analysis of factors associated with inadequate catch-up growth.

and 8.3 years. In the AGA subgroup, 2 of the 10 children that presented with short stature at age 10 (7 of whom were ELBW) had reached a normal height at 14 years (1 of them had received rhGH therapy at age 8.9 years) and 8 (6 of them ELBW) kept in short stature (1 of them started rhGH therapy at age 7.8 years, and 7 of them were not entitled to receive treatment due to normal responses in growth hormone stimulation tests).

Table 5 displays the results of the multiple logistic regression analysis conducted to study the association of neonatal clinical history with inappropriate catch-up growth in height at ages 2, 4, and 10. The analysis shows that the conditions of ELBW, SGA for height and preterm birth before 28 weeks of gestation were associated with inadequate catch-up growth in height at 2, 4, and 10 years. On the other side, SGA for both weight and height was associated with inadequate catch-up growth only at age 10, whereas preterm birth between 28 to 32 weeks of gestation was associated with inadequate catch-up growth only at ages 2 and 4. Additionally, multiple birth was not associated with inadequate catch-up growth at ages 2, 4 or 10 years.

5. Discussion

The terms "intrauterine growth restriction" (IUGR) and "small for gestational age" (SGA) newborn are not strictly equivalent concepts [30], since they are related to different chronological stages (fetal growth and anthropometric measurements at birth, respectively). Nevertheless, they refer to failure to reach the genetic growth potencial during the prenatal period as an adaptive response to an adverse uterine environment. In any way, both terms are used indistinctly in daily clinical practice in order to cluster those newborns whose weight and/or height at birth are equal to/below 2 standard deviations under the average of a reference population on the basis of gestational age and sex. In this case, the majority of children included in the so-called SGA group presented with a combined alteration in weight and height, whilst the proportion of children with exclusive weight or height disorder was slightly lower.

This definition requires a precise diagnosis of gestational age and the registration of anthropometric measurements after birth, whose values should be contrasted with reference standards for gestational age and sex. The choice of reference patterns is a determining factor in the assessment of newborn growth [31]. In fact, the variability of the anthropometric variables in relation to racial, genetic, social, environmental and maternal lifestyle factors make it advisable to use local or national growth reference charts. The charts from Lubchenco et al. [32], which were published in the 60s, have been widely used and are characterized by a contrasted clinical utility. At present, the most qualified local (Spanish) reference charts, which have been used in the present study, are the newborn (26–42 weeks of gestational age) weight and height charts from the anthropometric growth patterns of preterm from Carrascosa et al. [28].

Fetal development and intrauterine growth are complex processes in which continuous and harmonious cellular proliferation and differentiation take place. Multiple factors (maternal, fetal, placental and environmental) have been mentioned to have a negative impact on the fetus and set off a series of functional and structural adaptive changes that conclude in fetal growth restriction (in the so-called "thrifty phenotype hypothesis"). They are linked to different changes in hormone sensitivity and/or secretion that entails an increased risk of developing metabolic and/or endocrine disorders in adult life [33, 34]. In any way, most term newborns with previous intrauterine growth restriction manifest a compensatory growth (catch-up growth) after birth, mainly in the first year of life, that enables approximately 90% of the individuals to surpass the threshold of 2 SDs under the average in the reference population, or, in other words, to get normal height [2–4]. Even so, whenever this compensatory growth does not occur, a normal final height in adulthood is not likely to be reached. By knowing so, this event is considered one of the indications for rhGH therapy approved by the United States Food and Drug Administration (FDA), the European Medicines Agency (EMA) and the Growth Hormone Research Society, with the intention to boost the initial compensatory growth and/or to keep normal growth velocity [3, 35, 36].

The recent advances in obstetric and perinatal care have led to a considerable decrease in VLBW infants mortality; despite this, and owing to the potential sensorineural morbidity in this children, these patients are usually enlisted in follow-up programmes whose goal is the early detection of neurodevelopmental problems [1, 37]. The improvement of these programmes has eased the standardization of dietary and nutritional advices, and enabled growth monitoring in the first years of life. It also facilitates the analysis, as we performed in this study, of the evolution of anthropometric variables in VLBW infants [38].

The results obtained in this study confirm that, on one side, the VLBW newborns undergo a postnatal compensatory growth that is maximum during the first year of life, as it occurs in term newborns that are SGA. As a matter of fact, growth velocity during the first 12 months of life in VLBW was considerably higher than in the control group; this explains, to a great extent, the noticeably proportion of individuals in this group that reach normal height by age 2 years [39]. On the other side, this study remarks that VLBW infants have a lower rate and/or delay in the catch-up growth in height when comparing to that observed in full-term SGA infants [4, 16–18, 24, 25]. In point of fact, 50.6%, 21.1% and 12.9% of individuals, maintained short stature at age 2, 4 and 10, respectively; in other words, these individuals reached normal height in a similar percentage than that for full-term SGA infants at age 2. Additionally, barely 8.2% of children reached normal height between ages 4 to 10. Despite current data are inconsistent, these results are somehow congruent with those exposed by the different authors that previously noticed that catch-up in VLBW infants could be delayed [12, 15, 40–44]. Nevertheless, none of the authors cited has screened the influence of catch-up growth in weight, which is concurrent with the catch-up in height and, in accordance to the data collected, plays a decisive role [24, 25]. In effect, a great majority of individuals who present with normal height at age 2, 4 and 10 have gained an adequate catch-up growth in weight in the previous evaluations. For this reason, these individuals should follow a strict nutritional control in order to raise an issue on the prescription of nutritional supplements with the challenge to get weight recovery as fast as possible [26, 45–47].

The findings of our study have direct implications on clinical practice. First of all, the assessment and comparison of the patterns of catch-up height gain in AGA and SGA groups present only small variances in the age range under consideration, except at age 10. At age 10, only 1 out of the 10 children did not register normal height in the AGA group, whilst approximately 1 in 5 children in the SGA subgroup still had short stature. In other words, the lower rate of catch-up growth in VLBW infants is slightly further reduced or delayed in SGA infants. On the other hand, it is important to emphasize that 1 in 3 children get normal height in both the AGA and the SGA groups between ages 2 and 4 years. This fact suggests that the implementation of the recommendation of the EMA and the Growth Hormone Research Society to postpone the beginning of rhGH therapy until the age of 4 years would be more applicable than implementing the recommendation of the FDA, which recommends the beginning of treatment at age 2 years.

The analysis of catch-up growth in ELBW infants merits particular attention. First, we detected that the majority of children that had not attained normal height by age 10 years in both the AGA and the SGA subgroups were infants born with ELBW. Second, there was a noticeable amount of children in the AGA subgroup that were not considered for hormone therapy when the response to growth hormone stimulation test was normal, in accordance with the current recommendations of the FDA, the EMA and the Growth Hormone Research Society. This fact fully explains the reason why children in the AGA subgroup with short stature at age 10 years (the majority of them were VLBW) remained in the same situation at age 14 and, presumably, in adulthood. Since current guidelines do not give consideration to the option of beginning growth hormone therapy in AGA infants with normal GH secretion, we should reckon if these criteria should be revised in the case of children born with VLBW and, especially, those with ELBW.

The multiple logistic regression analysis corroborated that ELBW and EPT infants were at higher risk of inadequate catch-up in height at 2, 4, and 10 years of age; additionally, they have an increased risk of short stature in adulthood. These results sustain the hypothesis of a potential benefit from GH treatment, independently of the adequacy of their birth weight and/or length for gestational age [18, 48–50].

In conclusion, the growth pattern of children born preterm has particular features. Approximately 85% and 53% of VLBW and ELBW infants, respectively, will attain normal height by 4 years of age. In contrast, those individuals with short stature at age 4 years are not likely to attain normal height in childhood. Catch-up in weight appears to be a decisive factor for catch-up in height, and, on this basis, we recommend a rigorous nutritional follow-up in these individuals. If these measures do not help improve catch-up in height, they may be eligible for the establishment of rhGH therapy.

Author details

Teodoro Durá-Travé[1,2,3*], Isabel San Martín-García[2], Fidel Gallinas-Victoriano[2], María Malumbres-Chacón[2], Paula Moreno-González[2] and María Urretavizcaya-Martinez[2]

1 Department of Pediatrics, School of Medicine, University of Navarra, Pamplona, Spain

2 Department of Pediatrics, Navarra Hospital Complex, Pamplona, Spain

3 Navarra Institute for Health Research (IdisNA), Pamplona, Spain

*Address all correspondence to: tduratra@cfnavarra

References

[1] Raju TNK, Buist AS, Blaisdell CJ, Moxey-Mims M, Saigal S. Adults born preterm: A review of general health and system-specific outcomes. Acta Paediatr. 2017;106:1409-1437.

[2] Lee PA, Chernausek SD, Hokken-Koelega AC, Czernichow P, International Small for Gestational Age Advisory Board. International Small for Gestational Age Advisory Board consensus development conference statement: Management of short children born small for gestational age, April 24–October 1, 2001. Pediatrics. 2003;111:1253-61.

[3] Clayton PE, Cianfarani S, Czernichow P, Johannsson G, Rapaport R, Rogol A. Management of the child born small for gestational age through to adulthood: A consensus statement of the International Societies of Paediatric Endocrinology and the Growth Hormone Research Society. J Clin Endocrinol Metab. 2007; 2:804-810.

[4] Boguszewski MC, Mericq V, Bergada I, Damiani D, Belgorosky A, Gunczler P, et al. Latin American consensus: Children born small for gestational age. BMC Pediatr. 2008;11:66.

[5] Lemons JA, Bauer CR, Oh W, Korones SB, Papile LA, Stoll BJ, et al. Very low birth weight outcomes of the National Institute of Child health and human development neonatal research network, January 1995 through December 1996. NICHD Neonatal Research Network. *Pediatrics*. 2001; 107: E1.

[6] Gharib H, Cook DM, Saenger PH, Bengtsson BA, Feld S, Nippold TB, et al. American Association of Clinical Endocrinologists Growth Hormone Task Force 2003: American Association of Clinical Endocrinologists medical guidelines for clinical practice for growth hormone use in adults and children–2003 update. Endocr Pract 2003, 9: 64-73.

[7] Carrascosa A, Vicens-Calvet E, Yeste D, Espadero RM, Ulied A. Children born small for gestational age (SGA) who fail to achieve catch up growth by 2-8 years of age are short from infancy to adulthood. Data from a cross-sectional study of 486 Spanish children. Pediatr Endocrinol Rev. 2006; 4: 15-27.

[8] Argente J, Gracia R, Ibáñez L, Oliver A, Borrajo E, Vela A, et al. Spanish SGA Working Group: Improvement in growth after two years of growth hormone therapy in very young children born small for gestational age and without spontaneous catch-up growth: results of a multicenter, controlled, randomized, open clinical trial. J Clin Endocrinol Metab 2007, 92: 3095-3101.

[9] Arce Casas A, Iriondo Sanz M, Krauel Vidal J, Jiménez González R, Campistol Plana J, Poo Argüelles P, et al. Neurological follow-up of very low birth weight newborns at the age of two years (1998-1999). *An Pediatr* (Barc) 2003; 59: 454-461.

[10] Hernández González N, Salas Hernández S, García-Alix Pérez A, Roche Herrero C, Pérez Rodríguez J, Omeñaca Teres F, et al. Morbidity at 2 years in infants with a birth weight of < 1,500 g. *An Pediatr* (Barc) 2005; 62: 320-327.

[11] Saigal S, Stoskopf BL, Streiner DL, Burrows E. Physical growth and current health status of infants who were of extremely low birth weight and controls at adolescence. Pediatrics 2001; 108: 407-415.

[12] Hack M, Schluchter M, Cartar L, Rahman M, Cuttler L, Borawski E.

Growth of very low birth weight infants to age 20 years. Pediatrics 2003; 112: e30–e38.

[13] Finken MJ, Dekker FW, de Zegher F, Wit JM. Long-term height gain of prematurely born children with neonatal growth restraint: parallellism with the growth pattern of short children born small for gestational age. Pediatrics 2006; 118: 640-643.

[14] Niklasson A, Engstrom E, Hard AL, Albertsson-Wikland K, Hellstrom A. Growth in very preterm children: a longitudinal study. Pediatr Res. 2003; 54: 899-905.

[15] Farooqi A, Hägglöf B, Sedin G, Gothefors L, Serenius F. Growth in 10- to 12-year-old children born at 23 to 25 weeks' gestation in the 1990s: a Swedish national prospective follow-up study. Pediatrics 2006; 118: e1452–e1465.

[16] Euser AM, de Wit CC, Finken MJ, Rijken M, Wit JM. Growth of preterm born children. Horm Res. 2008;70:319-328.

[17] Hollanders JJ, van der Pal SM, van Dommelen P, Rotteveel J, Finken MJJ. Growth pattern and final height of very preterm vs. very low birth weight infants. Pediatr Res. 2017;82:317-323.

[18] Boguszewski MCS, Cardoso-Demartini A. Growth and growth hormone therapy in short children born preterm. Eur J Endocrinol. 2017;176:R111–R122.

[19] Lapillonne A, Griffin IJ. Feeding preterm infants today for later metabolic and cardiovascular outcomes. J. Pediatr. 2013, 162, S7–S16.

[20] Guellec I, Lapillonne A, Marret S, Picaud JC, Mitanchez D, Charkaluk ML, et al. Effect of intra- and extrauterine growth on long-term neurologic outcomes of very preterm infants. J Pediatr 2016; 175: 93-99.e91.

[21] Takeuchi A, Yorifuji T, Hattori M, Tamai K, Nakamura K, Nakamura M, et al. Catch-up growth and behavioral development among preterm, small-for-gestational-age children: A nationwide Japanese population-based study. Brain Dev 2019; 41: 397-405

[22] Kerkhof GF, Willemsen RH, Leunissen RW, Breukhoven PE, Hokken-Koelega AC: Health profile of young adults born preterm: negative effects of rapid weight gain in early life. J Clin Endocrinol Metabol 2012; 97: 4498-4506.

[23] Embleton ND, Korada M, Wood CL, Pearce MS, Swamy R, Cheetham TD. Catch-up growth and metabolic outcomes in adolescents born preterm. Arch Dis Child 2016; 101:1026-1031.

[24] Vohr BR, McKinley LT. The challenge pays off: early enhanced nutritional intake for VLBW small-for-gestation neonates improves long-term outcome. J Pediatr. 2003; 142:459-461.

[25] Yesinel S, Aldemir EY, Kavuncuoglu S, Yildiz H. Evaluation of growth in very low birth weight preterm babies. Türk Ped Ars.2014; 49:289-298.

[26] Toftlund LH, Halken S, Agertoft L, Zachariassen G. Catch-up growth, rapid weight growth, and continuous growth from birth to 6 years of age in very-preterm born children. Neonatology 2018;114:285-293

[27] Liu X, Biru Luo B, Wentao Peng W, Xiong F, Yang F, Wu J. Factors affecting the catch-up growth of preterm infants after discharge in China: a multicenter study based on the health belief model. Ital J Pediatr. 2019; 45:87

[28] Carrascosa A, Yeste D, Copil A, Almar J, Salcedo S, GussinyeM. Anthropometric growth patterns of preterm and full-term newborns (24-42 weeks' gestational age) at the Hospital

Materno-Infantil Vall D'Hebron (Barcelona, Spain) 1997-2002. An Pediatr (Barc). 2004; 60:406-16.11

[29] Durá Travé T, Garralda Torres I, Hualde Olascoaga J, Grupo Colaborador de Navarra. Longitudinal study of child growth in Navarre (1993-2007). *An Pediatr* (Barc). 2009; 70: 526-533.

[30] Wit JM, Finken MJJ, Rijken M, De Zegher F. Preterm growth restraint: A paradigm that unifies intrauterine growth retardation and preterm extrauterine growth retardation and has Implications for the small-for-gestational-age indication in growth hormone therapy. Pediatrics 2006; 117: e793–e795.

[31] Ayerza Casas A, Rodríguez Martínez G, Samper Villagrasa MP, Ventura Faci P. To born small for gestational age may depend on the growth curve used. Nutr Hosp. 2011; 26: 752-758.

[32] Lubchenco LO, Hansman C, Boyd E. Intrauterine growth in length and head circumference as estimated from live births at gestational ages from 26 to 42 weeks. Pediatrics 1966; 47: 403-408.

[33] Hales CN, Barker DJP. The thrifty phenotype hypothesis. Br Med Bull. 2001; 60:5-20.

[34] Vaag AA, Grunnet LG, Arora GP, Brons C. The thrifty phenotypehypothesis revisited. Diabetologia. 2012; 55:2085-2088.

[35] Gharib H, Cook DM, Saenger PH, Bengtsson BA, Feld S, Nippoldt TB, et al. American Association of Clinical endocrinologists medical guidelines for clinical practice for growth hormone use in adults and children-2003 update. Endocr Pract. 2003;9:64-73.

[36] Boguszewski MCDS, Cardoso-Demartini AA. Management of endocrine disease: Growth hormone therapy in short children born preterm. Eur J Endocrinol. 2017;176:R111-R122.

[37] Diez-López I, de Arriba-Muñoz A, Bosch-Muñoz J, Cabanas-Rodriguez P, Gallego-Gómez E, Martinez-Aedo Ollero MJ, et al.[Follow-up of the small-for-gestational-age child: clinical guide-lines] Spanish. An Pediatr (Barc). 2012; 76, 104.e1-7.

[38] López ID, Muñoz Ade A, Muñoz JB, Rodríguez PC, Gómez EG, Ollero MJ, et al. Follow-up of the small-for-gestational-age child: clinical guidelines. *An Pediatr* (Barc). 2012; 76: 104.e1-7.

[39] Olbertz DM, Mumm R, Wittwer-Backofen U, Fricke-Otto S, Pyper A, Otte J, et al. Identification of growth patterns of preterm and small-for-gestational age children from birth to 4 years – do they catch up? J. Perinat. Med. 2019; 47: 448-454

[40] Knops NB, Sneeuw KC, Brand R, Hille ET, den Ouden AL, WitJM, et al. Catch-up growth up to ten years of age in children born very preterm or with very low birth weight. BMC Pediatr.2005; 5:26.

[41] Sullivan MC, McGrath MM, Hawes K, Lester BM. Growth trajectories of preterm infants: birth to 12 years. J Pediatr HealthCare. 2008; 22:83-93.

[42] Bocca-Tjeertes IF, Kerstjens JM, Reijneveld SA, de WinterAF, Bos AF. Growth and predictors of growth restraint inmoderately preterm children aged 0 to 4 years. Pediatrics.2011; 128:e1187-94.

[43] Roberts G, Cheong J, Opie G, Garse E, Davis N, Duff J, et al. Growth of extremely preterm survivors from birth to18 years of age compared with term controls. Pediatrics.2013; 131:e439–e445.

[44] Finken MJ, Dekker FW, de Zegher F, Wit JM. Long-termheight

gain of prematurely born children with neonatal growth restraint: parallellism with the growth pattern of short children born small for gestational age. Pediatrics. 2018; 118:640-643.

[45] Liu X, Biru Luo B, Wentao Peng W, Xiong F, Yang F, Wu J. Factors affecting the catch-up growth of preterm infants after discharge in China: a multicenter study based on the health belief model. Ital J Pediatr. 2019; 45:87

[46] Japakasetr S, Sirikulchayanonta C, Suthutvoravut U, Chindavijak B, Nokdee S. Implementation of a nutrition program reduced post-discharge growth restriction in Thai very low birth weight preterm infants. Nutrients 2016; 8:820.

[47] Singhal A. Long-Term Adverse Effects of Early Growth Acceleration or Catch-Up Growth. Ann Nutr Metab 2017;70:236-240

[48] Boguszewski MC, Lindberg A, Wollmann HA. Three-year growth response to growth hormone treatment in very young children born small for gestational age-data from KIGS. J Clin EndocrinolMetab. 2014; 99:2683-2688.

[49] Berndt C, Schweizer R, Ranke MB, Binder G, Martin DD. Height, muscle, fat and bone response to growth hormone in short children with very low birth weight born appropriate for gestational age and small for gestational age. Horm Res Paediatr. 2014; 82:81-88.

[50] Qi W, Shen Q, Qiao Y, Wei Z, Wei Y, Fan T. The impact of recombinant human growth hormone on growth and development of low weight premature infants. Int J Clin Exp Med. 2016; 9:4983-4988.

Chapter 11

The Extremely Low Birth Weight Infant

Anet Papazovska Cherepnalkovski, Vesna Pavlov, Ivanka Furlan and Marija Bucat

Abstract

Extremely low birth weight infants (ELBW) are defined by birth weight of less than 1000 g and are frequently born at 27 weeks' gestation (GW) or younger. The neonatologists' efforts focused on improvement of intact survival rate, especially for those born at the frontiers of viability at 22/23 GW. Survival rates of >80% for the advanced gestations and > 50% for 23–24 GW have been reported. Higher gestational age and birth weight, female gender, better maternal education, and white race have been recognized as significant predictors of decreased morbidity in ELBW infants. Although the mortality rate has significantly contracted for this group with improved technology and better understanding of pathophysiology, the proportion of surviving infants without sequelae, has not improved as noticeably. We review the short and long-term morbidities in ELBW infants and compare own and literature data. We analyze some of the specific immediate problems for this group such as: respiratory problems, infection, thermoregulation, impaired glucose homeostasis and disturbed cardiovascular and excretory functions as well as late morbidities such as bronchopulmonary dysplasia, late-onset infections, central nervous system occurrences, retinopathy and anemia of prematurity. We also deal with preventive and therapeutic strategies for improved outcome in this sensitive group of patients.

Keywords: ELBW infants, survival, morbidities, outcomes, respiratory distress, bronchopulmonary dysplasia, retinopathy of prematurity

1. Introduction

Prematurity is a significant risk factor for survival of the neonate and is related to increased perinatal mortality and morbidity. Current minimal age of viability is considered to be 22–23 weeks' gestation with dispersed reports of survival earlier than this estimated gestational age (GA) [1].

Extremely low birth weight infants (ELBW) are defined by birth weight of less than 1000 g; also, are the youngest premature newborns typically born at 27 weeks' gestation or younger [1].

Attention has turned to the improvement of the intact survival rate of extremely low birth weight infants (ELBW), particularly of those born at the boundaries of current perinatal medicine. Survival rates to hospital discharge of above 80% have been reported in Canada, USA and Japan for the 25 GW [2–4]. Developed centers report on increase survival rates also for infants born at 23–24 GW [4] with significant variability in survival observed in resource limited centers [5, 6]. Factors found to be significantly positively correlated with improved survival and outcome of ELBW infants were: older gestational age [1, 5, 6], higher birth weight [1, 5–7], female gender [7], singleton birth [7], antenatal steroid use [1, 6–8], Apgar score at 5 min [1] and delivery by cesarean section (CS) [1, 6]. On the other hand, vaginal delivery in non-vertex presentation [1, 9, 10] placental abruption [1] and the existence of fetal growth restriction [11] have been recognized as adverse factors. Reports highlight birth weights of >750 g in association with better survival [1, 6, 12]. In our previous study, not only that we found a strong positive correlation of higher birth weights with survival, but also of broader head circumferences; the median head circumference was 2.5 cm larger for the survivors [12]. Apgar scores' median value 5 at the first minute were significantly positively associated with favorable outcome [12]. A significant correlation of caesarean section delivery with the outcome has been observed in studies [1, 6, 12], with a higher share of emergency cesarean sections in survivors [12] pointing out that CS is indeed a protective mode of delivery. However, indication of CS in pregnancies of less than 24 weeks is a matter of inclusive worldwide debate. To reach a conclusion, a nationwide survey is needed.

Although the mortality rate has significantly diminished with improved neonatal technologies, use of exogenous surfactant preparations and better understanding of pathophysiology of ELBW infants, the proportion of surviving infants without sequelae, such as chronic lung disease, cognitive delays, cerebral palsy and neurosensory deficits has not improved as noticeably [13, 14].

2. Specific problems in the ELBW infants

2.1 Thermoregulation

ELBW infants are particularly prone to heat loss immediately after birth due to high body surface area to weight ratio, thin skin, decreased brown fat tissue and decreased glycogen supply. Studies have found significant association of hypothermia to in-hospital mortality, respiratory distress syndrome, necrotizing enterocolitis (NEC), and intraventricular hemorrhage in low birth weight/preterm infants [15, 16]. A retrospective observational study performed at 29 Canadian Neonatal Networks' neonatal intensive care units encompassing 9833 infants born at <33 weeks' gestation showed U-shaped relationship between admission temperatures and adverse neonatal outcomes. Lowest rates of adverse outcomes have been associated with admission temperatures between 36.5 °C and 37.2 °C [15]. Thermal management is crucial for survival of the ELBW infants and includes interventions such as drying, heating under a radiant warmer, placing a hat on the head and plastic film over the body [16, 17]. Frequent monitoring of temperature should be done to avoid iatrogenic hyperthermia, especially when applying multiple interventions simultaneously (e.g. plastic bags + thermal mattresses) [16].

2.2 Respiratory distress syndrome

Respiratory distress syndrome (RDS) caused by surfactant deficiency is an early complication of extreme prematurity. Surfactant deficiency causes decreased pulmonary compliance, alveolar hypotension, and an imbalance between pulmonary ventilation and perfusion [17, 18]. Clinically marked by tachypnea, chest retractions, nasal flaring, cyanosis and grunting, this condition usually progresses to hypoventilation, hypoxemia and respiratory acidosis [17, 18]. RDS was recorded in 80% of babies born at 28 weeks' gestation and in 90% of those born at 24 weeks' gestation according to Vermont Oxford Network data during 2017 [18]. Common complications of RDS comprise air leak syndromes, bronchopulmonary dysplasia (BPD) and retinopathy of prematurity (ROP). Animal and synthetic surfactants have been widely used for the treatment of RDS which resulted with significant reduction in mortality. Also, a shift in practice has been noted towards non-invasive ventilation techniques such as continuous positive airway pressure CPAP [19]. Recent large trials showed a lower risk of chronic lung disease or death from early stabilization on CPAP with selective surfactant administration [20]. However, infants born at 23–24 weeks' gestation, may continue to have high need for intubation during initial stabilization.

The INSURE technique (Intubate-Surfactant-Extubate) for surfactant administration involves giving surfactant through an endotracheal tube while administering positive pressure inhalations, often with premedication. This method has been used since 1994 and efficacy has been replicated in many studies [21, 22]. LISA (Less Invasive Surfactant Administration) on the other hand, is a preferred new method that involves administering surfactant via a small intratracheal catheter, with the baby breathing spontaneously on CPAP or NIPPV support, without sedation [23, 24]. However, a recent study raised concerns over relatively low success rate of the first LISA attempt, often inadequate technical performance quality and recurrent desaturations [24].

Following the increasing use of CPAP, other non-invasive ventilation methods have been subjected to research, mostly nasal intermittent positive pressure ventilation (NiPPV) [25] and high-flow nasal cannula (HFNC). Trials have failed to show difference in rates of death and BPD when NiPPV was compared to CPAP [26, 27]. HFNC has been considered as an alternative non-invasive mode for post-extubating support [28]. Current mechanical ventilation (MV) tactics include shortening of duration of MV and the use of targeted volume ventilation (VT). VT results in shorter ventilation-time, fewer air-leaks and less BPD [17].

2.3 Cardiovascular problems

2.3.1 Patent ductus arteriosus

Up to 80% of ELBW infants have a clinically significant patent ductus arteriosus (PDA). As a consequence of the left-to-right systemic to pulmonary shunting various symptoms may appear, most notably, systolic murmur, hypotension, bounding pulses, decreased urine output, pulmonary hyperemia and edema, as well as and reduced mesenteric and cerebral perfusion [29]. Contrary to term newborn who exhibit spontaneous ductus closure in 90% at 48 hours, it occurs in only 30 to 35% of infants with BW < 1000 grams during the neonatal period [29].

The diagnosis is set by echocardiography, also Doppler ultrasound of the cerebral blood vessels in search for signs of diminished perfusion. Ideal management of the PDA in premature infants is still a topic of debate, despite more than three decades of active study [29, 30]. Indomethacin was the conventional drug of choice for ductus closure, but concerns regarding its negative effects on cerebral, renal and gastrointestinal perfusion have led to investigation of other agents such as ibuprofen [30]. A 2020 Cochrane review concluded equal effectiveness of ibuprofen and indomethacin in closing a PDA. However, in the light more favorable safety profile, ibuprofen was highlighted the drug of choice with an equal effectiveness of orogastric and intravenous administration [31]. Oral paracetamol was also supported by clinical studies as equally potent drug for ductus closure [32]. Surgical ligation should only be considered in the light of failed medicaments' treatment [17].

2.3.2 Variable hemodynamics

Blood pressure (BP) of preterm newborns is marked with wide range of observed values for every GA. It is generally accepted that lower BP values are seen with decreasing gestational age and birth weight. Usually, mean arterial blood pressure corresponds to the gestational age, but this relationship is less clear for the extremely premature infants [33]. The variations in BP are related to dynamic changes in physiology during neonatal transition and various disease processes in this group of patients. It has not been proven that institution of any kind of anti-hypotensive therapy, fluid bolus or dopamine could significantly influence the rise of BP 4–24 hours after birth. Therefore, it has been suggested not to rely on a single numerical BP cutoff value for predicting infants that could benefit from anti-hypotensive treatments [33].

Recent randomized controlled trial could not show differences in hemodynamic parameters, amplitude integrated EEG variables, clinical complications or brain ultrasound findings between groups of active, moderate or permissive BP treatment of patients ≤29 GW [34]. The last composite guideline for management of neonatal respiratory distress syndrome recommends treatment of hypotension when evidenced by signs of poor tissue perfusion such as oliguria or poor capillary return, rather than treating sole numerical values [17]. Dopamine has been found more efficient than dobutamine for treatment of systemic hypotension in preterm infants, while dobutamine and epinephrine could be opted for treatment of reduced ventricular function [35]. Hydrocortisone is an alternative medicament for treatment of hypotension in extremely preterm infants [36].

Hypovolemic shock should be managed by giving non-cross-matched O-Rhesus-negative blood or alternatively by administering an isotonic crystalloid solution; the proposed dose is 10–20 mL/kg [37]. Delayed cord clamping apart from expanding blood volume, was proven in clinical studies to yield multiple potential benefits for preterm infants such as improved neurodevelopmental outcomes, reduced blood transfusions, possible autologous transfusion of stem cells, and reduced incidence of intraventricular hemorrhage [38]. However, in infants who need immediate resuscitative measures, it is recommended that placental transfusion should be discontinued [37].

2.4 Central nervous system problems

Intraventricular hemorrhage (IVH) is an extravasation of blood in the brain that originates from the subependymal germinal matrix and advances into the ventricular system, most frequently occurring in the first 3 days of life [39]. The classical grading system of the extent of cerebral bleeding includes 4 grades of hemorrhages: grade I - confined to the germinal matrix, grade II – progression to the lateral ventricle without ventricle dilatation, grade III – blood in the ventricle results in ventricular dilatation, grade IV – periventricular hemorrhagic infarction. Our study group reported an incidence of IVH in almost a third of the ELBW cohort [12]. An inverse relationship exists between the incidence and severity of IVH and gestational age; the lowermost gestations and weights are most heavily affected.

IVH has been recognized as one of the crucial morbidities in ELBW infants, with serious potential short-term sequelae in survivors such as hemorrhagic periventricular infarction, post-hemorrhagic hydrocephalus or seizures, and in the long term, developmental delay, cerebral palsy, deafness, and blindness. [40]. A shift to milder forms of neurosensory impairment has been noted reflecting better practices in perinatal care [41]. Generally, a straightforward correlation exists between the IVH grade and its prognosis. However, close neurodevelopmental follow-up is also required for infants assigned to grades I and II IVH. Associations have been found between low-grade hemorrhages and reduced cortical volume at near term age [42]. Likewise, adverse neurodevelopmental outcomes for grades I and II IVH have been observed in follow up studies [41]. Forty four percent of ELBW children with grades III and IV intracranial hemorrhage present with disabling cerebral palsy (CP), and 45–85% of children with grade IV intracranial hemorrhage have mental retardation and CP at school age [43].

Periventricular leukomalacia (PVL) is damage to the periventricular white matter developed as a result of perinatal adverse insults such as hypoxia, hypo or hyper-perfusion, hypocarbia and chorioamnionitis combined with the defective cerebral vascular autoregulation in preterm infants. The estimated incidence of PVL is 4–15% in ELBW babies. We demonstrated an incidence of 19% in our ELBW cohort [44]. While strong correlation has been observed between diffuse cystic PVL and cerebral palsy, the clinical correlates of diffuse white mater injuries and localized cysts are not so clear-cut and might be related to a spectrum of behavioral/cognitive deficits [43].

2.5 Renal problems

Preterm infants exhibit increased sensitivity to impaired renal function. This is due to enhanced kidney maturation, fewer functional nephrons and higher renal filtration rate [45]. Acute kidney injury (AKI) in preterm infants can cause long-lasting renal damage leading to chronic kidney disease in adulthood [46]. Extremely premature infants are prone to developing AKI in the first days of life. Serum creatinine levels reflect maternal levels immediately after birth. Serum creatinine then picks, reaches a plateau in the first days of life, and declines thereafter. ELBW infants with AKI showed reduced survival until 36 weeks of post-menstrual age (PMA) [45]. Fluid status monitoring is a paramount. It involves daily monitoring of electrolytes, body weight, diuresis, blood pressure and insensible water loss.

2.6 Electrolyte imbalance

The ELBW infant is made up of 85% to 90% water, which is predominantly distributed in the extracellular space. During the first few postnatal days a weight loss of 10–20% is observed which is attributable to diuresis and can be intensified by iatrogenic causes such as radiant warmers or phototherapy. These developments in addition to the compromised renal function constitute a setting for frequent electrolyte abnormalities such as hypo/hypernatremia and hyperkalemia [47]. Disturbances of sodium are connected to the water flow and can either be presented with hypernatremia if significant amount of water is lost due to heating and phototherapy or with dilutional hyponatremia. Hyperkalemia, on the other hand, is a result of shifting from the intracellular to the extracellular compartment [47].

2.7 Impaired glucose homeostasis

Early hypoglycemia is a frequent occurrence in ELBW infants because of limited liver glycogen stores and immature endocrine mechanisms of blood glucose's control. In particular, ketogenesis and lipogenesis which lead to the production of alternative energy fuels, are limited for this group of patients, making them more dependent on glucose. Clinical conditions that are associated with hypoglycemia such as perinatal asphyxia, acidosis, sepsis and hypothermia are common [48]. Moreover, hypoglycemia in extremely preterm infants is rarely accompanied by symptoms typical for term counterparts such as jitteriness, lethargy, apnea or poor feeding.

Hyperglycemia is also observed in extremely premature infants and in those with intrauterine growth retardation (IUGR). This condition is usually the result of excessive glucose infusion rates, drug treatment by steroids or methylxanthines, or may reflect the immaturity of the regulatory mechanisms [48].

2.8 Infection

Early-onset neonatal infection (EOI), defined as one typically occurring in the first 72 hours of life, significantly contributes to the morbidity and mortality of ELBW infants with an estimated incidence of 26 per 1000 live ELBW births in US [49]. High index of suspicion of a possible intrauterine infection should be maintained in the presence of a premature birth. Current efforts are directed toward intrapartum antimicrobial prophylaxis and early neonatal infectious screening. Early-onset infection initiates with newborn's colonization with bacteria from the maternal genital tract, most commonly group B streptococcus, *E. coli* and Listeria [49]. Also, other Gram-positive or Gram-negative bacteria, as well as fungi and viruses can contribute to the microbial spectrum of EOI.

Late-onset sepsis (LOS) results from horizontal transmission of endogenous hospital flora and typically occurs after the first week of life. Frequent nosocomial pathogens are coagulase-negative staphylococci, Klebsiella and Pseudomonas species as well as methicillin-resistant *Staphylococcus aureus* (MRSA) and fungi [50, 51]. Many institutions, including ours follow a fluconazole prophylaxis protocol for the duration of the central catheters in order to reduce catheter-associated fungaemia [51]. Our institutions' low incidence of detection of fungal sepsis (3%) among LOS is attributable to strict adherence to this Candida-prophylaxis policy [44]. Predisposing factors for late-onset infections include: immaturity of the immune system, thin permeable skin and mucous membranes, ventilator care, parenteral nutrition, central venous catheters and tubes, overcrowded nursery, inadequate hand washing routine as well as exposure to extensive handling.

Neonatal infection in ELBW infants has been associated with poor neurodevelopmental and growth outcomes in early childhood according to results of a large-cohort follow-up study [14]. Symptoms of infection in preterm newborns often include: apnea, bradycardia and cyanosis, also lethargy and increased respiratory effort, symptoms being more pronounced with Gram-negative and fungal infections than with Gram-positive ones [49]. Treatment consists of first line therapy with ampicillin and gentamycin for EOI. If the mother's vaginal swab was positive for a Gram-negative bacterium such as *E. coli*, the protocol can be revised to cefotaxime and gentamycin. Vancomycin and gentamicin are used for treating LOS and may be adjusted according to microbial sensitivity of the hemoculture. When resistant septic shock is observed ceftazidime or imipenem should be urgently added. Fluconazole or amphotericin B are given for suspected or proven fungal infections.

2.9 Bronchopulmonary dysplasia

Bronchopulmonary dysplasia (BPD) was traditionally considered as oxygen and respirator-mediated injury related to prematurity. However, gentler ventilator techniques, prenatal corticosteroid therapy and treatment with surfactants have limited more severe lung injuries to infants of <1200 g BW and < 30 week' gestation [52]. BPD traditionally defined as a need for supplemental oxygen or ventilator support at 36 weeks' post menstrual age (PMA) occurs with an incidence of around 30% in ELBW infants [53].

In 2001, a new revised definition of BPD was devised by the National Institute of Child Health and Human Development (NICHD) categorizing the disease severity as mild, moderate, or severe based solely on oxygen dependency level at <32 GW. Mild BPD was defined by breathing room air at 36 weeks post menstrual age or discharge, moderate BPD equaled breathing <30% oxygen, and severe corresponded to breathing >30% oxygen or receiving positive pressure ventilation at PMA of 36 weeks. Radiographic findings were not included in the new definitions due to inconsistent interpretations and deficient availability at certain ages [52].

Infants with BPD were found to have higher rates of adverse neurodevelopmental outcomes and cognitive impairment in early childhood compared to those without BPD [53, 54]. At school age, children with BPD were recognized with growth impairment and academic difficulties [55]. Common rehospitalizations have been observed during the first 2 years of life, mostly as a consequence of respiratory illnesses including lower respiratory tract infections and RSV bronchiolitis [56]. RSV prophylaxis with palivizumab is included as standard care for BPD children in the first year of life.

2.10 Retinopathy of prematurity

Retinopathy of prematurity (ROP) represents interruption of the natural course of vascularization of the premature retina caused by oxygen exposure with consequent pathological compensation that results in abnormal neo-vascularization of the retina. Hence, prematurity and treatment with oxygen are the two main recognized risk factors for ROP.

Hyperoxia has been an enormous concern in the neonatal intensive care units, and the optimal oxygen saturation target ranges have been debated and explored in studies [57]. Results from several studies suggested possible harmful effect of oxygen saturation targets of 91–95%, on the contrary, lower target ranges of 85–89% resulted in increased mortality [57, 58]. Therefore, it has been recommended targeting saturations between 90 and 94% by setting alarm limits between 89 and 95%, though recognizing that ideal oxygen saturation targets are still unknown [17].

Variable incidence of retinopathy of prematurity has been reported in population-based studies due to variability in study designs and gestational ages of the included infants; reported incidences vary from 10–75% in different studies [59]. An incidence of 17.1% of severe ROP in the survivor's subcategory was reported by our group. The average number of blood transfusions for this group was 7 [44].

Severe ROP is defined by a unilateral or bilateral stage 4 or 5 disease or disease requiring laser/anti-vascular endothelial growth factor (anti-VEGF) monoclonal antibody treatment, at least unilaterally. The timing of onset of ROP depends on both the gestational and the chronological age, whereas the diseases' incidence and severity are inversely proportional to both birth weight and gestational age [59]. Apart from oxygen, suggested adverse impacts that might predispose to retinopathy of prematurity are intrauterine infection, hyperglycemia, neonatal infection, probably due to systemic inflammation, being born small for gestational age, and also repeated blood transfusions [59, 60].

Current joint recommendation of the relevant American expert societies outlines that indirect ophthalmoscopy screening for ROP should be commenced by 31 weeks PMA for infants born at 22–27 weeks and repeated in scheduled intervals thereafter. Also, all infants of <1500 g and < 30 weeks' gestation, and at-risk infants >30 weeks' gestation ought to be included in the ROP screening process [61].

Current treatment options include laser photocoagulation, intraocular injection of anti-VEGF treatment and vitrectomy. Parallel to the increased survival of the most immature infants, the number of survivors with severe ROP has also increased. However, blindness has become a rare consequence of the most severe disease cases. Infants with ROP exhibit other ophthalmological problems such as myopia, strabismus and astigmatism [59]. Apart from visual disturbances, ROP alone or in association with other problems of the premature infants can lead to neurodevelopmental difficulties and lower academic performances [54, 55].

2.11 Anemia of prematurity

Anemia of prematurity (AOP) is a condition specific to premature infants caused by a combination of physiologic reasons such as depleted iron stores, shorter life span of erythrocytes, immature erythropoietic response, vitamin B12 and folate deficiencies as well as rapid postnatal growth, combined with iatrogenic causes observed in frequent phlebotomies for laboratory studies. Treatment of anemia consists of transfusions with erythrocyte concentrates.

Early administration of erythropoietin in the first week of life has not proven to significantly reduce the need for blood transfusions, but instead increases the risk of severe ROP [62]. Positive association has been found between anemia in the first week of life and the number of required blood transfusions with ROP development [60]. The proposed mechanism of progressing ROP is the replacement of hemoglobin F with hemoglobin A during blood transfusion which sharply increases oxygen availability to the retina [63].

Recommended transfusion thresholds are the following: hemoglobin (Hb) 12 g/dL /hematocrit (HTC) 36% for severe cardiopulmonary disease, Hb 11 g/dL /HCT 30% when dependent on oxygen and Hb 7 g/dL/HCT 25% when clinically stable beyond 2 weeks of age [17]. To decrease the risk of transfusion-related infection, a single donors' unit of packed red blood cells should be used, divided into several satellite bags to be used for the same patient for several weeks [64].

Other problems of the ELBW spectrum include: apnea of prematurity, gastrointestinal problems, feeding intolerance, hyperbilirubinemia, necrotizing enterocolitis, inguinal hernias, total parenteral nutrition-associated cholestatic jaundice as well as postnatal growth restriction [65].

3. Conclusion

The mortality rate of ELBW infants significantly diminished with improved technology and improved neonatal practices, however there are still many issues to be covered for optimal complete approach to these patients that would reduce not just the immediate, but also the long-term consequences. A multidisciplinary approach to treatment and follow up of these children is necessary, with special focus of the most sensitive areas of care such as neurodevelopmental, cognitive, auditory, visual, respiratory, speech and language, behavioral and emotional. Providing a family-centered care and structuring of appropriate data basis is necessary.

Conflict of interest

The authors declare no conflict of interest.

Author details

Anet Papazovska Cherepnalkovski[1,2*], Vesna Pavlov[2], Ivanka Furlan[2] and Marija Bucat[2]

1 University Department of Health Studies, University of Split, Split, Croatia

2 Department of Neonatology, University Hospital of Split, University Clinic for Gynecology and Obstetrics, Split, Croatia

*Address all correspondence to: anet.cherepnalkovski@gmail.com

References

[1] Ogawa M, Matsuda Y, Kanda E, et al. Survival rate of extremely low birth weight infants and its risk factors: case-control study in Japan. ISRN Obstet Gynecol. 2013; 873563. DOI: 10.1155/2013/873563

[2] Canadian Neonatal Network. 2019 Annual Report. [Internet]. 2019. Available from: http://www.canadianneonatalnetwork.org/Portal/LinkClick.aspx?fileticket=lsGgJQ_EDJ8%3d&tabid=39 [Accessed: 2020-11-21]

[3] Itabashi K, Horiuchi T, Kusuda S, et al. Mortality rates for extremely low birth weight infants born in Japan in 2005. Pediatrics. 2009;123(2):445-450. DOI: 10.1542/peds.2008-0763

[4] Stoll BJ, Hansen NI , Bell EF et al. Eunice Kennedy Shriver National Institute of Child Health and Human Development Neonatal Research Network. Trends in Care Practices, Morbidity, and Mortality of Extremely Preterm Neonates, 1993-2012. JAMA. 2015;314(10):1039-1051. DOI: 10.1001/jama.2015.10244

[5] Kalimba E M, Ballot D E. Survival of extremely low-birth-weight infants. South African Journal of Child Health. 2013;7(1):13-16. DOI:10.7196/SAJCH.488

[6] Trotman H, Lord C. Outcome of extremely low birthweight infants at the University Hospital of the West Indies, Jamaica. West Indian Med J. 2007;56(5):409-413. PMID: 18303752

[7] Tyson JE, Parikh NA, Langer J, et al. Intensive care for extreme prematurity--moving beyond gestational age. N Engl J Med. 2008; 358(16):1672-81. DOI: 10.1056/NEJMoa073059

[8] Carlo WA, McDonald SA, Fanaroff AA, et al. Association of antenatal corticosteroids with mortality and neuro developmental outcomes among infants born at 22 to 25 weeks' gestation. JAMA. 2011; 306(21):2348-2358. DOI: 10.1001/jama.2011.1752

[9] Deulofeut R, Sola A, Lee B, et al. The impact of vaginal delivery in premature infants weighing less than 1,251 grams. Obstetrics and Gynecology. 2005;105(3):525-531. DOI: 10.1097/01.AOG.0000154156.51578.50

[10] Görbe E, Chasen S, Harmath A, et al. Very-low-birth weight breech infants: short-term outcome by method of delivery. Journal of Maternal-Fetal and Neonatal Medicine. 1997;6(3):155-158. DOI: 10.1002/(SICI)1520-6661(199705/06)6:3<155::AID-MFM7>3.0.CO;2-K

[11] Ott WJ. Small for gestational age fetus and neonatal outcome: reevaluation of the relationship. Am J Perinatol. 1995;12(6):396-400. DOI: 10.1055/s-2007-994506

[12] Bucat M, Papazovska Cherepnalkovski A, Furlan I, et al. Novorođenčad ekstremno niske rodne mase (Extremely Low Birth Weight Infants) [Croatian]. Pediatr Croat. 2018;62(Supl I):15-21.

[13] Gargus RA, Vohr BR, Tyson JE, et al. Unimpaired outcomes for extremely low birth weight infants at 18 to 22 months. Pediatrics. 2009;124(1):112-121. DOI: 10.1542/peds.2008-2742

[14] Stoll BJ, Hansen NI, Adams-Chapman I, et al.; National Institute of Child Health and Human Development Neonatal Research Network. Neurodevelopmental and growth impairment among extremely low-birth-weight infants with neonatal infection. JAMA. 2004;292(19):2357-2365. DOI: 10.1001/jama.292.19.2357

[15] Yanyu L, Prakesh S S , Xiang Y Y, et al., Canadian Neonatal Network. Association between admission temperature and mortality and major morbidity in preterm infants born at fewer than 33 weeks' gestation. JAMA Pediatr. 2015;169(4):e150277. DOI: 10.1001/jamapediatrics.2015.0277

[16] McCall EM, Alderdice F, Halliday HL, et al. Interventions to prevent hypothermia at birth in preterm and/or low birthweight infants. *Cochrane Database Syst Rev.* 2018;12;2(2):CD004210. DOI: 10.1002/14651858.CD004210.pub5

[17] Sweet DG, Carnielli V, Greisen G, et al. European Consensus Guidelines for the Management of Neonatal Respiratory Distress Syndrome - 2019 Update. Neonatology 2019;115(4):432-450. DOI: 10.1159/000499361

[18] Najafian B and Khosravi M H (January 13th 2020). Neonatal Respiratory Distress Syndrome: Things to Consider and Ways to Manage. In IntechOpen: DOI: 10.5772/intechopen.90885. Available from: https://www.intechopen.com/books/update-on-critical-issues-on-infant-and-neonatal-care/neonatal-respiratory-distress-syndrome-things-to-consider-and-ways-to-manage [Accessed: 2020-11-21]

[19] Szyld E, Aguilar A, Musante GA, et al. Delivery Room Ventilation Devices Trial Group. Comparison of devices for newborn ventilation in the delivery room. J Pediatr. 2014; 165(2): 234-9.e3. DOI: 10.1016/j.jpeds.2014.02.035

[20] Rojas-Reyes M X, Morley C J, Soll R. Prophylactic versus selective use of surfactant in preventing morbidity and mortality in preterm infants. Cochrane Database Syst Rev. 2012;(3):CD000510. DOI: 10.1002/14651858.CD000510.pub2

[21] Werder H, Robertson B, Greisen G et al. Surfactant therapy and nasal continuous positive airway pressure for newborns with respiratory distress syndrome. Danish-Swedish Multicenter Study Group. N Engl J Med 1994;331(16):1051-1055. DOI: 10.1056/NEJM199410203311603

[22] Dani C, Corsini I, Bertini G, et al. Effect of multiple INSURE procedures in extremely preterm infants. J Matern Fetal Neonatal Med. 2011;24(12):1427-1431. DOI: 10.3109/14767058.2011.572203

[23] Kribs A , Roll C , Göpel W, et al. , NINSAPP Trial Investigators Collaborators. Nonintubated Surfactant Application vs Conventional Therapy in Extremely Preterm Infants: A Randomized Clinical Trial. JAMA Pediatr. 2015;169(8):723-730. DOI: 10.1001/jamapediatrics.2015.0504

[24] De Kort E, Kusters S, Niemarkt H, et.al. Quality assessment and response to less invasive surfactant administration (LISA) without sedation. Pediatr Res. 2020;87(1):125-130. doi: 10.1038/s41390-019-0552-z

[25] Bhandari V, Gavino RG, Nedrelow JH, et al. A randomized controlled trial of synchronized nasal intermittent positive pressure ventilation in RDS. J Perinatol. 2007;27(11):697-703. DOI: 10.1038/sj.jp.7211805

[26] Meneses J, Bhandari V, Alves JG. Nasal intermittent positive-pressure ventilation vs nasal continuous positive airway pressure for preterm infants with respiratory distress syndrome: a systematic review and meta-analysis. Arch Pediatr Adolesc Med. 2012;166(4):372-376. DOI: 10.1001/archpediatrics.2011.1142

[27] Kirpalani H, Millar D, Lemyre B, et al., NIPPV Study Group. A trial comparing noninvasive ventilation strategies in preterm infants. N Engl

J Med. 2013;369(7):611-620. DOI: 10.1056/NEJMoa1214533

[28] Collins CL, Holberton JR, Barfield C, Davis PG. A randomized controlled trial to compare heated humidified high-flow nasal cannulae with nasal continuous positive airway pressure postextubation in premature infants. *J Pediatr.* 2013;162(5):949-54.e1. DOI: 10.1016/j.jpeds.2012.11.016

[29] Clyman RI, Couto J, Murphy GM. Patent ductus arteriosus: are current neonatal treatment options better or worse than no treatment at all? Semin Perinatol. 2012;36(2):123-129. DOI: 10.1053/j.semperi.2011.09.022

[30] Van Overmeire B, Smets K, Lecoutere D, et al. A comparison of ibuprofen and indomethacin for closure of patent ductus arteriosus. N Engl J Med. 2000;343(10):674-681. DOI: 10.1056/NEJM200009073431001

[31] Ohlsson A, Walia R, Shah SS. Ibuprofen for the treatment of patent ductus arteriosus in preterm or low birth weight (or both) infants. Cochrane Database Syst Rev. 2020;2(2):CD003481. DOI: 10.1002/14651858.CD003481.pub8

[32] Dani C, Lista G, Bianchi S, et al. Intravenous paracetamol in comparison with ibuprofen for the treatment of patent ductus arteriosus in preterm infants: a randomized controlled trial. Eur J Pediatr. 2020; https://doi.org/10.1007/s00431-020-03780-8. Online ahead of print.

[33] Batton B, Li L, Newman NS, et al.; Eunice Kennedy Shriver National Institute of Child Health and Human Development Neonatal Research Network. Evolving blood pressure dynamics for extremely preterm infants. J Perinatol. 2014;34(4):301-305. DOI: 10.1038/jp.2014.6

[34] Pereira SS, Sinha AK, Morris JK, et al. Blood pressure intervention levels in preterm infants: pilot randomized trial. Arch Dis Child Fetal Neonatal Ed. 2019;104(3):F298-F305. DOI: 10.1136/archdischild-2017-314159.

[35] Subhedar NV, Shaw NJ. Dopamine versus dobutamine for hypotensive preterm infants. Cochrane Database Syst Rev. 2003; 3(3):CD001242. DOI: 10.1002/14651858.CD001242

[36] Ibrahim H, Sinha IP, Subhedar NV. Corticosteroids for treating hypotension in preterm infants. Cochrane Database Syst Rev. 2011;12(12):CD003662. DOI: 10.1002/14651858.CD003662.pub4

[37] Perlman JM, Wyllie J, Kattwinkel J, et al.: Part 7. Neonatal resuscitation: 2015 International Consensus on Cardiopulmonary Resuscitation and Emergency Cardiovascular Care Science with treatment recommendations. Resuscitation 2015; 132(16 Suppl 1):S204–S241. DOI: 10.1161/CIR.0000000000000276

[38] Bayer K. Delayed Umbilical Cord Clamping in the 21st Century: Indications for Practice. Adv Neonatal Care. 2016 Feb;16(1):68-73. DOI: 10.1097/ANC.0000000000000247

[39] Dolfin T, Skidmore MB, Fongk W, et al. Incidence, severity and timing of subependymal and intraventricular hemorrhages in preterm infants born in a perinatal unit as detected by serial real-time ultrasound. Pediatrics. 1983;71(4):541-546. PMID: 6835737

[40] Bolisetty S, Dhawan A, Abdel-Latif M, et al. Intraventricular hemorrhage and neurodevelopmental outcomes in extreme preterm infants. Pediatrics. 2014; 133(1):55-62. DOI: 10.1542/peds.2013-0372

[41] Adams-Chapman I, Heyne RJ, DeMauro SB, et al. Neurodevelopmental Impairment Among Extremely Preterm Infants in the Neonatal Research Network. Pediatrics.

2018;141(5):e20173091. DOI:10.1542/peds.2017-3091

[42] Vasileiadis GT, Gelman N, Han VK, et al. Uncomplicated intraventricular hemorrhage is followed by reduced cortical volume at near-term age. Pediatrics. 2004; 114(3):e367–e372. DOI: 10.1542/peds.2004-0500

[43] Extremely Low Birth Weight NICU Graduate Supplement to the Critical Elements of Care for the Low Birth Weight Neonatal Intensive Care Graduate (CEC-LBW). [Internet]. 2004. Available at: https://depts.washington.edu/dbpeds/ELBW-NICU-Graduate.pdf [Accessed: 2020-11-21]

[44] Papazovska Cherepnalkovski A, Bucat M, Furlan I, et al. Extremely Low Birth Weight Infant, late morbidities and health outcomes. Pediatr Croat. 2018; 62 (Supl I): 22-27.

[45] Lee CC, Chan OW, Lai MY, et al. Incidence and outcomes of acute kidney injury in extremely-low-birth-weight infants. PLoS One. 2017;12(11):e0187764. DOI: 10.1371/journal.pone.0187764

[46] Brenner BM, Chertow GM. Congenital oligonephropathy and the etiology of adult hypertension and progressive renal injury. Am J Kidney Dis. 1994;23(2):171-175. PMID: 8311070

[47] Lorenz JM, Kleinman LI, Markarian K. Potassium metabolism in extremely low birth weight infants in the first week of life. J Pediatr. 1997;131(1 Pt 1):81-86. DOI: 10.1016/s0022-3476(97)70128-8

[48] Mitanchez D. Glucose Regulation in Preterm Newborn Infants. Horm Res 2007;68:265-271 DOI: 10.1159/000104174

[49] Simonsen KA, Anderson-Berry AL, Delair SF, Davies HD. Early-onset neonatal sepsis. Clin Microbiol Rev. 2014;27(1):21-47. DOI: 10.1128/CMR.00031-13

[50] Lollis TR, Bradshaw WT. Fungal prophylaxis in neonates: a review article. Adv Neonatal Care. 2014;14(1):17-23. DOI: 10.1097/ANC.0000000000000048

[51] Cetinkaya M, Ercan TE, Saglam OK, et al. Efficacy of Prophylactic Fluconazole Therapy in Decreasing the Incidence of Candida Infections in Extremely Low Birth Weight Preterm Infants. Am J Perinatol. 2014;31(12):1043-1048. DOI: 10.1055/s-0034-1371358

[52] Jobe AH, Bancalari E. Bronchopulmonary dysplasia. Am J Respir Crit Care Med. 2001;163(7):1723-1729. DOI: 10.1164/ajrccm.163.7.2011060

[53] Natarajan G, Pappas A, Shankaran S, et al. Outcomes of extremely low birth weight infants with bronchopulmonary dysplasia: impact of the physiologic definition. Early Hum Dev. 2012;88(7):509-515. DOI: 10.1016/j.earlhumdev.2011.12.013

[54] Schmidt B, Asztalos EV, Toberts RS, et al. Impact of bronchopulmonary dysplasia, brain injury and severe retinopathy of prematurity on the outcome of extremely low-birth-weight infants at 18 months. JAMA. 2003;289(9):1124-1129. DOI: 10.1001/jama.289.9.1124

[55] Short EJ, Klein NK, Lewis BA, et al. Cognitive and academic consequences of bronchopulmonary dysplasia and very low birth weight: 8-year-old outcomes. Pediatrics. 2003;112(5):e359. DOI: 10.1542/peds.112.5.e359

[56] Doyle LW, Ford G, Davis N. Health and hospitalizations after discharge in extremely low birth weight infants. Semin Neonatol. 2003;8(2):137-145. DOI: 10.1016/S1084-2756(02)00221-X

[57] Carlo WA, Finer NN, Walsh MC, et al. Target ranges of oxygen saturation in extremely preterm infants. N Engl J Med. 2010;362(21):1959-1969. DOI: 10.1056/NEJMoa0911781

[58] Sola A, Golombek S, Bueno MT, et al. Safe oxygen saturation targeting and monitoring in preterm infants. Can we avoid hypoxia and hyperoxia? Acta Paediatr. 2014;103(10):1009-1018. DOI: 10.1111/apa.12692

[59] Hellström A, Smith LE, Dammann O. Retinopathy of prematurity. Lancet. 382(9902):1445-57. DOI: 10.1016/S0140-6736(13)60178-6.

[60] Lundgren P, Athikarisamy SE, Patole S, et al. Duration of anaemia during the first week of life is an independent risk factor for retinopathy of prematurity. Acta Paediatr. 2018; 107(5):759-766. DOI: 10.1111/apa.14187

[61] Fierson WM; American Academy of Pediatrics Section on Ophthalmology, American Academy of Ophthalmology, American Association for Pediatric Ophthalmology and Strabismus, American Association of Certified Orthoptists. Screening examination of premature infants for retinopathy of prematurity. Pediatrics 2018 Dec;142(6):e20183061. DOI: 10.1542/peds.2018-3061.

[62] Aher SM, Ohlsson A. Early versus late erythropoietin for preventing red blood cell transfusion in preterm and/or low birth weight infants. Cochrane Database Syst Rev 2020;2(2):CD004865. DOI: 10.1002/14651858.CD004865.pub4.

[63] Stutchfield CJ, Jain A, Odd D, et al. Foetal haemoglobin, blood transfusion, and retinopathy of prematurity in very preterm infants: a pilot prospective cohort study. Eye (Lond). 2017;31(10):1451-1455. DOI: 10.1038/eye.2017.76

[64] Strauss RG, Villhauer PJ, Cordle DG. A method to collect, store and issue multiple aliquots of packed red blood cells for neonatal transfusion. Vox Sang. 1995; 68(2):77-81. DOI: 10.1111/j.1423-0410.1995.tb02557.x

[65] Repa A, Lochmann R, Unterasinger L, et al. Aggressive nutrition in extremely low birth weight infants: impact on parenteral nutrition associated cholestasis and growth. PeerJ. 2016;4:e2483. DOI: 10.7717/peerj.2483

Chapter 12

Haemodynamic Changes during Preterm Birth Treatment

Szymon Bednarek, Małgorzata Głogiewicz, Rafał Adamczak and Mariusz Dubiel

Abstract

The well-being of the fetus depends on the efficiency of its circulatory system and the proper maternal-fetal exchange. Hemodynamic changes can occur due to disturbance of fetal and maternal homeostasis, malformations, pregnancy pathology, and medications. Preterm labor directly affects maternal-fetal haemodynamics, both due to uterine contractions and medications used to inhibit it. Research on maternal-fetal haemodynamics in preterm labor is currently focused mainly on the safety of the used tocolytics. In this chapter, we will discuss the basic principles of fetal haemodynamics, ultrasound methods of maternal-fetal circulation assessment, and the influence of preterm labor on maternal-fetal haemodynamics, with particular emphasis on medications used in threatening and progressive preterm labor.

Keywords: preterm labor, maternal-fetal haemodynamics, doppler

1. Introduction

During pregnancy, the maternal body undergoes significant hemodynamic changes to ensure normal fetal growth. On average, maternal cardiac output can increase up to 30%–45%, resulting mostly from the intensified metabolism, increased circulating blood mass, the appearance of an accessory placental circulatory system, and finally, a gradual increase in body weight during pregnancy. Although blood volume increases, the systemic blood pressure in a healthy mother undergoes no significant changes. This is mainly due to a decrease in total peripheral vascular resistance, primarily at the arteriolar level. The mammalian placenta is also important for the regulation of both the maternal and fetal circulations. Adequate uterine blood flow is critical to fetal growth and development [1]. Fetal heart undergoes functional changes: throughout gestation, the fetal myocardium becomes more compliant and making ventricular filling less dependent on atrial contraction. Both the increase in size and the maturational changes lead to a tremendous increase in cardiac output [2].

IntechOpen

2. Maternal-fetal circulation

The primary heart and vascular system appear in the middle of the third week of development. On about 22nd-23rd day, the heart begins its systolic action.

Oxygenated blood, rich in nutrients, flows through the umbilical vein from the placenta to the portal sinus. The portal sinus is a wide L-shaped vessel at the terminal end of the umbilical vein, connecting two main vessels termed the right and left intrahepatic portal veins perfusing the right and left hepatic lobes. It then goes into the ductus venosus. The ductus venosus originated from the portal sinus as the latter turned at an almost right angle into the right lobe of the liver. The ductus venosus is a branchless, hourglass-shaped vessel that ascends steeply in the direction of the diaphragm. The blood flow in the ductus venosus is regulated by the sphincter mechanism. The blood then flows in the inferior vena cava and enters the right atrium of the heart. Most of the blood from the inferior vena cava is directed to the secondary septum through the oval foramen to the left atrium. There it mixes with a relatively small amount of poorly oxygenated blood returning through the pulmonary veins from the lungs. The blood from the left atrium flows into the left ventricle and leaves it through the ascending aorta. The arteries that supply the heart, head, neck and upper limbs receive well-oxygenated blood. The small amount of well-oxygenated blood from the inferior vena cava that remains in the right atrium of the heart mixes with the poorly oxygenated blood from the superior vena cava and coronary sinus and flows into the right ventricle. This blood leaves the right heart through the pulmonary trunk. Due to the high pulmonary vascular resistance during fetal life, blood flow through the lungs is low. About 10% of the blood flows to the lungs and most of it flows through the arterial duct to the fetal aorta. The blood returns to the placenta through the umbilical arteries [3, 4].

3. Vascular flow testing using Doppler ultrasonography

Doppler examination assessing the vascular flow of the maternal-fetal circulation is an important diagnostic tool in the assessment of the well-being of the fetus. The analysis of vascular flows is also used to make decisions about the further duration of pregnancy. It is often a pregnancy complicated by diseases that threaten the life of the mother and the fetus. Due to the high risk of iatrogenic prematurity, the experience of the person performing the ultrasound examination is extremely important, taking into account the factors that may affect the parameters of the vascular flow wave. Overinterpretation of the Doppler results may expose both parents and the perinatological team to unnecessary stress, medical activities and costs [5, 6].

The safety of ultrasound examinations is based on the degree of fetal exposure, which depends on the amount and duration of ultrasound examinations and the energy used for the examination. It takes into account the control of the thermal and mechanical index and the superior principle of using the lowest dose of energy that allows correct imaging - ALARA (as low as reasonably achievable). The term thermal index describes the quotient of the power lost to the reference power that increases the tissue temperature by 1 °C. The mechanical index describes the amplitude of the ultrasound wave. Ensuring the safety of ultrasound examination is only possible through excellent knowledge of anatomy and embryology, as well as regular index control when changing the settings of the ultrasound machine.

The table contains the most frequently assessed vascular flows along with their correct imaging.

Vessel	Visualization	Doppler sample volume (mm)	Insonation angle	Flow velocity/ waveforms
Umbilical artery	Free loop of the umbilical cord, without fetal breathing movements	2–3	<30°	4–6 waveforms
Middle cerebral artery	Cross-section of the brain, visualization of the Willis circle, mapping on the proximal side of the transducer, Doppler gate in the 1/3 proximal course of the vessel, as little pressure as possible on the fetal head - high risk of change of intracranial pressure and flow velocity	2–3	<30°	3–10 waveforms
Ductus venosus	Sagittal or transverse section of the fetus	0,5–1	<30°	3–6, velocity > 30 cm/s
Uterine arteries	Measurement on the right and left side of the patient, after visualizing the junction with the iliac vessels, cephalic direction	2	<30°	3–6, velocity > 50 cm/s

The special structure of the fetal uteroplacental, umbilical and cerebral circulation ensures a constant vascular flow in the fetus, independent of the mother's heart cycle. This system gradually develops in the utero-fetal circulation. The significant effect of this phenomenon consists not only in the gradual increase in the end-diastolic velocity of the flow wave, but also in the accompanying decrease in pulsation, which is the difference between the components of the maximum systolic and end-diastolic velocity.

The correct shape of the flow wave of both the fetal middle cerebral artery and the umbilical cord artery is not characterized by the disappearance of the flow wave or its inversion. It is one of the disparities in the fetal circulatory system that does not give a compensatory break in the heart's work. If it occurs, it is called absent flow or reverse flow. Both of these phenomena are among the alarm signals of poor fetal condition [7].

3.1 Mistakes in Doppler examination

Due to incomplete bone calcification, the head of a premature fetus is susceptible to pressure. Excessive pressure with the transducer may indicate the disappearance of the end-diastolic wave in the assessed fetal middle cerebral artery [7, 8].

The assessment of the vascular flow spectrum should cover several fetal heartbeat cycles. One of the reasons for doing this are the breathing movements of the fetus, which can disrupt the normal flow spectrum. Similar phenomena can be observed when a pregnant woman breathes too deeply. In order to verify the correctness of the vascular flow, a patient should be asked to shorten her breath or even temporarily stop breathing.

Incorrect parameters of the ultrasound device settings may falsify the Doppler measurements.

Corticosteroids administered to the mother to stimulate the maturation of the fetal lungs in the event of impending preterm labor may temporarily "improve" the flow waves. In that case, it is reasonable to repeat the Doppler examination approximately 48 hours after administering the medications [7, 9].

4. Medications used in the preterm labor

The use of medications should take place primarily in compliance with the principles of patient safety and the minimum risk of side effects. The problem of therapy in pregnancy is related to the limited possibility of testing the effects of the medication on the pregnant woman and the fetus, and often the lack of consent to perform such tests. Therefore, medications used in pregnancy often have limited indications and are administered taking into account the individual risks and benefits of therapy. The pharmacological action of the medication in the fetus must take into account the kinetics of its transformations in the mother's organism as well as in the placenta. The distribution of the medication and its metabolism in the mother's body determine its availability to the fetus. Since pregnancy involves profound physiological and biochemical changes, the metabolism of many medications is also significantly altered. Data from animal studies suggest that the rate of metabolism of medications in the liver decreases during pregnancy and their availability to the fetus may be greater than expected. The transfer of the medication from the mother's body to the fetus takes place from arterial blood through the intervillous spaces to the fetal capillaries in the villi and further through the umbilical vein.

Despite the fact that the placenta is treated as a specific protective barrier for the fetus, it has little ability to metabolize medications. Many medications can reach the fetus in the form of metabolites, often more toxic [10]. The safety of the use of tocolytics is still a significant perinatological problem. The duration of tocolysis should be short enough to allow the full effect of steroid therapy on the fetus, with the least negative impact on the health of the mother and child [11].

The most commonly used medications that inhibit uterine contractions are discussed below, with particular emphasis on their effects on the circulatory system of the mother and the fetus.

4.1 Calcium channel blockers – nifedipine

Nifedipine contains the formula of a short- and long-acting 1,4-dihydropyridine calcium channel blocker. It prevents contraction of calcium-dependent myocytes and their vessels by blocking the influx of calcium into smooth muscle cells. The second possible vasodilatory mechanism is the inhibition of pH-dependent calcium influx by inhibiting smooth muscle carbonic anhydrase. Nifedipine is used to treat high blood pressure and chronic stable angina. At therapeutic sub-toxic concentrations, it has little effect on myocardium and conducting cells. Inhibition of calcium influx lowers smooth muscle contraction, which causes dilation of the coronary and systemic arteries, increased oxygen delivery to the muscle tissue, reduced total peripheral resistance, blood pressure and afterload.

The most common side effect of nifedipine reported by mothers is headache associated with a transient reduction in blood pressure after initiating therapy. The second common effect is tachycardia. In addition, dizziness, drowsiness, nausea, a sharp drop in blood pressure, slurred speech and weakness may occur. One in ten patients may experience palpitations and hot flushes. Severe side effects, such as myocardial infarction, maternal dyspnea, patient hypoxia, severe maternal hypotension with intrauterine fetal death, atrial fibrillation were also observed during nifedipine therapy. Pulmonary edema has been reported in a group of pregnant patients after taking nifedipine.

It is not recommended for use in patients with twin pregnancies due to the more frequent occurrence of dyspnea. It is absolutely contraindicated in the group of patients with heart disease, maternal hypertension and intrauterine infection. Dyspnea occurring in twin pregnancy is explained by a reduced blood flow and the degree of lung ventilation due to the higher elevated diaphragm dome [11–15]. Nifedipine has no effect on motor activity, heart rate and blood flow in the fetus. The occurrence of side effects is not related to the level of this medication in the patient's blood serum, so there is no need to adjust its dose based on body weight, body mass index (BMI) or gestational age [14].

In a study carried out on laboratory animals, the effect of nifedipine on the normal development of pregnancy was assessed. After administration of three and thirty times higher doses of nifedipine than recommended for humans, dilatation of blood vessels, increased vascularization of the uterus and placenta, and trophoblast hyperplasia were observed in both groups. Higher placental weights were seen in the higher dose group, but this had no effect on fetal survival or an increased risk of birth defects. Fetal weight did not differ from the control group at the lower dose, but statistically significantly lower weight was reported for the group with the higher dose of the drug. As expected, there were changes in the uterine muscle and collagen structure of the cervix during tocolysis. The authors concluded that the use of nifedipine in pregnancy in acceptable doses should not have a negative impact on the condition of fetuses and newborns, and that this therapy often improves the prognosis [16].

The optimal dose of nifedipine is still being determined. The starting dose in most studies was 10 mg either orally or sublingually. If uterine contractions were maintained, the dose was repeated every 15–20 minutes, until a dose of 40 mg was obtained in the first hour. Then, maintenance therapy is 20 mg every 6–8 hours for two to three days [14].

In a comparative study of nifedipine and another tocolytic combined with steriodotherapy, no significant risk to the fetuses was observed [17].

4.2 Beta-adrenergic receptor agonists

Ritodrine stimulates the beta-2-adrenergic receptor, increasing the level of cAMP and decreasing the concentration of intracellular calcium, which in turn leads to the relaxation of uterine smooth muscles and a reduction in the frequency of uterine contractions.

Terbutaline is a relatively selective bronchodilator with little or no effect on alpha-adrenergic receptors. It appears to have a greater effect on stimulating the beta receptors of the bronchi, vessels and smooth muscle, including the uterus (beta-2 receptors), than at the heart receptors (beta-1). This drug relaxes smooth muscles and inhibits uterine contractions, but it can also have a stimulating effect on the heart and central nervous system.

The mechanism of action is based on the stimulation of beta-adrenergic receptors in intracellular adenylate cyclase, the enzyme that catalyses the conversion of adenosine triphosphate (ATP) to cyclic adenosine 3‘, 5'-monophosphate (c-AMP). Elevated levels of c-AMP are associated with relaxation of bronchial smooth muscles and inhibition of the release of immune system mediators, especially from mast cells.

Fenoterol stimulates beta-2 receptors in the lungs and causes bronchial smooth muscle relaxation, bronchodilation and increased air flow. Symptoms of overdose are chest pain, dizziness, dry mouth, fatigue, flu-like symptoms, headaches, heart abnormalities, high or low blood pressure, high blood glycemia, insomnia, muscle spasms, nausea, nervousness, rapid heartbeat, seizures and tremors.

4.3 Prostaglandin synthesis inhibitors – indomethacin

As an analgesic and antipyretic drug, indomethacin inhibits the secretion of prostaglandins involved in the pain reaction, fever and inflammation. Symptoms of overdose: nausea, vomiting, severe headache, dizziness, confusion or lethargy. There have been reports of paraesthesia, numbness and convulsions.

4.4 Magnesium sulfate

Magnesium sulfate reduces striated muscle contraction and blocks neuromuscular transmission, reducing the release of acetylcholine. In addition, magnesium inhibits the inflow of calcium, enhancing the relaxing effect of vascular smooth muscles [12]. It is currently treated as a mild tocolytic. Used in fetal neuroprotection in preterm labor below 32 weeks of pregnancy.

4.5 Oxytocin receptor antagonist – atosiban

It is a competitive antagonist of human oxytocin at the receptor level. In rats and guinea pigs, atosiban has been observed to bind to oxytocin receptors, reducing the frequency of contractions and the tension of the uterine muscles, thereby reducing uterine contractions. Atosiban has also been observed to bind to vasopressin receptors, reducing its effect. In animals, atosiban had no effect on the cardiovascular system. In women at risk of preterm labor, atosiban, at the recommended doses, prevents uterine contractions and induces a resting state of the uterus. Uterine relaxation following atosiban administration is rapid, uterine contractions are significantly reduced within ten minutes, and uterine quiescence of less than four contractions per hour is achieved and stable for twelve hours.

In women at risk of preterm labor receiving atosiban by intravenous infusion (300 micrograms per minute for six to twelve hours), steady-state plasma concentrations were reached within one hour of starting the infusion.

The use of atosiban below 24 and above 33 weeks of pregnancy is contraindicated. There was no evidence of fetal toxicity. Small amounts of the drug are excreted into breast milk, no effect of the drug on breastfeeding has been acknowledged.

The most common side effects of treatment with this preparation include nausea, headache and dizziness, hot flushes and an increase in heart rate [18].

4.6 Medications that relax the uterine muscles

Scopolamine (hyoscine) is an alkaloid. Along with its derivatives, it resembles atropine and has a similar effect, but with a greater influence on the nervous system. Hyoscine belongs to a group of medications called parasympatholytics. The action of cholinolytic medications is to block the stimulation of cholinergic receptors (activated by acetylcholine). Hyoscine acts on muscarinic receptors and relaxes smooth muscles of the gastrointestinal, biliary and urogenital tract.

Side effects may include dry mouth, atonic constipation, increased urination disorders, urinary retention, decreased sweat secretion, increased heart rate (tachycardia), hypotension, and visual disturbances [12, 18].

Drotaverine inhibits the activity of the phosphodiesterase IV enzyme, which leads to an increase in the concentration of cAMP and a further cascade of intracellular reactions that result in the relaxation of the muscle cell. It may also have calcium channel blocking abilities.

The relaxant effect affects the smooth muscles of the gastrointestinal tract, urogenital system, cardiovascular system and bile ducts and is stronger than that of papaverine. It is used in the case of contraction of smooth muscles of both nervous and muscular origin. Side effects are rare and similar to scopolamine [12, 18].

5. Effect of preterm labor and its treatment on maternal-fetal hemodynamics

5.1 Patient's body position

Khatib et al. analyzed changes in vascular flow in the fetal circulation when changing the left lateral to supine position in pregnant women in the third trimester. Test time was approximately fifteen minutes. The authors noted a statistically significant decrease in the value of the pulsation index in the middle cerebral and umbilical artery, as well as a decrease in the maximum systolic velocity of the middle cerebral artery and the systolic-diastolic index of the umbilical artery [19]. It is most likely related to the symptom of brain sparring of the fetal circulation. As can be seen from the above studies, the mechanisms of circulatory centralization are not only activated by the pathological condition, but also by a stressful situation for the fetus, such as changing the position from a comfortable left-lateral or vertical position to a supine position, limiting the correct placental-fetal flow. The mechanism of fetal circulation centralization protects the fetus in a situation of persistent limited blood flow. Vascular resistance in the cerebral circulation is reduced, which allows blood flow to the brain to be increased.

Katwijk and Wladimiroff analyzed changes in the value of flows in the umbilical artery when the body position changes. When changing the patient's body position from vertical to lying, they noted an increase in the umbilical artery pulsation and resistance index, regardless of the gestational age, and this is explained by the flow mechanism of a lock [20].

Kinsella et al. in the group of twenty pregnant women in the third trimester did not observe any changes in the flow in the fetal umbilical artery when the patient's body position was changed [21].

Similarly, Armstrong et al. in the group of twenty-five full-term pregnant women qualified for elective cesarean section did not observe changes in vascular flow depending on the different positions of the patient's body. The authors assume that the degree of compression of the inferior vena cava and aorta in different body positions is not significant enough to disturb the vascular flow in the umbilical artery, or that these changes are so subtle that Doppler devices are unable to capture them [22].

Marx et al. monitored the vascular flow in the umbilical cord in various body positions in the early stage of labor. The systolic-diastolic index of the umbilical artery was significantly higher in the supine position compared to the left-lateral position of the patient, which in turn led to an increase in vascular resistance in the umbilical artery [23].

Inferior vena cava syndrome most often occurs in the third trimester of pregnancy, when a large weight of the pregnant uterus presses on the inferior vena cava, especially in the supine position, which disturbs the maternal-fetal flow and may lead to fainting, and consequently the fetus to hypoxia. Ryo et al. undertook studies to determine the risk of inferior vena cava syndrome in the second trimester of pregnancy and its consequences for the fetus. In a group of ninety Japanese pregnant women between the twenty-fourth and twenty-seventh weeks of pregnancy, they assessed umbilical artery flow and its relationship with uteroplacental flow.

There were no changes in the umbilical artery resistance index during the five-minute supine position of the patient [24].

In a study by Qu et al. on a group of fifty pregnant women between the twenty-seventh and forty weeks of gestation, no changes in the umbilical artery flow values were found when the patient's body position was changed [25], similarly to Backe et al. [26], while Sorensen et al. did not report changes in the systolic-diastolic index in patients with normal blood pressure [27].

Kinsella et al. and Witter and Besinger did not find statistically significant changes in uterine artery flows depending on the patient's body position and the duration of the study [21, 28].

In the group between thirty-seven and forty weeks of pregnancy, Qu et al. observed a statistically significant increase in the resistance index in the uterine arteries after changing the position of the pregnant woman [25].

Sohn et al. proved that uterine flow clearly decreases in the sitting and standing position of the pregnant woman, which is associated with an increase in vascular resistance. In the conclusions, the authors emphasize that apart from uterine contractions, there are also other factors influencing uterine flow, which may be important in the monitoring of fetuses with limited growth rate [29]. In another work, the author presents the concept of selecting a safe position of the patient's body based on the results of measurements of vascular flows in the maternal-placental circulation [30]. Similar conclusions were presented by Easterling et al. in each trimester of pregnancy [31], as well as by Ryo et al. [24].

5.2 The influence of tocolytics on vascular flows

In the study by Bednarek et al. on the safety of tocolytic medications in preterm labor, mean values of vascular flow measurements before the initiation of therapy that inhibits premature uterine contraction and at least one day after their initiation, subjected to statistical analysis, did not show significant changes in most of the parameters studied. The changes mainly concerned the systolic-diastolic index in the umbilical artery, where its decrease was noted, the peak systolic velocity in the middle cerebral artery increased, and the pulsation index decreased. The patients' therapy mainly included nifedipine. The lack of statistically significant changes in the value of vascular flows may indirectly confirm the safety of this medication and the lack of negative impact on the well-being of the mother and the fetus. No patients experienced life-threatening or health-threatening symptoms, and the reported side effects were mainly periodic headache during the first day of therapy and transient reddening of the skin. There was no significant decrease in blood pressure in patients undergoing treatment. This significantly increases the benefits associated with the use of this therapy, especially in relation to therapy with beta-mimetics, especially fenoterol.

Cornette et al. analyzed the effect of nifedipine on the values of vascular flow in the cerebral and placental-fetal circulation. They found no statistically significant changes in the vascular flow of the fetal middle cerebral artery, umbilical cord, uterine arteries and ductus venous. The study was conducted in pregnant women between the thirty-fifth and thirty-seventh week of gestation in a group of fifteen healthy pregnant women, after administering 20 milligrams of nifedipine orally and assessing vascular flow one hour after dosing. The authors emphasize the mechanisms counteracting the disturbance of the uterine circulation despite the significant reduction of maternal afterload under the influence of nifedipine, which means that in healthy pregnant women with normal arterial pressure, trophoblast invasion lowers uterine vascular resistance to such an extent that administration of nifedipine, which has the ability to lower peripheral vascular resistance, is no longer able to lower uterine resistance. Adverse effects of nifedipine have been reported in the situation of significantly lowered blood pressure in pregnant women, therefore it is important that the use of this medication as an inhibitor of uterine contractions ought to be considered only in pregnant women with normal blood pressure [32].

The study by Lima et al. was based on the administration of nifedipine in a dose of 20 milligrams sublingually every twenty minutes to a pregnant woman with uterine contraction, until the activity subsided. Thereafter, 20 milligrams of nifedipine was orally administered every six hours, until a total dose of 120 milligrams per day. Vascular flow in the fetal and maternal circulation was assessed before the initiation of nifedipine, five and twenty-four hours after the initiation of the therapy. Five and twenty-four hours after the initiation of the therapy, there was no change in the resistance index from pre-treatment measurements, while a decrease in the resistance index in the fetal central artery was observed between five and twenty-four hours after the initiation of the therapy.

The value of the peak systolic velocity of the middle cerebral artery was also analyzed. In the Lima study, there was a decrease after five hours, while comparing the measurements before and 24 hours after starting the treatment, no statistically significant changes were noted [33]. In the study by Bednarek et al., the peak systolic velocity of the middle cerebral artery increased statistically significantly after the initiation of the therapy. It is noteworthy, however, that the measurements were made at least twelve hours after the initiation of the therapy. Similarly, Grzesiak et al. reported a decrease in the peak systolic velocity in the middle cerebral artery, with no changes in the remaining parameters during the day after the initiation of oral nifedipine therapy [34].

The special structure of the fetal uteroplacental, umbilical and cerebral circulation ensures constant vascular flow independent of the heart cycle. This system gradually develops in the utero-fetal circulation. A significant effect of this phenomenon consists not only in the gradual increase in the velocity of the end-diastolic flow wave, but also in the accompanying decrease in the pulsation index, which is the difference between the components of the maximum systolic velocity and the end-diastolic velocity [33].

Similarly, Guglu et al. observed a decrease in the pulse index of the central cerebral artery one day after the initiation of nifedipine therapy. The authors note that nifedipine reduces blood pressure while keeping the maternal heart rate unchanged. Moreover, they acknowledged a decrease in resistance in the uterine circulation. The mechanism of increased resistance in the umbilical artery with an accompanying decrease in the pulse index in the central artery of the brain prevents diastolic changes in the fetal heart [35, 36]. It is noteworthy that the maternal-fetal circulation has mechanisms that protect the fetus against changes in flow that may be a real threat to its well-being.

Beta-memetic therapy is now used much less frequently in suppressing preterm labor. Despite the lack of obvious adverse effects on vascular flow in the fetal circulation, side effects in the mother are significant enough to minimize this method of treatment [37–39]. In a study with ritodrine, an increase in the pulse index in the middle artery of the fetal brain was noted, with a decrease in the pulse index in the umbilical artery [40]. Friedman et al. claim that therapy with ritodrine does not increase the resistance to placental circulation, does not lead to fetal hypoxia, changes in the fetal heart rate or preload on the fetal heart, but shortens the systolic fraction of the heart, which may lead to an increase in vascular resistance in the fetal circulation or reduce contractility of the heart muscle [41, 42]. Similarly, terbutaline increases vascular flow through the fetal heart, thus increasing its load [43]. Beta-agonist therapy should be limited as much as possible due to the side effects of these medications on both the mother and the fetus.

Oxytocin receptor blockers are a new class of tocolytic drugs. The oxytocin antagonist atosiban has less side effects than beta-agonists [44]. Atosiban crosses the placenta. Drug concentrations in the fetal circulation do not increase with longer infusion rates, suggesting that the drug does not accumulate in the fetus. Atosiban has the best maternal and fetal safety profile; however, its costs are considerable. Maternal heart rate and blood flow in (R-UtA/L-UtA) were not altered significantly during atosiban administration. No significant changes in FHR as well as Doppler parameters (resistance index, pulsality index, peak systolic velocity) in umbilical artery and middle cerebral artery were recorded after 24/48 hours of tocolytic treatment. The mean values of cerebroplacental ratio (CPR) remained unaltered during treatment. Detailed evaluation of fetal cardiac function parameters (E/A, SF, MPI) calculated independently for both ventricles, revealed no significant changes over the time [45].

Tocolytic treatment with atosiban is associated with elevation of oxidative stress markers after a 48 hours administration. This effect of atosiban may reduce its potency as a tocolytic agent and therefore should be considered with respect to its clinical use, especially because of its connection with the occurrence of premature birth [46].

Indomethacin used as a substance inhibiting premature uterine contractile activity does not negatively affect the cerebral flow in the fetus, however, it should be remembered that long-term therapy with non-steroidal anti-inflammatory medications may lead to blood flow disorders in the arterial duct [47, 48].

Intravenous magnesium sulfate is also allowed in the treatment of preterm labor. Keeley et al. analyzed the effect of this medication on vascular flow and found a decrease in the flow velocity in the fetal middle cerebral artery and an increase in flow velocity in the uterine arteries. There were no disturbances in the flow in the umbilical artery. During the study, the blood circulation was normalized, which the authors associate with the beneficial effects of magnesium sulphate also on the fetus and the tocolytic effect [49]. This is also confirmed by the studies of Pezzati et al., who assessed the fetal and neonatal circulation in the first hours of life of children in the therapy of magnesium sulphate and ritodrine [50].

When analyzing the safety of tocolytic medications, it should be remembered that in most patients, steroid therapy is started parallel to stimulate the fetal respiratory system. In the study by Bednarek et al. no significant haemodynamic changes were found after steroid therapy, however, other authors observed a transient decrease in the pulse index of the fetal middle cerebral artery [51, 52]. It cannot be ruled out that these differences result from the different tocolitics analyzed. Corticosteroids administered to the mother to stimulate the maturation of the fetal lungs in the event of impending preterm labor may temporarily "improve" the flow waves. In such a situation, it is reasonable to repeat the Doppler examination approximately 48 hours after administration [34].

Brar et al. reported lower efficacy of tocolysis in patients with abnormal flows in the maternal-fetal circulation before the therapy, which increases the risk of preterm labor [53].

Summing up, it should be emphasized that drugs inhibiting uterine contractions do not have a significant, long-term and permanent effect on the vascular flow of the maternal-fetal circulation. When considering the efficacy of tocolysis, other factors disrupting normal vascular flow should be taken into account, which may reduce the effectiveness of tocolytic drugs and increase the risk of preterm labor.

5.3 Preterm labor ended with cesarean section

Nakayi et al. analyzed the vascular flow of the uterine arteries on the third, sixth and ninth day after cesarean section. They found no significant changes in the resistance index in these vessels [54].

The assessment of uterine artery flow seems to be useful in vaginal bleeding in puerperal patients after cesarean section, as one of the complications of this operation may be rupture of the intraoperatively developed pseudoaneurysm of the uterine artery [55].

5.4 Infection in preterm labor

Caroll et al. assessed the flow in the middle cerebral and umbilical arteries of fetuses and in the uterine arteries of patients with premature rupture of the membranes with or without intrauterine infection. They found no changes in vascular flow, which means that Doppler examination is not useful for monitoring the developing intrauterine infection associated with premature drainage of amniotic fluid [56].

Different results were obtained by Yücel et al. They analyzed vascular flows in patients after premature drainage of amniotic fluid with histopathologically confirmed placental inflammation. The researchers proved that an increase in the systolic-diastolic index in the uterine artery can be considered as a marker of developing intrauterine infection [57].

5.5 Ultrasound features of the cervix shortening

Bednarek et al. observed no statistically significant changes depending on the length of the cervix. Similar results were established by Klemm et al. analyzing uterine flows after radical trachelectomy. There were no changes in the uterine arterial resistance index in relation to the control group [58].

The three-dimensional evaluation of the cervical circulation accounts for a new diagnostic possibility. Samutchaikij et al. established reference values for certain measurements of the cervical vascular bed, and De Diego et al. analyzed three-dimensional images of the cervix in patients at risk of preterm labor. The authors found differences in the parameters of cervical vascularization in patients with preterm labor in comparison to asymptomatic patients with a comparable length of the cervix. It is possible that three-dimensional ultrasound will become a practical tool for the actual assessment of cervical insufficiency [59, 60].

5.6 Pregnancy duration and vascular flows

The study by Bednarek et al. involved the division of the study group into preterm labor below and above 32 weeks of pregnancy. Vascular flow differences were found in the umbilical artery. The pulsation, resistance and systolic-diastolic index values were higher in the younger group. Similar conclusions were presented by Chanprapaph et al. in the analysis of measurements in over three hundred healthy pregnant women. This phenomenon should be explained by the progressive increase in end-diastolic velocity with increasing gestational age, which directly translates into a decrease in the pulsation index. The authors draw attention to the fact that the value of the systolic-diastolic index above three, in a pregnancy above the thirtieth week, is more often associated with complications of low fetal body weight and birth disorders - the presence of meconium in the amniotic fluid, cesarean section and worse birth condition of the newborn [61–64].

Mari and Deter draw attention to the parabolic shape of the curve of changes in the flow rates of the central artery of the brain, the values of which are maintained in newborns until the first month of life. The curves established by the authors are applicable to the monitoring of fetuses with low body weight [65].

Degani found a clear decrease in the value of the middle cerebral artery pulsation index after the thirty-sixth week of pregnancy, which is related to the compensation mechanism that protects the fetus against a progressive decrease in oxygen tension [66].

Gadelha da Costa et al. assessed the increase in fetal middle cerebral artery resistance index up to the twenty-sixth week of pregnancy, and then a decrease to the period of full-term pregnancy [67, 68].

The lack of vascular changes in the uterine arteries in pregnant women with pre-term labor confirms the assumption that the assessment of the flow of these vessels is justified in pregnancies with placental abnormalities, such as intrauterine growth restriction, arterial hypertension or diabetes [69, 70].

6. Summary

Research on maternal-fetal haemodynamics in preterm labor is currently focused mainly on the safety of the used tocolytics. The reduction of the use, and often the elimination of beta-agonists, undoubtedly increased the safety of the mother and the fetus. The above literature review proves that despite some influence of medications on maternal-fetal blood flow values, tocolysis does not significantly disturb haemodynamics. However, it is worthwhile to remember about safety rules during ultrasound examinations with the use of Doppler technique.

Author details

Szymon Bednarek, Małgorzata Głogiewicz, Rafał Adamczak and Mariusz Dubiel*
Department of Obstetrics and Gynecology, Nicolaus Copernicus University, Bydgoszcz, Poland

*Address all correspondence to: profdubiel@gmail.com

References

[1] Zhao H, Wong R, Doyle T, Nayak N, Vreman H, Contag C, Stevenson D. Regulation of Maternal and Fetal Hemodynamics by Heme Oxygenase in Mice, Biology of Reproduction, Volume 78, Issue 4, 1 April 2008, Pages 744-751.

[2] Van Mieghem T, Deprest J, Verhaeghe J. Fetal and maternal hemodynamics in pregnancy: new insights in the cardiovascular adaptation to uncomplicated pregnancy, twin-to-twin transfusion syndrome and congenital diaphragmatic hernia. Facts Views Vis Obgyn. 2011;3(3):205-213.

[3] Moore K. et al. Embriologia i wady wrodzone. Edra Urban&Partner. Wrocław. 2013.

[4] Mavrides E, Moscoso G, Carvalho JS, Campbell S, Thilaganathan B. The anatomy of the umbilical, portal and hepatic venous systems in the human fetus at 14-19 weeks of gestation. Ultrasound Obstet Gynecol. 2001 Dec;18(6):598-604. doi: 10.1046/j.0960-7692.2001.00581.x. PMID: 11844197.

[5] Robson SC. Assessment of hemodynamics usin Doppler ultrasound. Ultrasound Obstet Gynecol. 2000;15:456-459.

[6] Maulik D. Doppler Ultrasound in Obstetrics and Gynecology. Springer, Berlin, Heidelberg 2005.

[7] Dubiel M, Bednarek S, Bernard P. Najczęstsze błędy w badaniu dopplerowskim w ciąży. Ginekologia po dyplomie 2015; 17(6): 62-78.

[8] Vyas S, Campbell S, Bower S, Nicolaides K. Maternal abdominal pressure alters fetal cerebral blood flow. Brit J Obstet Gynaecol.1990;97:740-747.

[9] Thuring A, Malcus P, Maršál K. Effect of maternal betamethasone on fetal and uteroplacental blood flow velocity waveforms. Ultrasound Obstet Gynecol. 2011;37(6):668-672.

[10] Kostowski W. red. Farmakologia. Podstawy farmakoterapii. PZWL. Warszawa. 1998.

[11] Wielgoś M, Bomba-Opoń A. Tokoliza w porodzie przedwczesnym – aktualne wytyczne. Ginekol Pol 2014; 85(05):332-334.

[12] http://www.drugbank.ca/drugs/DB01115

[13] Gáspár R, Hajagos-Tóth J. Calcium channel blockers as tocolytics: principles of their actions, adverse effects and therapeutic combinations. Pharmaceuticals 2013, 6, 689-699.

[14] Conde-Agudelo A, Romero R, Kusanovic J P. Nifedipine for the menagement of preterm labor: a systematic review and metaanalysis. Am J Obstet Gynecol. 2011 February; 204(2):134.

[15] Bednarek S, Lauda-Świeciak A, Latoch I, Skórczewski J, Ludwikowski G, Dubiel M, Bręborowicz GH. The influence of nifedipine in pre-term labour therapy on blood flow parameters in fetus middle cerebral, umbilical artery and in maternal uterine arteries. APM 2016; 22(1): 48-52.

[16] Richichi J, Vasilenko P. The effects of nifedipine on pregnancy outcome and morphology of the placenta, uterus, and cervix during late pregnancy in the rat. Am J Obstet Gynecol. 1992 Sep;167(3):797-803.

[17] de Heus R, Mulder EJ, Derks JB, Visser GH. The effects of the tocolytics atosiban and nifedipine on fetal movements, heart rate and blood flow. J Matern Fetal Neonatal Med. 2009 Jun;22(6):485-490.

[18] http://bazalekow.mp.pl

[19] Khatib N, Weiner Z, Beloosesky R, Vitner D, Thaler I. The effect of maternal supine position on umbilical and cerebral blood flow indices. Eur J Obstet Gynecol Reprod Biol. 2014 Apr;175:112-114.

[20] van Katwijk C, Wladimiroff JW. Effect of maternal posture on the umbilical artery flow velocity waveform. Ultrasound Med Biol. 1991;17(7):683-685.

[21] Kinsella SM, Lee A, Spencer JA. Maternal and fetal effects of the supine and pelvic tilt positions in late pregnancy. Eur J Obstet Gynecol Reprod Biol. 1990 Jul-Aug;36(1-2):11-17.

[22] Armstrong S, Fernando R, Columb M, Jones T. Cardiac index in term pregnant women in the sitting, lateral, and supine positions: an observational, crossover study. Anesth Analg. 2011 Aug;113(2):318-322.

[23] Marx GF, Patel S, Berman JA, Farmakides G, Schulman H. Umbilical blood flow velocity waveforms in different maternal positions and with epidural analgesia. Obstet Gynecol. 1986 Jul;68(1):61-64.

[24] Ryo E, Okai T, Kozuma S, Kobayashi K, Kikuchi A, Taketani Y. Influence of compression of the inferior vena cava in the late second trimester on uterine and umbilical artery blood flow. Int J Gynaecol Obstet. 1996 Dec;55(3):213-218.

[25] Qu LR, Kan A, Masahiro N. Fetal circulation in relation to various maternal body positions. Zhonghua Fu Chan Ke Za Zhi. 1994 Oct;29(10):589-591, 635-6.

[26] Backe B, Brodtkorb CJ, Giltvedt J, Kvernes S, Brubakk AO, Torp H, Angelsen BA. Fetal and maternal aortic flow in two different maternal positions. An investigation with combined Doppler-velocimetry and ultrasonic multiple array. Ultrasound Med Biol. 1983 Nov-Dec;9(6):587-593.

[27] Sorensen TK, Hendricks S, Easterling TR, Carlson KL, Benedetti TJ. Effect of orthostatic stress on umbilical Doppler waveforms in normal and hypertensive pregnancies. Am J Obstet Gynecol. 1992 Sep;167(3):643-647.

[28] Witter FR, Besinger RE. The effect of maternal position on uterine artery flow during antepartum fetal heart rate testing. Am J Obstet Gynecol. 1989 Feb;160(2):379-380.

[29] Sohn C, Kesternich P, Fendel H. The effect of body position on uterine blood flow in the 3d trimester of pregnancy. Ultraschall Med. 1989 Feb;10(1):10-14.

[30] Sohn C Fendel H, Billet P, Werdin R, Kesternich P, Schonlau H. Changes in uterine circulation in relation to body position in pregnancy. Z Geburtshilfe Perinatol. 1987 Sep-Oct;191(5):169-173.

[31] Easterling TR, Schmucker BC, Benedetti TJ. The hemodynamic effects of orthostatic stress during pregnancy. Obstet Gynecol. 1988 Oct;72(4):550-552.

[32] Cornette J, Duvekot J, Roos-Hesselink J, Hop W, Steegers E. Maternal and fetal haemodynamic effects of nifedipine in normotensive pregnant women. BJOG. 2010 Dec 24.

[33] Lima MM, Souza AS, Diniz C, Porto AM, Amorim MM, Moron AF. Doppler velocimetry of the uterine, umbilical and fetal middle cerebral arteries in pregnant women undergoing tocolysis with oral nifedipine. Ultrasound Obstet Gynecol. 2009 Sep;34(3):311-315.

[34] Grzesiak M, Ahmed RB, Wilczynski J. 48-hours administration

of nifedipine in spontaneous preterm labor - Doppler blood flow assessment of placental and fetal circulation. Neuro Endocrinol Lett. 2013;34(7):687-692.

[35] Guclu S, Gol M, Saygili U, Demir N, Sezer O, Baschat AA. Nifedipine therapy for preterm labor: effects on placental, fetal cerebral and atrioventricular Doppler parameters in the first 48 hours. Ultrasound Obstet Gynecol. 2006 Apr;27(4):403-408.

[36] Guclu S, Saygili U, Dogan E, Demir N, Baschat AA. The short-term effect of nifedipine tocolysis on placental, fetal cerebral and atrioventricular Doppler waveforms. Ultrasound Obstet Gynecol. 2004 Dec;24(7):761-765.

[37] Grzesiak M, Hincz P, Forys S, Ahmed RB, Wilczynski J. 48-hours administration of fenoterol in spontaneous preterm labor - Doppler blood flow assessment of placental and fetal circulation. Neuro Endocrinol Lett. 2013;34(6):553-558.

[38] Grzesiak M, Forys S, Sobczak M, Ahmed RB, Wilczynski J. 48-hours administration of fenoterol in spontaneous preterm labor - does it affect fetal preload? Neuro Endocrinol Lett. 2013;34(6):549-552.

[39] Faber R, Ruckhäberle KE, Robel R. Comparison of Doppler ultrasound assessment of utero-placento-fetal perfusion in normal pregnancies and in those with threatened premature labor. Zentralbl Gynakol. 1993;115(1):27-32.

[40] Gokay Z, Ozcan T, Copel JA. Changes in fetal hemodynamics with ritodrine tocolysis. Ultrasound Obstet Gynecol. 2001 Jul;18(1):44-46.

[41] Friedman DM, Blackstone J, Young BK, Hoskins IA. Fetal cardiac effects of oral ritodrine tocolysis. Am J Perinatol. 1994 Mar;11(2):109-112.

[42] Park YK, Hidaka A. Effect of left-lateral position on maternal hemodynamics during ritodrine treatment in comparison with supine position. Nihon Sanka Fujinka Gakkai Zasshi. 1991 Jun;43(6):655-662.

[43] Grzesiak M, Ahmed RB, Wilczynski J. Doppler evaluation of blood flow in fetal inferior vena cava during 48-hours Atosiban administration in spontaneous preterm labor. Neuro Endocrinol Lett. 2013;34(8):787-791.

[44] Fabry I, Paepe P, Kips J, Bortel L. The influence of tocolytic drugs on cardiac function, large arteries, and resistance vessels. European Journal of Clinical Pharmacology, Springer Verlag, 2011, 67 (6), pp.573-580.

[45] Grzesiak M, Wilczynski J. Preliminary report of 48-hours Atosiban administration in spontaneous preterm labor - Doppler blood flow assessment of placental and fetal circulation. Neuro Endocrinol Lett. 2013;34(7):681-686.

[46] Grzesiak M, Gaj Z, Kocyłowski R, Suliburska J, Oszukowski P, Horzelski W, von Kaisenberg C, Banach M. Oxidative Stress in Women Treated with Atosiban for Impending Preterm Birth. Oxid Med Cell Longev. 2018 Dec 2;2018:3919106.

[47] Parilla BV, Tamura RK, Cohen LS, Clark E. Lack of effect of antenatal indomethacin on fetal cerebral blood flow. Am J Obstet Gynecol. 1997 Jun;176(6):1166-1169; discussion 1169-71.

[48] Pacifici GM. Clinical pharmacology of Ibuprofen and indomethacin in preterm infants with patent ductus arteriosus. Curr Pediatr Rev. 2014;10(3):216-237.

[49] Keeley MM, Wade RV, Laurent SL, Hamann VD. Alterations in maternal-fetal Doppler flow velocity waveforms in preterm labor patients undergoing

magnesium sulfate tocolysis. Obstet Gynecol. 1993 Feb;81(2):191-194.

[50] Pezzati M, Giani T, Gambi B, Dani C, Bertini G, Biagiotti R, Rubaltelli FF. Influence of maternal magnesium sulphate and ritodrine treatment on cerebral blood flow velocity of the preterm newborn. Acta Obstet Gynecol Scand. 2001 Sep;80(9):818-823.

[51] Piazze J, Anceschi MM, Cerekja A, Cosmi E, Meloni P, Alberini A, Pizzulo S, Argento T, Cosmi EV. The combined effect of betamethasone and ritodrine on the middle cerebral artery in low risk third trimester pregnancies. J Perinat Med. 2007;35(2):135-140.

[52] Bednarek S. Wpływ tokolityków na wartości prędkości przepływu krwi w tętnicy środkowej mózgu u płodu i w krążeniu matczyno-łożyskowym - rozpr. dok. CMUMK. Bydgoszcz. 2015.

[53] Brar HS, Medearis AL, DeVore GR, Platt LD. Maternal and fetal blood flow velocity waveforms in patients with preterm labor: prediction of successful tocolysis. Am J Obstet Gynecol. 1988 Oct;159(4):947-950.

[54] Nakai Y, Imanaka M, Nishio J, Maeda T, Ozaki A, Sun TT, Ogita S. Uterine blood flow velocity waveforms during early postpartum course following caesarean section. Eur J Obstet Gynecol Reprod Biol. 1997 Aug;74(2):121-124.

[55] Kulkarni SS, Teoh WH, Sia AT, Nair S. Ruptured uterine artery pseudoaneurysm: an overlooked cause of late postpartum haemorrhage. Acta Anaesthesiol Belg. 2013;64(4):159-162.

[56] Carroll SG, Papaioannou S, Nicolaides KH. Doppler studies of the placental and fetal circulation in pregnancies with preterm prelabor amniorrhexis. Ultrasound Obstet Gynecol. 1995 Mar;5(3):184-188.

[57] Yücel N, Yücel O, Yekeler H. The relationship between umbilical artery Doppler findings, fetal biophysical score and placental inflammation in cases of premature rupture of membranes. Acta Obstet Gynecol Scand. 1997 Jul;76(6):532

[58] Klemm P, Tozzi R, Köhler C, Hertel H, Schneider A. Does radical trachelectomy influence uterine blood supply? Gynecol Oncol. 2005 Feb;96(2):283-286.

[59] Samutchaikij T, Pitukkijronnakorn S, Panburana P. Normal reference of cervical blood perfusion in pregnancy. J Med Assoc Thai. 2014 Apr;97(4):369-373.

[60] De Diego R, Sabrià J, Vela A, Rodríguez D, Gómez MD. Role of 3-dimensional power Doppler sonography in differentiating pregnant women with threatened preterm labor from those with an asymptomatic short cervix. J Ultrasound Med. 2014 Apr;33(4):673-679.

[61] Chanprapaph P, Wanapirak C, Tongsong T. Umbilical Artery Doppler Waveform Indices in Normal Pregnancies. Thai Journal of Obstetrics and Gynaecology June 2000, Vol. 12, pp. 103-107.

[62] Hendricks SK1, Sorensen TK, Wang KY, Bushnell JM, Seguin EM, Zingheim RW. Doppler umbilical artery waveform indices--normal values from fourteen to forty-two weeks. Am J Obstet Gynecol. 1989 Sep;161(3):761-765.

[63] Erskine RL, Ritchie JW. Umbilical artery blood flow characteristics in normal and growth-retarded fetuses. Br J Obstet Gynaecol. 1985 Jun;92(6):605-610.

[64] Gadelha-Costa A, Spara-Gadelha P, Filho FM, Gadelha EB. Hemodynamic changes in the fetal arteries during

the second half of pregnancy assessed by Doppler velocimetry. Eur J Obstet Gynecol Reprod Biol. 2007 Jun;132(2):148-153.

[65] Mari G, Deter RL. Middle cerebral artery flow velocity waveforms in normal and small-for-gestational-age fetuses. Am J Obstet Gynecol 1992; 166: 1262-1270.

[66] Degani S. Evaluation of fetal cerebrovascular circulation and brain development: the role of ultrasound and Doppler. Semin Perinatol. 2009 Aug;33(4):259-269.

[67] Gadelha-Costa A, Spara-Gadelha P, Filho FM, Gadelha EB. Hemodynamic changes in the fetal arteries during the second half of pregnancy assessed by Doppler velocimetry. Eur J Obstet Gynecol Reprod Biol. 2007 Jun;132(2):148-153.

[68] Gadelha Da Costa A, Mauad Filho F, Spara P, Barreto Gadelha E, Vieira Santana Netto P. Fetal hemodynamics evaluated by Doppler velocimetry in the second half of pregnancy. Ultrasound Med Biol. 2005 Aug;31(8):1023-1030.

[69] Hofstaetter C, Dubiel M, Gudmundsson S, Marsal K. Uterine artery color Doppler assisted velocimetry and perinatal outcome. Acta Obstet Gynecol Scand. 1996 Aug;75(7):612-619.

[70] Simanaviciute D, Gudmundsson S. Fetal middle cerebral to uterine artery pulsatility index ratios in normal and pre-eclamptic pregnancies. Ultrasound Obstet Gynecol. 2006 Nov;28(6):794-801

Chapter 13

Preterm Birth and Inflammation

Melinda Matyas

Abstract

Half of all preterm births are caused or triggered by an inflammation at fetal-maternal interface. The sustained inflammation that preterm neonates are exposed is generated by maternal chorioamnionitis, premature rupture of membranes. This inflammation will facilitate the preterm labor, but also plays an important role in development of disease like: bronchopulmonary dysplasia, necrotizing enterocolitis, retinopathy of prematurity, intraventricular hemorrhage and periventricular leukomalacia. Preterm neonates have immature immune system. The fragile co-regulation between immune defense mechanisms and immunosuppression (tolerance) is often disturbed at this category of patients. They are at high risk of sepsis due to this imbalance between the defense and suppression mechanisms but also several injuries can contribute to the onset or perpetuation of sustained inflammation. They experience altered antigen exposure in contact with hospital-specific germs, artificial devices, drugs, nutritional antigens, and hypoxia or hyperoxia. This is more significant at extremely preterm infants less than 28 weeks of gestation as they have not developed adaptation processes to tolerate maternal and self-antigens.

Keywords: preterm birth, inflammation, chorioamnionitis, premature rupture of membranes

1. Introduction

Preterm birth defined as birth before 37 weeks of gestation will have impact on newborns outcome not just immediately but long term. Around 70% of preterm births are spontaneous and are produced by premature rupture of membranes and preterm labor. In 50% of cases the preterm birth associates different form of inflammation, chorioamnionitis and maternal infection. The aim of this chapter is to present the impact of maternal inflammation and/or infection on their preterm health.

2. Preterm birth and preterm neonate particularities

Preterm birth according to the World Health Organization (WHO) is defined as birth before 37 completed weeks of gestation. In 2010, 14.9 million babies were born preterm, accounting for 11.1% of all births worldwide. In European countries, preterm birth represents approximately 5% of all births, while in certain African countries this ratio is around 18% [1]. Preterm birth represent the leading cause of childhood mortality in children under 5 years of age [2]. The high economic burden is generated by the neonatal intensive care, often followed by ongoing health care needs and a significant emotional impact experienced by families [3].

Preterm birth may occur spontaneously or based on a medical indication. About one third of all preterm births have a medical indication, determined by maternal or fetal risk factors, which are higher than the benefits generated by the continuation of pregnancy and include preeclampsia or diabetes mellitus [4]. Approximately 70% of preterm births are spontaneous, caused by premature rupture of membranes, preterm labor [4]. Preterm labor in about half of the cases is associated with inflammatory syndrome, with sustained inflammation. Preterm labor has a complex etiology; it can be induced by many factors: infection or inflammation, utero-placental hemorrhage, placental ischemia, uterine overdistension or stress [5]. Maternal risk factors with a role in triggering preterm labor are numerous: extreme ages of the mother, high body mass index (BMI), multiple gestation, assisted reproductive technologies, history of preterm birth, and low socioeconomic status [4]. Race is also an important risk factor; African-Americans are at higher risk of preterm birth than other ethnic groups [5].

Preterm birth is an important cause of morbidity and mortality in the newborn. The pathologies induced by preterm birth are both acute and chronic. Chronic diseases may have a long-term impact on the health of preterm neonates, affecting their neurodevelopmental outcome in variable degrees.

The main acute disorders associated with preterm birth are: respiratory distress, cerebral hemorrhage, periventricular leukomalacia, necrotizing enterocolitis (NEC), while the most frequent chronic diseases with an impact on the development and long-term prognosis of newborns are: bronchopulmonary dysplasia, retinopathy of prematurity, periventricular leukomalacia, and abnormal neurological development.

Prematurely born adults will have an increased risk of hypertension at adult age, diabetes mellitus and obesity [4].

The evolution of preterm infants is dependent on sex. Some studies showed that at the age of 2 years, chronic respiratory and neurological complications were more frequent among male compared to female preterm newborns [6].

Cytokines play an important role in initiating and regulating labor. Labor occurs under pro-inflammatory conditions with the participation of cytokines. In this pro-inflammatory environment, a three-step process takes place, which is characterized by uterine contractility, cervical ripening and membrane activation/rupture [7].

There will be a considerable release of interleukin IL-1 β, IL-6 and IL-8, and tumor necrosis factor alpha (TNF-α). These pro-inflammatory substances will be released by stromal cells as well as monocytes and neutrophils that invade the myometrium and the cervix during labor. IL-1β and TNF-α will cause myometrial contraction through calcium influx in myometrial smooth muscle cells. Myometrial contraction is also stimulated by prostaglandins: $PGF_{2\alpha}$ and PGE_2.

Chemotactic activity and cytokine production differ in the case of premature rupture of membranes compared to term rupture of membranes. In the decidua, leukocyte infiltration occurs during labor. The number of neutrophils that infiltrate the decidua is much higher in the case of preterm labor with associated infection. In addition to neutrophils, the number of macrophages also increases, but this increase is present in both term and preterm labor [8].

Nuclear factor kB (NF-kB), which plays a role in the synthesis of prostaglandins and the regulation of matrix metalloproteinase (MMP) expression, thus influencing myometrial contraction and cervical ripening, should also be mentioned.

Chorioamnionitis is an inflammation caused by bacterial infections in the fetal membrane. This may induce different severe disorders in newborns, such as necrotizing enterocolitis, cerebral palsy or patent ductus arteriosus. These complications will have an immediate and long-term impact on the evolution of the neonate [9].

Inflammatory mediators will reach the fetus through the amniotic fluid or by transmission through the umbilical cord [10].

3. Inflammation effect on preterm neonate

3.1 Effects on the lung

The inflammatory cytokines that reach the amniotic fluid will have an effect on the development of the fetal lung. Chorioamnionitis is an important risk factor for bronchopulmonary dysplasia. In neonates whose mothers had increased cytokine levels in the amniotic fluid: IL-8, IL-8, IL-1β and TNF-α, severe forms of bronchopulmonary dysplasia were more frequent. The pathological examination of the placenta can provide important information about the placental inflammatory process. Among our cases, we had a patient with a severe form of bronchopulmonary dysplasia, with oxygen requirements until the age of 4 months, without a history of severe respiratory distress, but with abscess areas, extensive inflammation evidenced by the pathological examination of the placenta and umbilical cord (**Figures 1** and **2**). The mother showed no clinical symptoms, but inflammatory syndrome and premature rupture of membranes were evidenced 14 days prior to labor [11].

Although there are meta-analyses showing a weak association between inflammation and bronchopulmonary dysplasia, animal studies have revealed significant inflammation in the lungs after endotoxin injection in preterm lambs [12]. Inflammatory mediators have effects on the regulation of angiogenesis, morphogenesis and cell growth in the lungs [13].

Bronchopulmonary dysplasia is more frequent in extreme preterm neonates. It may have a long-term effect on respiratory function during childhood or even adulthood. These children at school age will have an increased risk to develop asthma phenotype. Treatments used in bronchopulmonary dysplasia can also have adverse effects that will be validated in the medium or long term. Thus, prolonged use of corticoids in severe disease forms can have an impact on neurological

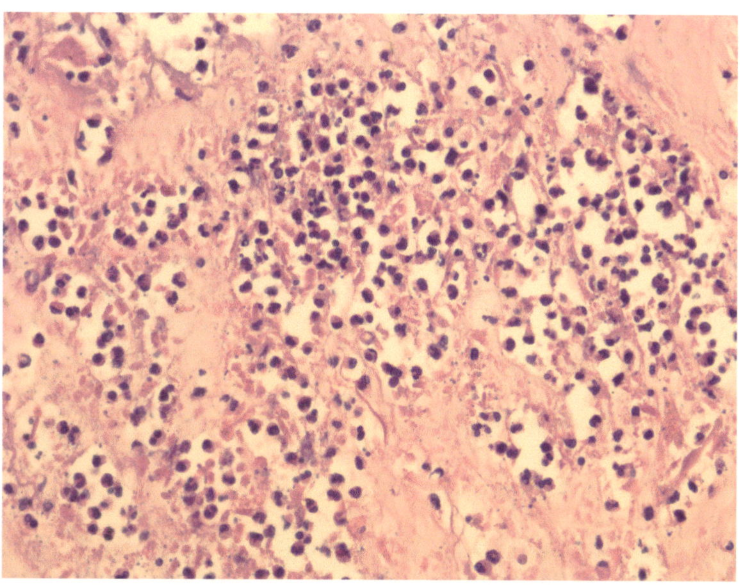

Figure 1.
Amniotic membrane inflammation [11].

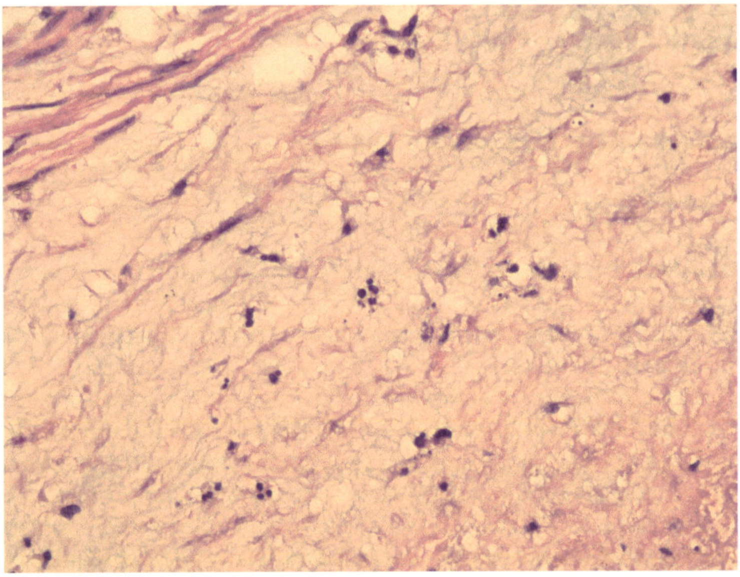

Figure 2.
Inflammation in the umbilical cord [11].

development; prolonged use of diuretics may influence auditory bone development in the newborn [11]. Studies have shown airway obstruction in prematurely born children or adults with a history of BPD [14]. Other factors favoring the development of the disease in preterm infants are delivery by cesarean section, infections, antibiotic therapy. The risk of infections increases with the decrease of gestational age. Humoral and cellular immunity is not prepared for extrauterine life in newborns with small gestational age.

Recent research has highlighted a correlation between microbiota and immunity, i.e. the presence of a lung - intestine axis regarding mucosal status.

Multivariate logistic regression analysis of a neonatal cohort (2527 neonates with BPD and 12826 unaffected controls) revealed that neonatal sepsis is a risk factor for BPD. Breast milk and probiotics play a role in reducing BPD incidence in preterm infants [15].

In BPD, there are changes in pulmonary vascularization, the number of alveoli, the reduction of septation, the simplification of alveolar structure with an impact on gas exchanges.

In the lungs, there is an inflammatory process mediated by pro-inflammatory cytokines, inflammation being maintained by mechanical ventilation, oxygen administration and infection. The cytokine level will depend on the duration of mechanical ventilation, tidal volume and the type of ventilation used.

Preterm neonates with BPD have in their cord blood a high level of Th17 compared to unaffected newborns [16]. A study analyzing the serum of newborns with BPD revealed high levels of Il-6, IL-8 and granulocyte–colony stimulating factor (G-CSF) in the first week of life [17].

3.2 Effects of inflammation on the heart

Inflammation in the fetal period, particularly in the case of preterm neonates, will act on an immature, developing heart.

The process of formation, development of cardiomyocytes continues until the time of birth.

Currently, it is known that inflammation, cytokine release are correlated with the occurrence of pulmonary hypertension, which will have an effect on the right ventricle and will induce systolic and diastolic dysfunction. However, studies have demonstrated that maternal inflammation will have an effect on the fetal and subsequently neonatal heart. Hyperoxia induced by inflammation will affect left ventricular structure, causing systolic and diastolic dysfunction.

Extrauterine growth restriction is correlated with adaptation difficulties, limitations of physical activity in former extreme preterm infants. This limitation can be generated by a degree of heart failure in former extreme preterm neonates and by their insufficient growth due to inadequate energy intake [15].

In adults, cardiac dysfunction induced by massive cytokine release as part of an inflammatory process or associated with sepsis has been described [18].

3.3 Effects of inflammation on the intestine

Due to its immaturity, the preterm neonatal intestine is at high risk for lesions caused by inflammation.

The risk factors for inflammatory lesions are represented by: immaturity of the mucosal barrier, immune cell dysfunction, low motility, reduced secretion of IgA and peptides with an antimicrobial role, high risk of dysbiosis and bacterial colonization.

Maternal chorioamnionitis determines a higher incidence of late sepsis in preterm newborns. The major intestinal consequence of maternal chorioamnionitis, chronic ischemia during pregnancy, antibiotic exposure is represented by necrotizing enterocolitis [19].

Pro-inflammatory mediators are important triggers in the development of the disease. Cyclooxygenase and platelet activating factors play a role in the inflammatory pathogenesis of NEC. The role of TLR4 receptors in NEC has been described. TLR4 recognize lipopolysaccharides and activate NF- κB, triggering the pro-inflammatory cascade. Enterocyte apoptosis is induced. The bacterial signal mediated by TLR4 causes mucosal lesions and allows the passage of bacteria into circulation. In mesenteric vessels, TLR4 will interact with bacteria, determining increased nitric oxide production, with severe vasoconstriction and reduced intestinal perfusion [20, 21].

The intestinal microbiota has an influence on immunity in both the intestine and the entire body.

Inflammation in NEC is caused by dysbiosis in the intestine and the exaggerated inflammatory response to this imbalance of the intestinal flora.

3.4 Effects of inflammation on the kidney

Nephrogenesis occurs until the gestational age of 34–36 weeks. The intrauterine inflammatory process will have an effect on renal function. Inflammation has an effect on the nephrogenesis process. Animal studies have demonstrated that the number of nephrons is up to 25% smaller in the case of exposure to hyperoxia and concomitant inflammation [22].

The reduced number of nephrons will have an impact on long-term renal function during childhood and adulthood, and it will favor the development of arterial hypertension at adult age.

3.5 Effects of inflammation on the central nervous system

Besides the impact on the pulmonary parenchyma, the inflammatory process in the intrauterine period also affects neurological development. Fetal inflammation, as well as inflammation in the neonatal period due to infections can have consequences on the brain, causing lesions of the white matter, inducing periventricular leukomalacia, cerebral palsy, respectively.

The increased levels of IL-1 β, IL-6 and particularly TNF-α will exert a toxic effect on developing oligodendrocytes, but will also have a toxic effect at neuronal level. Experimental animal models have revealed the evolution of neurological lesions in time. MRI studies have evidenced long-term cerebral changes during adult life in animal models exposed to inflammation in the intrauterine period. Although there are no data about preterm infants exposed to inflammatory syndrome in the intrauterine period, it is important to consider the fact that some authors have reported cases of autism as an effect of persistent inflammation in the fetal period, or schizophrenia as an effect of latent inflammation [23].

Inflammation will induce lesions directly in the oligodendrocytes and neurons, but also indirectly, through the activation of microglial cells with the release of proinflammatory cytokines, followed by neuronal and oligodendrocytes damage [24].

The ELGAN study showed that a high level of inflammatory markers during the first month of life will entail a high risk of decrease in the intelligence quotient (IQ) and executive functions [25].

The imbalance of the intestine – brain axis has an important role in neurocognitive development. Many studies describe the role of this imbalance. In its activity, endocrine, metabolic, immune and neural factors play an important role, but they have not yet been completely elucidated.

4. Conclusion

Preterm birth represents a public health problem. Inflammation during pregnancy has effects on the fetus and subsequently, on the newborn. Inflammatory mediators in the amniotic fluid induce lesions in the lung and the central nervous system.

A non-invasive respiratory approach and the limited use of invasive respiratory support will prevent severe forms of bronchopulmonary dysplasia. Enteral feeding with breast milk will have a beneficial effect on the reduction of NEC incidence, the reduction of the incidence of sepsis, BPD and ROP, as well as on the reduction of the risk for bronchial asthma during childhood and young adulthood. In the long term, implementing individualized therapeutic measures will allow a better management of each case, the decrease of fetal and neonatal mortality, and optimal neurological development.

Appendices and nomenclature

BMI	body mass index
NEC	necrotizing enterocolitis
TNF-α	tumor necrosis factor α
IL 1β	interleukin 1 β
NF kB	nuclear factor kB
G-CSF	granulocyte colony stimulating factor

Author details

Melinda Matyas
Iuliu Hatieganu University of Medicine and Pharmacy, Cluj Napoca, Romania

*Address all correspondence to: melimatyas@yahoo.com

References

[1] Blencowe H, Cousens S, Oestergaard M.Z, Chou D, Moller A.B, Narwal R, Adler A, Vera Garcia, C, Rohde S, Say L, Lawn J.E. National, regional, and worldwide estimates of preterm birth rates in the year 2010 with timetrends since 1990 for selected countries: a systematic analysis and implications. 2012.Lancet 379, 2162-2172.

[2] Harrison M.S, Goldenberg R.L. Global burden of prematurity. 2015. Semin. FetalNeonatal Med.

[3] Howson C.P, Kinney M.V, Mcdougall L, Lawn J.E. Born too soon: preterm birth matters. 2013.Reprod. Health 10 (Suppl. 1), S1.

[4] Rubens C.E, Sadovsky Y, Muglia L, Gravett M.G, Lackritz E, Gravett C.Prevention of preterm birth: harnessing science to address the global epidemic. 2014.Sci. Transl. Med. 6, 262sr5.

[5] Goldenberg R.L, Culhane J.F, Iams J.D, Romero R. Epidemiology and causes of preterm birth. 2008.Lancet 371, 75-84.

[6] Peacock J.L, Marston L, Marlow N, Calvert S.A, Greenough A. Neonatal and infant outcome in boys and girls born very prematurely. 2012. Pediatr. Res. 71,305-310.

[7] Rinaldi S.F, Catalano R.D, Wade J, Rossi A.G, Norman J.E. 15-epi-lipoxinA4 reduces the mortality of prematurely born pups in a mouse model ofinfection-induced preterm birth. 2015. Mol. Hum. Reprod. 21, 359-368.

[8] Hamilton S, Oomomian Y, Stephen G, Shynlova O, Tower C.L, Garrod A, Lye S.J, Jones R.L. Macrophages infiltrate the human and rat decidua during term and preterm labor: evidence that decidual inflammation precedes labor. 2012.Biol. Reprod. 86, 39.

[9] Been J.V, Lievense S, Zimmermann L.J, Kramer B.W, Wolfs T.G. Chorioamnionitis as a risk factor for necrotizing enterocolitis: a systematic review and meta-analysis. 2013. J. Pediatr. 162, 236-242 (e2).

[10] [10]Adams Waldorf K.M, Mcadams R.M. Influence of infection during pregnancy on fetal development. 2013. Reproduction 146, R151–R162.

[11] [11]MatyasM, BlagaL, Hasmasanu M, Zaharie G. Severe form of bronchopulmonary dysplasia. Obstetrics and Gynecology, LXVII, no3.2019

[12] Kramer B.W, Kramer S, Ikegami M, Jobe A.H. Injury, inflammation, and remodeling in fetal sheep lung after intra-amniotic endotoxin. 2002. Am. J. Physiol.Lung Cell. Mol. Physiol. 283, L452–L459.

[13] Mcadams R.M, Vanderhoeven J, Beyer R.P, Bammler T.K, Farin F.M, Liggitt H.D, Kapur R.P, Gravett M.G, Rubens C.E, Adams Waldorf K.M. Choriodecidual infection down regulates angiogenesis and morphogenesis pathways in fetal lungs from *Macaca nemestrina*. 2012. PLoS One 7, e46863.

[14] Vollsaeter M, Roksund O.D, Eide G.E, Markestad T, Halvorsen T. Lung function after preterm birth: development from mid-childhood to adulthood. 2013. Thorax 68, 767-776.

[15] Härtel C, Pagel J, Spiegler J et al Lactobacillus acidophilus/ Bifidobacterium infantis probiotics are associated with increased growth of VLBWI among those exposed to

antibiotics. 2017.Sci Rep 7: 5633. https://doi.org/10.1038/s41598-017-06161-8

[16] Gleditsch DD, Shornick LP, Van Steenwinckel J et al. Maternal inflammation modulates infant immune response patterns to viral lung challenge in a murine model. 2014.Pediatr Res 76:33-40. https://doi.org/10.1038/pr.2014.57

[17] Leroy S, Caumette E, Waddington C, et al. A time-based analysis of inflammation in infants at risk of bronchopulmonary dysplasia. 2018. J Pediatr 192:60-65.e1. https://doi.org/10.1016/j.jpeds.2017.09.011

[18] Sergi C, Shen F, Lim DW et al Cardiovascular dysfunction in sepsis at the dawn of emerging mediators. 2017. Biomed Pharmacother 95:153-160. https://doi.org/10.1016/j.biopha.2017.08.066

[19] Matyas M, Urda A, Crivii CB, Hasmasanu M, Ighian I, Budusan A, Manea AM, Boia M, Zaharie G. The impact of risk factors on the evolution of VLBW preterm infants with necrotizing enterocolitis. 2019.Jurnalul pediatrului, Vol. XXII, Nr. 85-86, January-June 2019

[20] Hodzic Z, Bolock AM, Good M. The role of mucosal immunity in the pathogenesis of necrotizing enterocolitis.2017.Front Pediatr 3(5):40

[21] Hackam D, Caplan M. Necrotizing enterocolitis: pathophysiology from a historical context. 2018.Semin Pediatr Surg 27:11-18

[22] Modena AB, Fieni S. Amniotic fluid dynamics. 2004.ActaBiomedica de l'Ateneo Parmense, In, pp 11-13

[23] Meyer U, Feldon J, Dammann O, Schizophrenia and autism: both shared and disorder-specific pathogenesis via perinatal inflammation? 2011. Pediatr. Res.69, 26r–33r.

[24] Burd I, Balakrishnan B, Kannan S. Models of fetal brain injury, intrauterine inflammation, and preterm birth. 2012. Am. J. Reprod. Immunol. 67, 287-294.

[25] Kuban KCK, Joseph RM, O'Shea TM, et al Circulating inflammatory-associated proteins in the first month of life and cognitive impairment at age 10 years in children born extremely preterm. 2017.J Pediatr 180:116-123.e1. https://doi.org/10.1016/j.jpeds.2016.09.054

Section 4

Caesaren Section Community

Chapter 14

Approaches at Community Level for Care of the Preterm Neonates in Low-Income Countries

Pontius Bayo and Juliet Ajok

Abstract

The survival of preterm babies has significantly improved over the last several decades in the high-income countries because of the availability of Neonatal Intensive Care Units (NICU's) in both large and small hospitals, presence of specially trained physicians, nurses, and other health care personnel with easy access to sophisticated equipment. However, the bigger public health advances that saw improvements in socio-economic status of the populations, improvements in education and sanitation conditions and reductions in malnutrition and rates of infectious diseases were probably the main reasons for this improved survival rates for preterm neonates. Low in-come countries are currently highest bearers of the burden of preterm morbidity and mortality. The current preventive and care interventions do not reach all the neonates and their mothers, the coverage has remained low, access is poor and the quality of care is low. The aim of this chapter is to propose ideas on how the current preterm neonatal care interventions can be adapted for community scale up through community-based health system structures like community health workers to improve survival of neonates who have been delivered from home or after they have been discharged from hospital.

Keywords: preterm, communities, low in-come countries, access, coverage

1. Introduction

Globally, about 15 million neonates are born preterm, the majority of which are in Sub-Saharan Africa [1]. The survival of these pre-term babies depends on which part of the world they are born from [1]. This chapter is meant for neonatal care deliverers in third world economies where subsistence farming managed by women is the backbone, where women engaged in other occupations are scarce, majority of the populations are in the lowest economic quantiles, access to quality education and health services are poor, access to family planning information and services is low and where teenage pregnancy rates have remained notoriously high. Such are the economies that present the highest numbers of preterm births in the global records and yet also present poor health systems with high rates of home deliveries and high rates of perinatal deaths [2]. The knowledge, expertise and the technology required for the preterm babies to survive is limited in these economies.

The survival of preterm babies has significantly improved over the last several decades in the high-income countries because of the availability of Neonatal

Intensive Care Units (NICU's) in both large and small hospitals, presence of specially trained physicians, nurses, and other health care personnel with easy access to sophisticated equipment [3]. However, the bigger public health advances that saw improvements in socio-economic status of the populations, improvements in education and sanitation conditions and reductions in malnutrition and rates of infectious diseases were probably the main reasons for this improved survival rates for preterm neonates [4]. The countries in low-resource regions are currently at different stages of economic growth and health system development and will see similar improvements at some point. But strengthened political will, increased community participation in and awareness of their health are necessary for larger strides in the desired improvements. Strategic research focused on prevention of preterm births and implementation of innovative interventions at the community level is also crucial.

There is need for programmatic innovation to close the gaps in coverage, equity and quality of care left by the health facility based preterm neonatal care interventions and focus on integration and scale up. Health care packages can be linked through the lifetime of individuals (adolescent, woman, mother, newborn and child) and across health levels in the system (at home, primary health care center, district/regional hospitals) using the continuum of care principle.

2. The exaggerated risk of death for the preterm newborns at the community level

Birth and the succeeding few days present the highest risk of death to any newborn in the human lifespan because of the delicate needs of body temperature regulation, glycemic control, and a clean environment to prevent infection. Preterm infants, however, are at an exaggerated risk of dying compared to their full-term counterparts as they are not able to adequately regulate their body temperature, have poor suckling reflex for adequate feeding, and also have poor lung maturity for adequate lung expansion and are therefore, prone to respiratory distress syndrome and infection [5, 6]. These medical complications may be managed with relative ease in the health care facility setting and this makes the difference in survival for the preterm newborns in the different economies.

Most health facilities in the developing world still lack the appropriate technology and skills to save preterm neonates, and it is worse at the community level where the health systems lack community structures for continued care at home after hospital discharge or to access care for those delivered from home. The death of a preterm baby is thus, considered inevitable by both the healthcare system and the families in these economies, yet many of them could be saved with simple interventions that can be rendered and/or continued at the community level [7]. The majority (>80%) of preterm babies are born between 32–37 weeks of gestation and can survive without the need for sophisticated medical care [8]. This chapter aims to highlight the key medical needs of the preterm neonates and how community health structures can be re-aligned to offer simple interventions to support their survival at home in developing countries. It is an attempt to contribute to the efforts towards achieving SDG goal 3 target of reducing neonatal mortality to at least 12 per 1,000 live births [9].

3. The rationale for a community approach in the developing economies

The risk factors for preterm births are ripe in the developing economies where access to health care is poor. Young and advanced maternal age, low maternal body mass, short inter-pregnancy intervals, gender-based violence, infections such as urinary tract infections, malaria, bacterial vaginosis, HIV, and syphilis are still very common in these countries and are associated with preterm births. Lifestyle behaviors such as excessive physical work, smoking and excessive alcohol consumption have also been associated with preterm births and are common practices in these developing countries [10].

The numbers of preterm births are therefore, higher in these countries and yet survival is poor, as most of these births take place at home, some of the traditional practices of neonatal care simply heighten neonatal infection rates such as application of substances on the cord, the knowledge to detect danger signs is limited and referral pathways are also limited. Well planned and coordinated interventions at community level would argument health system programs to reduce neonatal mortalities in these countries. However, before such interventions are designed and implemented, there is need to assess the contextual newborn care practices at the household level and understand the beliefs attached to these practices. This helps to inform the cultural feasibility and therefore, acceptability of the intervention as well as to define the delivery platform within the local health system.

4. Which of the following preterm neonatal issues can be resolved at the community level?

This chapter is not in any way to replace actions/interventions at the health facilities in any country but to emphasize preventive, health promotive and essential care actions that are possible at the community level to increase survival in contexts where access to health care is poor. It is, therefore, important for it to be clear to the reader that preterm neonates have multiple issues, some of which may not be alienable at the community level. Some of these issues are pointed out here for emphasis, and it is prudent that each case is assessed carefully and independently.

1. *Severe infections*: Most preterm neonates will die once they get severe infections; therefore, prophylactic antibiotics may be necessary for all preterm neonates.

2. *Respiratory Distress Syndrome*: Preterm neonates born before 32 weeks of gestation have immature lungs that lack surfactant in the alveoli and thus have poor lung expansion. Antenatal corticosteroid injections to women in preterm labor has proved helpful in reducing the risk of RDS [11].

3. *Jaundice*: The preterm neonate's liver is not able to metabolize bilirubin adequately and the brain is at higher risk of damage as the blood–brain barrier is also poorly developed to offer protection.

4. *Intraventricular hemorrhage*: This is the most common cause for brain damage and is often related to the RDS and hypotension.

5. *Necrotizing enterocolitis*: Formula feeding seems to increase the risk tenfold as opposed to those neonates who are breast fed.

6. *Anemia*: This may show up a few weeks after birth because of delayed red blood cell production by the immature bone marrow.

5. The medical and socio-economic challenges while caring for preterm newborns at the community level

Developing countries can reduce their neonatal mortality rates significantly by offering appropriate care to preterm neonates through regular breast feeding, optimum body temperature maintenance, cord, and skin care, as well as early detection and treatment of infections. However, multiple technical, social, and economic challenges exist which might render these elements of care difficult at the community level.

5.1 Care of pre-term babies at the community level may be complex and stressful for parents compared to at the health facility with the support of the health care providers and availability of appropriate equipment

Parents and care takers at home not only require the knowledge about the needs of pre-term babies over and beyond those of the term babies, what medical complications to anticipate and how to prevent them but they also need social structures to support them provide the care to their babies and help with other domestic chores.

Some of the difficulties may vary according to context influenced by culture and traditions. Kangaroo mother care (KMC) for example, has promise to support preterm neonates at home and prevent occurrence of most of the above medical complications, however, its practice has remained low [12]. The traditional way of carrying neonates at the back makes KMC an odd intervention and shameful for mothers to practice [13]. Most communities are aware of the need for warm care for neonates and already have traditional ways of providing it e.g., putting a lamp or a charcoal stove in the room where the neonate sleeps, smearing the body of the neonate with special oils etc. This has made it difficult for KMC to receive social approval in such communities. It has been reported in some studies that community members have accused mothers practicing KMC of using their chests to hide stolen property [14]. This kind of stigmatizing comments from the community members does not only make the mothers fear to practice KMC but also limits the participation of the male partners. It has also been reported that close relatives may generally support and help mothers practicing KMC with household chores, but they are likely to overly subject the mothers to a lot of questions.

Certain traditional practices and norms increase risk of infection among preterm babies such as many care takers in the community not willing to wash hands before handling the neonates, large number of people visiting the mother and the neonate insisting on carrying the baby without washing the hands. Families, therefore, go through a lot of psychological stress from forces within the communities that takes away their confidence while taking care of preterm neonates. The healthcare systems must address this through providing adequate and coordinated information and education.

5.2 Gender roles place mothers of preterm babies in responsibility of household chores with limited assistance from the male partners

Beyond the complexity of detecting medical complications and offering the care needed to prevent them, the mothers in the developing world have additional burden placed on them by gender norms within the societies. It has already been noted that the care for preterm neonates is labor intensive and time consuming and yet in most settings gender roles place the mothers in positions where they receive minimum assistance from their male partners towards household chores. The mothers must cook for their husbands and the other children at home, clean up the house, produce food from the gardens besides having to look after themselves [15].

5.3 Feeding challenges as pre-term babies have a poor suck reflex and insufficient suck-swallow coordination

Pre-term neonates have a poor coordination of the hunger-satiety cues, they also tire easily at suckling and may sleep off without effective feeding [16]. Unfortunately, their mothers do not usually recognize this challenge especially when the neonates tire and sleep off, the mothers tend to believe that they are full. In some communities, mothers use undesirable feeding options when the neonates are not able to suckle adequately such as giving sugar water instead of expressed breast milk [17]. Different breast-feeding methods for these pre-term neonates needs to be taught to their mothers and regular close monitoring implemented.

5.4 Health systems failure to create consistent awareness and education on pre-term neonatal care at the community level

The health care systems have no clear strategies to promote preterm neonatal care at community level, for example, most mothers learn about KMC from health workers for the first time only after giving birth in the hospital [13]. Preterm labor and pre-mature neonates are not subjects discussed with the mothers during antenatal period. Peer -to- peer information sharing has been noted to be a major source of trusted information that most mothers relied on to care for pre-term neonates [13]. The mothers are, therefore, not mentally ready about what to expect and feel overwhelmed with anxiety once confronted with the demands of the preterm baby. Health systems that have community health structures such as village health teams (VHTs) or community health workers (CHWs), these have program specific trainings in most settings and pre-term neonatal care at community level is usually not one of the priorities. For example, the personnel are trained as community drug distributors for childhood illnesses, breastfeeding supporters, and as safe motherhood volunteers while others promote malaria prevention. Most health systems lack evidence informed policy and standard guidelines for pre-term neonatal care at the community level.

The education needs of parents being discharged from hospital need to be carefully assessed to empower them to take care of pre-term neonates at home and be provided with a discharge plan based on the needs of the pre-term neonate, their competencies and availability of resources for care. These educational needs are likely to change over time to information regarding growth and development. Health systems, therefore, need to design and adapt parental support structures at the community level that are dynamic at the different stages of baring a pre-term neonate.

5.5 Financial constraints for professional home care and health promotion

A structured coordinated home care by health care professionals would provide parents an opportunity of support in their own physical environment making use of their own social support networks. However, the human resources to provide this and the supplies required is often lacking in the developing world.

It is difficult for most families in the developing world to afford materials that are required for the desired practice especially among the poorest communities. They often lack the basic supplies such as warm clothes for keeping the baby warm, no adequate clean water and sanitation facilities at the homesteads, as well as inadequate maternal nutrition often compounds the situation. In one study, mothers reported lack of funds to buy fuel (charcoal and paraffin) and oil to smear the baby or for accessing healthcare when the neonate gets sick [18].

Health systems would need to make commitments for an institutionalized approach of home care for pre-term neonates and act on the roles and obligations towards achieving agreed goals and rights. Decisions and actions towards financial obligations need to be based on evidence and rights. There is also be need to have clear accountability frame works for any financial commitments for home based care for pre-term neonates including institutionalized monitoring and evaluation systems that facilitate learning and progress.

6. Resources available at the community level to support care of pre-term neonates in low-income countries

6.1 There are traditional birth attendants (TBAs) in communities who continue to attend births from home

Mothers in rural areas in the developing world continue to rely on TBAs for assistance at birth and advise on postnatal newborn care. The knowledge, attitudes, and practices of these TBAs needs constant evaluation by the health systems. It has been demonstrated in some studies that mothers prefer to follow the tradition and are heavily influenced by these local TBAs and family pressure [19].

6.2 There are community-based health structures composed of voluntary community health workers (CHWs) monitored by the health systems in most developing countries

As already stated above, most of these community structures are established for specific programs. Integrating the knowledge and safe practices for newborn care into the existing activities of the VHTs/CHWs can stimulate a structured newborn care at community level under the supervision of the health systems. There has been successful home-based neonatal care programs [20], and this can be scaled up for preterm neonates.

6.3 There are locally known signs to identify pre-term neonates

Community members such as Traditional birth attendants (TBAs) can correctly identify preterm neonates with features such as 'baby at birth is very small', 'not able to suckle', 'skin is wrinkled' and 'inability to open eyes at birth [21].

6.4 There is some knowledge about how to look after pre-term babies

The need to give the pre-term babies extra-care is known to many community members such as keeping them warm, encouraging adequate feeding and keeping the environment clean. For example, warmth is generated from the different sources in different societies including covering the babies with many clothes, lighting charcoal stoves under the bed where the baby is laid and providing hot water jerrycans [22].

7. Essential preterm prevention and care packages at the community level in low-income countries

The essential neonatal care packages exist in literature but there is a gap between this wealth of knowledge and practice. There is need to adapt the interventions and care packages tested in randomized trials to local settings especially when strongly held beliefs and cultural barriers exist against the scientific mechanisms of the interventions. The extend of the adaptation may depend on survival benefit and affordability of the intervention.

7.1 Prevent preterm births

Preventive strategies in low-income countries should focus on risk reduction and this includes preconception interventions through to interventions during pregnancy. The interventions need to be packaged and delivered through coordinated community health structures involving trained CHWs and VHTs. During preconception period, communities need to be educated and empowered to improve adolescent and preconception nutrition, strengthened family planning information, education and methods delivery system at community level; prevent gender based violence, prevention, and management of sexually transmitted infections (STIs) at community level, preventive strategies for control of malaria infections through use of insecticide treated mosquito nets and cessation of smoking and excessive alcohol consumption.

During pregnancy, mothers need to be supported, monitored, and supervised by CHWs to attend ANC through multiple home visits to ensure targeted care for women with increased risk for preterm birth.

7.2 Community -health facility linkages to ensure health facility births under skilled care

Access to health care is a major obstacle for many women in developing countries. Women and their families have been encouraged to have a birth preparedness plan which needs to clearly identify health facility for birth, means of transport to the facility, a skilled health care provider, a companion from home, financial support, clothes to provide warmth for the neonate and person(s) to continue giving support looking after other children while away. This preparedness should be monitored through the community health structures such as the village health teams (VHTs) or community health workers (CHWs) who need to be facilitated to conduct home visits to all pregnant women in their catchment areas.

Deliveries under skilled care is crucial to correctly identify preterm neonates, ensure their birth weights are determined, early and exclusive breast feeding is established, and resuscitation done if required. The referral pathways need to be established through linkages with the VHTs and/or CHWs for mothers and neonates who have delivered from home.

7.3 Thermal care

Community health structures can be organized to VHTs and CHWs to support women through postnatal home visits to establish adequate thermal care for their preterm neonates. Every neonate needs thermal care by simple actions such as drying and wrapping, warming up the room the neonates are in, covering the head with a cap, delaying the first bath, and using warm water for bathing [23]. Preterm babies will require kangaroo mother care which involves placing the preterm neonate on the chest of the mother or other attendant for a direct, continuous skin-to-skin contact to provide stable warmth and encouraging exclusive breast feeding. These techniques can be taught to mothers and other family members and reinforced through regular supervision and monitoring by VHTs/CHWs.

7.4 Early breast feeding

Breast milk is particularly important for preterm neonates not just for nutrition but for their immunological and neurological development. Preterm neonates have ineffective suckling reflex that leads poor breast feeding; they need support with expressed breast milk fed using a cup or a spoon. Again, community health structures established through VHTs/CHWs can support mothers to establish early and effective breast feeding for preterm neonates through education, supervision, and monitoring.

7.5 Hygiene at birth and after birth

Preterm neonates have a heightened risk for sepsis usually because of poor cord care and unhygienic conditions during and after birth [3]. Mothers continue to have home births under unhygienic conditions; health systems need to acknowledge this and be able to provide clean birth kits at community level for births that are likely to take place at home. Awareness needs to be created among mothers and close relatives about hand washing prior to handling a neonate and avoid separating mother and baby especially when there is no need.

Different communities in developing countries apply different substances at the cord and different cultural beliefs are attached to the practice. Chlorhexidine has been proven to be effective in preventing neonatal cord sepsis and there are suggestions that a policy of using it at community level might eliminate use of harmful products.

7.6 Resuscitation

About 5–10% of all babies will need support to initiate breathing at birth and fortunately 80% of these can survive with just basic resuscitation with a bag and a mask [23]. Traditionally this has been a function of health facilities but whether resuscitation training can be conducted to birth attendants plus CHWs at community level to equip them with skills to identify infants with apnea and how to stimulate and perform basic manual ventilation needs further study. Considering that many mothers continue to give birth at home, basic ventilation with bags and face masks at community level is a skill worth considering at that level.

8. Strategic research agenda

Despite the wealth of information on the risk factors for preterm birth and care interventions in the health facilities, there is need to further study how these interventions can be adapted for difficult settings or at the community level. Effective interventions such as KMC are not practiced widely at community level and factors that affect its utilization at scale needs to be understood. Strategic implementation research focused on adapting existing interventions to specific contexts with an aim to increase coverage, reduce cost and improve access. Research can also focus on developing new approaches including behavior change interventions to prevent preterm births, calling on the communities to their moral obligation to participate in improving their own health.

Community members need to be mobilized, educated and awareness be created in organized groups such as women groups, youth groups etc. The modalities for these mobilization strategies need to be studied. The rational choice and the motivation for individuals to participate in a collective behavior change program might be influenced by many factors including social trust, relationship networks, and social norms etc., that can promote collective social response [24]. Individuals can be pushed to change their behaviors and be forced to participate in collective community responses after personal constraints and experiences or such behavior change can be a result of external pressure and supervision from social norms [25]. Some studies show that government support and guidance can also influence individuals participation in collective actions through organizing them, policy guidance and financial support.

Author details

Pontius Bayo[1*] and Juliet Ajok[2]

1 St. Mary's Hospital Lacor, Gulu, Uganda

2 University Research Co., Jinja, Uganda

*Address all correspondence to: pontiusby@gmail.com

References

[1] Blencowe H, Cousens S, Chou D, Oestergaard M, Say L, Moller A, et al. Born too soon: the global epidemiology of 15 million preterm births. Reprod Health 2013;10 Suppl 1:S2-S2.

[2] Saifon Chawanpaiboon M, Joshua PV, Ann-Beth Moller M, Pisake Lumbiganon P, Max Petzold P, Daniel Hogan P, et al. Global, regional, and national estimates of levels of preterm birth in 2014: a systematic review and modelling analysis. Lancet Global Health, Vol 7, Iss 1, Pp e37-e46 (2019) 2019(1):e37.

[3] Lawn JE, Davidge R, Paul VK, von Xylander S, de GJ, Costello A, et al. Born too soon: care for the preterm baby. Reprod Health 2013;10 Suppl 1:S5-S5.

[4] Darmstadt GL, Shiftman J, Lawn JE. Advancing the newborn and stillbirth global agenda: priorities for the next decade. Arch Dis Child 2015 02/02;100:s13-s18.

[5] Waiswa P, Kallander K, Peterson S, Tomson G, Pariyo GW. Using the three delays model to understand why newborn babies die in eastern Uganda. Tropical Medicine & International Health 2010 08;15(8):964-972.

[6] Charsha DS. Gently Caring: Supporting the First Few Critical Hours of Life for the Extremely Low Birth Weight Infant. Crit Care Nurs Clin North Am 2009;21(–):57-65.

[7] Noguchi LM, Reeves MF. Department: Simple interventions can save newborn lives. Journal of Midwifery and Women's Health 2005;50(–):351-352.

[8] Blencowe H, Bhutta Z, Althabe F, Lawn J, Howson C. I044 Born Too Soon: a Global Action Report for 15 Million Preterm Births. INTERNATIONAL JOURNAL OF GYNECOLOGY AND OBSTETRICS 2012:S171.

[9] Bongaarts J. World Health Organization Health in 2015: From MDGs, Millennium Development Goals, to SDGs, Sustainable Development Goals Geneva: WHO Press, 2016. 212 p. $60.00 (pbk.). Population and Development Review 2016(3):575.

[10] Dean SV, Mason E, Howson CP, Lassi ZS, Imam AM, Bhutta ZA. Born too soon: care before and between pregnancy to prevent preterm births: from evidence to action. Reprod Health 2013;10 Suppl 1:S3-S3.

[11] DARMSTADT GL, BHUTTA ZA, COUSENS S, ADAM T, WALKER N, DE BERNIS,Luc, et al. Evidence-based, cost-effective interventions : how many newborn babies can we save? Lancet (British edition) 2005(9463):977.

[12] CHARPAK N, RUIZ-PELAEZ J. Resistance to implementing Kangaroo Mother Care in developing countries, and proposed solutions. Acta paediatrica (Oslo) 2006(5):529.

[13] Lydon M, Longwe M, Likomwa D, Lwesha V, Chimtembo L, Donohue P, et al. Starting the conversation: community perspectives on preterm birth and kangaroo mother care in southern Malawi. J Glob Health 2018 06;8(1):010703-010703.

[14] Kambarami RA, Mutambirwa J, Maramba PPP. Caregivers' perceptions and experiences of `kangaroo care' in a developing country. Trop Doct 2002(3):131.

[15] Leonard A, Mayers P. Parents' lived experience of providing kangaroo care to their preterm infants. 2008.

[16] Oras P, Blomqvist YT, Nyqvist KH, Gradin M, Rubertsson C, Hellström-Westas L, et al. Breastfeeding Patterns in Preterm Infants Born at 28-33 Gestational Weeks. J Hum Lact 2015 08;31(3):377-385.

[17] COOPER PA. The Challenge of Reducing Neonatal Mortality in Low- and Middle-Income Countries. Pediatrics (Evanston) 2014 01/01;133(1):4-6.

[18] Gondwe KW, Brandon D, Yang Q, Malcom WF, Small MJ, Holditch-Davis D. Emotional distress in mothers of early-preterm infants, late-preterm infants, and full-term infants in Malawi. Nurs Outlook 2020;68(1):94-103.

[19] Kumar S, Dansereau EA, Murray CJL. Does distance matter for institutional delivery in rural India? Appl Econ 2014 11/20;46(33):4091-4103.

[20] August F, Pembe AB, Mpembeni R, Axemo P, Darj E. Effectiveness of the Home Based Life Saving Skills training by community health workers on knowledge of danger signs, birth preparedness, complication readiness and facility delivery, among women in Rural Tanzania. BMC Pregnancy & Childbirth 2016 06/02;16:1-12.

[21] World HO. Born too soon: the global action report on preterm birth. 2012.

[22] WAISWA P, NYANZI S, NAMUSOKO-KALUNGI S, PETERSON S, TOMSON G, PARIYO GW. 'I never thought that this baby would survive; I thought that it would die any time': perceptions and care for preterm babies in eastern Uganda. TM & IH Tropical medicine & international health 2010 01/01;15(10):1140-1147.

[23] Requejo J, Merialdi M, Althabe F, Keller M, Katz J, Menon R. Born too soon: care during pregnancy and childbirth to reduce preterm deliveries and improve health outcomes of the preterm baby. Reprod Health 2013;10 Suppl 1:S4-S4.

[24] Ostrom E, Ahn TK. The Meaning of Social Capital and Its Link to Collective Action. Handbook of Social Capital: The Troika of Sociology, Political Science and Economics 2009:17-35.

[25] Yang L, Ren Y. Moral Obligation, Public Leadership, and Collective Action for Epidemic Prevention and Control: Evidence from the Corona Virus Disease 2019 (COVID-19) Emergency. International Journal of Environmental Research and Public Health 2020 04/01;17(2731):2731-2731.

Chapter 15

In the Crossing of Politics With Science: Medical Arguments on the High Rate of Cesarean Sections in Rio de Janeiro, Brazil

Jaqueline Ferreira

Abstract

Brazil is the second country with the highest rate of cesarean sections in the world. Most of these procedures are without medical reasons, representing risks for the mother and baby. Obstetric doctors are appointed as the main responsible for this index. The reasons given are for financial reasons or for the convenience of predictable and planned births, and in these cases, cesarean sections are performed without sufficient clarification to pregnant women about their risks and their real need. In this context, there is a constant conflict between doctors and social movement activists in favor of the humanization of childbirth. The purpose of this paper is to analyze from an anthropological point of view the arguments that doctors use to defend themselves against these accusations. Through participant observation at scientific events and meetings of representatives of medical entities, it was found that obstetricians argue that they are based on "medical evidence" and accuse humanized childbirth activists of being based on "ideology". These arguments reflect the current political context in Brazil marked by intolerance and the advance of neoconservatism.

Keywords: cesarean section, anthropology, obstetricians, medical evidence, humanization of childbirth

1. Introduction

This study is anchored in the field of Anthropology of Biomedicine, which addresses an area of anthropological investigation focused on the influence of sociocultural aspects in the biomedical theories and practices. In this view, it is important to recognize that medicine is a cultural system as subject to anthropological analysis as any other context [1, 2]. Likewise, studies in unusual fields like Bruno Latour and Steve Woolgar's [3] in laboratory helped to put under perspective the production of scientific facts as topics of investigation in the social sciences.

In this line of reasoning, diagnostic and therapeutic interventions bring to the light political, economic and commercial issues in their ethical, clinical and philosophical dimensions. Such questions have lived up debates in Sociology of Science and Anthropology of Biomedicine with questionings like: What are the meanings and effects of these interventions on intimacy? How is the health/illness process reconfigured in the daily life of the individuals in face of such interventions? How do health professionals remodel their practices and their relations with sick individuals in front of these new technological and scientific resources? Which is the accessibility and the ethical and cultural consequences of the intense development of these scientific technologies for the societies and the individuals? From the point of view of the Foucauldian notions of biopolitics and biopower, the debates show that the biotechnologies constantly use hegemony, inequality, and subordination to create social consumption in order to control both individuals and collectives. It is with this view that this study approaches the positioning of entities representing the physicians of Rio de Janeiro, Brazil on the excessive number of cesarean sections in the country, in counterpoint to the position of activists for humanized childbirth. The goal is to understand how the physicians conduct their discourses and practices concerning the contemporary issues on childbirth medicalization, specifically the C-section.

In Brazil, the rate of C-sections is considered way above any existing parameter. The World Health Organization (WHO) recommends a rate of 15% of C-sections in the country, although a slight increase can be presently observed in part of the developed countries [4]. In the United States, for instance, there was an increase from 20.7% in 1996 to 31.1% in 2006 [4]. In Brazil, current data indicate a rate of 53% of C-sections on the total labors in the country, existing a distinction between the rate for those conducted in the public sector (46%) when compared to those accomplished in the private health sector (88%), being considered that there is a "cesarean epidemic" in the country [5, 6].

The WHO recognizes that there is an "actual cesarean culture in the country, even when considering that local particularities make the definition of a unified goal difficult [4]. Thus, the organization advocates for the need to reduce C-sections in the country, claiming that this procedure "can cause significant, sometimes permanent complications, as well as sequelae or death" in mothers and babies.

Several works try to identify the causes of these high rates and the focus is always on the physicians. A great number of inquiries accuse them of carrying through procedures like C-sections because they are better remunerated [7]. Others point equally to the preference of physicians for carrying through procedures in schedules and days marked according to their own comfort [8, 9].

These arguments have been used also by the feminist activists for humanized childbirth to accuse the doctors of carrying through an excessive medicalization of labor in which the cesarean is the major representative. They also emphasize that the doctors do not privilege the autonomy of the women, do not appreciate their experience and do not respect all their citizenship rights related with the choice of their way of labor [10]. The activists claim that the doctors must respect the female physiology of the childbirth, not interfering unnecessarily, recognizing the social and cultural processes of labor and birth, providing emotional support to the woman and her family, facilitating the mother–child bond, and assuring her autonomy when choosing the way and the place where the childbirth will be carried through: at the hospital or at home. In the same way, they claim that the doctors must inform the woman on all the procedures [11–13].

There are several works dedicated to study the point of view of women on the cesarean childbirth [14, 15]. However, the medical reasons are little studied. Thus, this study will focus on the medical perspective. The universe of the study that will be presented here regards to the medical representatives of Federal Council of Medicine of Rio de Janeiro [16].

In Brazil, the agencies that inspect, regulate, and promote the doctors activities are the Federal and the Regional Councils. The Federal Council of Medicine é based in the Brasília, F.D. and has jurisdiction over the whole Brazilian territory. However, in each region, it works in partnership with the Regional Councils of Medicine (RCM). There are several RCMs in the country, as it is the case of Rio de Janeiro, the CREMERJ. The CREMERJ exists for 60 years and is formed by 42 council members who represent the several medical specialties.

The RCMs watch for the ethical principles of the profession in all Brazilian regions. They are autarchies with autonomy in their administration, keeping their own view, values, and financial management. For such, they make available information, documents, resolutions, and publications. In order to accomplish their activities, all doctors must be registered at the RCM of their state, being them, therefore, crucial for the exercise of the activity. Trying to enclose all professionals and specialties, the RCMs are subdivided to address each sector of medicine. They are the Chambers and Commissions, aimed to the medical specialties and other activities of the doctors, like clinic manager or health entrepreneur. Everything is inspected by the Council.

The regional councils are places of the medical elite with a political and scientificist aura. They assume the mission of appreciating the profession and they have the power to entitle or exclude doctors carrying through an ethical analysis of medicine. This leads us to the power of the medical class as already mentioned by Freidson: "The origin of the control of Medicine on its own work is, therefore, of a clear political character, involving the aid of the State in the establishment and preservation of the preeminence of the profession" ([17], p43).

Despite the advances, there still are huge gaps related to the strongly corporatist character of the profession. In this sense, the debate promoted by CREMERJ concerning the c-sections is exemplary. In this case, there is a straight confrontation with feminist militants who, to a large extent, are represented by the classic "enemies" of the profession, midwives and nurses. Not less relevant is the character of gender that historically crosses the childbirth medicalization, as the feminist militants are females and the medical representatives of CREMERJ are mostly males [18].

One of the tasks of CREMERJ is to develop events and debate meetings aimed to promote good medical practices. For this research, it was accomplished a participant observation of the "Symposium Childbirth and Abortion" (29 and 30 March, 2019), promoted by the entity between 29 and 30 of March [19]. It was also made the documental analysis of news published in its website, of documents produced by it and statements of its members to the media.

It is worth highlighting that the debate on C-section versus normal childbirth is quite polarized in the country. It has opposing political partisan contours: the ultraconservative right and the progressive left. It should be made here a brief retrospect of the current Brazilian context that livens up this debate.

2. The political context in Brazil and the political-ideological polarizations around the cesarean and the humanized childbirth

Brazil suffered a coup in 2016 that removed the first female president elected of the country, Dilma Rousseff, under the accusation of corruption. This event was followed by neoliberal transformations that increasingly decreased the accountability of the State in the addressing of social problems. Consequently, there was a reduction of investments in the public sector and the wellbeing of the population was delegated to private organizations. Unemployment and poverty increased enormously, social rights historically acquired were lost and unions and social movements have demobilized.

The media, strongly aligned with the interests of the elites, demonized the left movements and parties, which had progressive agendas and advocated for human rights. In this way, the country has been crossing a period in which intolerances result in aversion to the differences, to the minorities and that are manifested in hostile discourses. Souza [20] tries to interpret this phenomenon to the light of the values crucial to the democratic regime:

> *This way takes us to think on the discursivation of antagonistic relations in the present Brazilian society, on the dichotomist and hierarchized way of materializing the force relations underlying these discursive practices. To put in question the hatred discourse concerns, overall, to the limits of the rights of liberty of speech; to the way how the relation I/other is engendered; to the way how the freedom and equality values circulate in our society. It concerns, therefore, to think on dignity and human rights. ([20], p930)*

In this context, the progressive agendas are accused of being "ideological", as they are often associated with totalitarian states, intense critics of capitalism. In these "intolerances", we observe that the expression "ideology" is loaded with derogatory meanings.

Also, the neoconservative agendas based on religious values oppose to the rights to gender equality, to sexual diversity and to reproductive rights. This way, the debate around normal or cesarean childbirth became an expression of ideological differences between liberals and conservatives. In 2018, in the electoral period that elected the candidate Jair Bolsonaro, identified as extreme-rightist, there were many controversies around this issue, as his speeches indicated that he would put at risk any agenda related with reproductive rights in counterpoint to the speeches of former-president Luis Inácio da Silva (Lula) and former-president Dilma Roussef, from leftist parties.

It should be highlighted that the coup that removed President Dilma Rousseff was strongly supported by the medical entities, among them the CREMERJ, which claimed the doctors to be involved in the pro-impeachment movement under the slogan "corruption is bad for health". One of accusations to the government of the female President was her arbitrary attitudes regarding decisions in the health fields without inviting the doctors to the debate [21].

Jair Bolsonaro and his family have openly advocated for the limitation of abortion and criticized the movements for childbirth humanizing. The current board of CREMERJ openly advocates for the same positions: against the abortion and questions the advocacy for the reduction of cesareans. The fact is that the current board is openly rightist and conservative, like the counselor representing the obstetricians and one of the major representatives of the Symposium. He assumed in an interview to BBC News Brazil that the new board "was openly elected with a more conservative agenda". According to him, "most of the people are from the right. Then, ideologically, we are closer to Bolsonaro", claims the gynecologist, adding having voted and made campaign for Bolsonaro [22].

The counselor has assumed his views in several articles published in the media and in the CREMERJ bulletin, in which he questions the scientific validity, the financing and the "conflict of ideological interests" that permeate the debates on abortion and C-sections [22–24]. On the other hand, he accuses the activists of competing with the doctors: "nurses and doulas want this field of work", illustrating the historical competitions of gender and professional categories around the medicalizing of childbirth.

The CREMERJ representatives question the benefits of the normal labor and the World Health Organization international goals to decrease C-sections. According to

DOI: http://dx.doi.org/10.5772/intechopen.97635

them, an "excessive autonomy of the woman" and non-doctors in the follow up of the childbirth would be harmful to the baby, as the scientific medical knowledge is what must prevail in this event.

In counterpoint, the activists who fight for the childbirth humanizing recognize the C-section relevance, but they argue that when it is not well used, it puts mothers and babies at risk, killing or resulting in sequelae. For instance, Talíria Petrone, the left member of the House of Representatives who participated in the event analyzed in this work, says: "I don't see that it's something ideological, from the left or from the right. It's a matter of rights. We cannot leave the context where we are. There is a polarization in which there is a political line that denies and excludes rights; and another one that defends rights historically acquired", says the activist, who claims to personally advocate the conquests of the left governments, especially those from the Workers Party (PT) and the former-president Lula.

One of the criticisms of the feminist activists for the humanizing childbirth to the doctors, especially to the representatives of CREMERJ, is based on their closeness to Jair Bolsonaro's family. During the last presidential elections, for instance, the vice-president of the entity took a picture with one of Bolsonaro's sons mimicking a "gun", and that was emblematic of his presidential campaign. The picture circulated widely in the social networks and was quite criticized on the Internet and representatives of human rights movements; a female doctor shared the idea of adhesion to the guns, and consequently the discourse of hatred and violence that accompanies it. The reply of CREMERJ board when asked on this fact is that "people have the right to vote on those they want". "The democratic" position is highlighted by the board of the entity in many events, like the one that will be analyzed next. It is worth highlighting that the current president consistently emphasizes that this is the first non-partisan" and "non-ideological" management "of CREMERJ, in a clear reference to previous boards that "showed a trend to the left".

2.1 The abortion symposium

The symposium Childbirth and Abortion was a privileged space of observation to know the medical arguments in favor of C-section and for the refusal of the accusation to the category for its high rates in the country.

The first day of the event was exclusively dedicated to the subject of Childbirth, while the second focused on the subject Abortion. There were around 40 people in the audience, most of them female obstetricians and young residents in obstetrics. Most of the speakers were male and their conferences approached mainly technical issues on childbirth and legal resolutions. Concerning the female speakers, one was a pediatrician and spoke about the advocacy of cesareans for the sake of the newborn wellbeing, and a female resident in obstetrics reported an aggression that she suffered in a shift. The other women were an attorney general who addressed "obstetric violence" and two federal representatives who debated on cesarean and humanized childbirth.

The female federal representatives invited by CREMERJ are from opposing political parties, one from the left and the other from the right. This choice of CREMERJ was explained by its directors as on purpose in order to show the "opening of the entity to the democratic debates".

The representative from the right, Janaína Paschoal, is known for her ultraconservative positions and speeches, in full agreement with President Jair Bolsonaro. Her conference was entitled: "The obstinacy for the normal childbirth leads women to death". Her argument was that women with low purchasing power and who wish to have a cesarean are not able to have it in the public sector. According to her, poor women need to comply with what is offered in "public health", motivated by the "mantra of the epidemic of cesarean". According to the federal representative, these women also have the right to what we call in Brazil as "cesarean upon request", that is, the woman being able to choose previously her way of childbirth, in this case the cesarean, and denying this right to the women is violence: "these are almost torture-like situations", and many of them and/or the babies end up dying. The federal representative assumed that she was based on accounts she had access to as a lawyer during the presidential campaign of Jair Bolsonaro, as well as in conversations with the Obstetrician Counselor of CREMERJ, openly adept of Bolsonaro.

On the other hand, the leftist representative Talíria Petrone, militant of the issues related to tackling violence against woman and for reproductive rights, spoke on "Normal childbirth as a social conquest and women's freedom". Her speech was clearly against the cesarean, accusing its trivialization when childbirth is approached as a good. According to her, the medical knowledge cannot intervene with the choices of the woman in relation to her body and denying information to her is the most serious element that we have in the health scopes.

The debate that followed was intense, with aggressive reactions from the audience to the leftist representative, being often necessary the intervention of the organizers to calm down the people. These two antagonistic and polarized positions reflect the existing conflicts in Brazil on the excessive childbirth medicalization and the humanized childbirth. In this context, it has been significant the position of the medical entity of Rio de Janeiro, CREMERJ, which has been making a strong opposition to the activists for the humanized childbirth with the argument that they are not based on "scientific evidence", but rather on "ideologies". The symposium was especially marked by this conflict.

2.2 Scientific evidence x ideologies: categories in dispute

The main argument of CREMERJ doctors in the symposium in favor of the cesarean concerns the evolutive process. In this sense, the obstetrician counselor speech was the highlight of the event. It was based on an article authored by him and colleagues published in 2011 in the *Arch Gynecol Obstet* under the title "The history of vaginal birth" [25]. One of the images presented in the Symposium is from the abovementioned paper and compares the pelvis of female primates and modern western woman. The abstract of the paper illustrates the authors' position:

> *Vaginal delivery, as known today, is a still unfinished product, originated hundreds of million years ago, much before mammals evolved on land. In this article, we will discuss the way in which our direct ancestors were born over the eons until the present day, focusing on the factors that presented substantial changes in how birth occurred, in relation to our earlier ancestors. The history begins with the first amniotes around 300 million years ago and ends with the appearance of the first Homo sapiens around 160,000 years ago. ([25], p1)*

It follows the paper's argument showing that the evolution of species gave origin to a narrowing of the birth canal in women in the post-industrial era. This way, modern women may face more difficulties in childbirth and the use of more efficient procedures to give birth, i.e., a cesarean, is justified. The rationale that the maternal pelvic dimensions are subject to the powerful competitive demands of reproduction and locomotion is widely accepted in the biomedical literature. According to this reasoning, the two-legged phenomenon associated to the erect position and, later, to the alimentary changes, caused evolutive transformations that modified the dimensions of the females pelvis [26–28].

The evolutionist ideas have been accepted by the scientific community since the 1940s, receiving criticisms more in the field of human sciences than in the biological sciences. This way, this argument is strongly used as undisputed scientific evidence, justifying the increasing childbirth medicalization.

The speech of the obstetrician counselor during the event follows in defense of the cesarean, highlighting "scientific evidence":

> *It is a duty of the obstetrician to be updated on the best medical evidence. Episiotomy is recommended in selected cases. The C-section has several relative and absolute indications and a Guideline from 2019 of the American College of Obstetricians and Gynecologists (ACOG) showed that, in the current level of knowledge, it cannot be said that there is a safer childbirth. There is no scientific evidence that the vaginal childbirth is better that the cesarian in situations when there is no indication for it: over 39 weeks.*

The symposium continued with the entity's representatives accusing the advocates of humanized childbirth of following an "ideological" trend and that it does not fulfill the scientific canons. These arguments, especially the most emphatic views of counselor were applauded by most of the public.

The fact is that in the opposition evidence x ideology related with the indication of C-sections or not specifically addressed in this symposium, it can be observed that the evidence can be aimed and used in accordance with non-scientific interests. Let us consider the speech of the two federal representatives: Janaína Paschoal advocates for the incentive to cesareans under the rationale that women depending on the public health network want to have it and they cannot because of a "stubbornness for the normal childbirth". Her speech was challenged by one female doctor in the audience only, an activist of humanized childbirth, with the argument that if women had as much difficulty to have cesareans, there would not be as many unnecessary C-sections in the country. This, as well as any reference on the high rates of this procedure in the country, did not have any reaction from the pro-cesarean audience.

On the other hand, the speech of the leftist representative, grounded on the advocacy of the humanized childbirth, condemning the excessive medicalization of childbirth, raised violent reactions. One particular aspect mentioned by her – "Women know how to give birth and children know how to be born", which insinuates that the doctor would be a mere supporting actor in the birth process, resulted in intense and aggressive reactions both from the audience and from the speeches that followed, accusing it of being an "ideological position". Other speakers reassumed this issue bringing "scientific evidence" of how the doctors are necessary in childbirth, given the modifications that the female physiology has been suffering with the evolutive process and the fact that childbirth is an unexpected event. A female doctor, member of CREMERJ council, emphasized that a safe childbirth can only be the one attended by doctors, when is an integrated and up-to-date team, as well as available material and human resources. In turn, the childbirth "adventure" (referring to the humanized labor) would be the one when the parents are suspicious due to so many disagreeing information, with rejected and questioned protocols and medical recommendations in "an alternative and ideological" environment.

Since childbirth passed from the hands of midwives to the doctors', it was redefined by biomedicine as a medicalizing event with the promise from the obstetric science to foresee and minimize its risks. Although a large body of feminist literature has criticized the biomedical field with the argument that this weakens the women in labor and makes a pathological event of a normal one, the biomedical language of risk within a "technical-scientific" model emphasizing the specialist and based on evidence knowledge, predictability and control are dominant. To minimize the risk, the childbirth must, therefore, be managed by specialists, constantly monitored and subject to a series of investigations to investigate disfunctions and anomalies [29].

In turn, for the activists, the humanized childbirth is resistance to this model. In its conception, the woman's body cannot be object of a medical technology. It is about an alternative approach for the birth in which the woman in labor is the center of the process. This contrasts strongly with a technocratic model of childbirth in which the woman in labor and her body are predominantly presented as objects of the medical specialist. However, the humanized labor activists try to be substantiated in scientific evidence as a way to legitimize their discourse in favor of the change in practices [30]. But this approach coexists with the discourse of the biomedical risk, as the humanized childbirth assumes equally medicalized and surveillance technologies [31].

On the other hand, the literature has shown that the biomedical argument of "risk" for the raised incidence of C-sections in Brazil does not agree with the reality of its clientele: middle-class women, with better prenatal assistance, good health, and nutrition. Thus, it is evident that other medical reasons besides the scientific ones act in this context. Besides the factors already described in this study, like medical comfort and remuneration, other authors equally point the fear of lawsuits in case of problems in the childbirth with the mother and the baby, reduction of the stress for having to wait long hours for the normal childbirth, what would increase the "risk" and, overall, the total control on the process:

> *It is unquestionable that the doctors have to deal with an ambiguity: they manage a physiological process that in most cases, as they recognize, would end well, regardless of their presence. The resource to the risk concept justifies the presence of the doctor in the assistance to the childbirth, but it also conditions their behavior, favoring the intervention. ([32], p434)*

This is in opposition to Freidson [17], who says that the medical practice is made of uncertainties. In fact, everything indicates that the doctors wish to control their diagnostic practices and therapeutical procedures. Aiming to reduce its uncertainties, the Evidence-based Medicine medical movement was inaugurated in Canada in 1980. In this sense, evidence would be scientific proofs based on experimentation. This way, the doctors must be guided in their daily practice for the use of the best updated evidence for decision making in their practice [33].

For Uchôa and Camargo [34], Evidence-based Medicine is liable to criticism. Using Fleck's study [35] as a starting point that reports how the facts are collectively constructed in accordance with a thought style, the authors claim:

> *We have chosen the hypothesis that the supposed adhesion to the transmutation of the "art" dimension of the medical practice – recognition and appreciation of the doctor's individual experience – to the scientific one (formal logical validation to the medical knowledge) does not happen as a "natural" result of the cumulative and linear technoscientific progress, but as an option of the category for, at the same time, diminishing the degree of uncertainty of their choices and reaffirming their autonomy and social status. We start from the assumption that the decisions and judgments of the doctors in interaction with the other "social worlds" which determine, support, and develop their "thought style" also determine what is considered as valid knowledge: the scientific fact. ([34], p2241)*

Thus, according to the authors, evidence would be, for the doctors, another way of normatization of health, becoming sick, and living experiences.

Other fields of knowledge have also been dedicated to claim that science is not neutral nor exempt of values and that it presents judgments of political, economic, and even moral order. As Kuhn said [36]: "Science is a historical phenomenon and it can only be understood in its historical dimension". According to the author, a philosopher of science, it must be considered the historical, sociological, and psychological aspects in the analysis of the scientific practice, and even a certain subjectivity and "irrationality", which ultimately have a decisive role in the imposing of certain theories in the detriment of others.

That is, science is only science when surrounded by the border of uncertainty, doubt. Despite being cumulative, the scientific knowledge is always provisional and relative. Nonetheless, the scientist's common sense is peculiar, distinct from the ordinary person's, but equally influenced by ideological factors. In our context, we can exemplify by relativizing the term "humanizing".

"Humanization" is a term used for many decades by exponents of obstetrics in Brazil and the international scope. For them, interventions like narcosis and forceps "have humanized the assistance to childbirths" [37, 38], that is, the increasing medicalization of the childbirth assumes here a humanizing function.

On the other hand, as already mentioned, in the current Brazil the word "ideology" became an accusation category related with totalitarian regimes. This is what we observed when the obstetricians of the mentioned event referred to the ideas advocating normal labor as "ideological", when medicine only works with evidence. This makes a strong reference to the common sense in which the term is used as a set of ideas or world views of a certain group guided by social actions of political matrix.

This way, we observe that "scientific evidence" and "ideologies" are categories in dispute by activists for the humanized childbirth and obstetricians in search of legitimacy of their discourses and practices. In this sense, this paper assumes that the issues linked with medicalization of the childbirth, having the cesarean as the main protagonist, bring to the surface scientific and political issues. Thus, we can say that the arguments of CREMERJ doctors in relation to C-sections are also permeated by ideologies.

3. Conclusions

Entities like CREMERJ mirror quite well the thought of the medical category, as well as have the power to influence it. When doctors use their power and establish conditions and limits for their practices and teaching, we are in face of ideologization of practices and knowledge. Even with the pretext of fighting ideologies where they must not intervene, these doctors end up acting and thinking under ideological premises, becoming themselves the target of what they fight.

The scientific work is limited by the scientists' non-scientific ideologies. On behalf of the religion that he/she may profess or beliefs, a scientist can curtail in research, suppressing research topics and problems that oppose his/her religious beliefs. Or, on behalf of a certain political-partisan option, even a social scientist can make harmful corrections of interpretation so that it does not collide with his/her non-scientific ideas. This does not imply that these influences can affect the technical and formal rigor of the scientific research in itself, because the interference happens previously, in the choice of topics and in the definition of investigation problems.

From the anthropological point of view, the data here presented searched for an exercise of understanding the positions of doctors in face of the accusation of being the major accountable ones for the "C-sections epidemic" in Brazil. In their defense, they are grounded on "scientific evidence" supporting that the childbirth is a totally liable to medicalization and that the interference of non-medical professionals, midwives and obstetric nurses, and their techniques, are grounded on "ideologies". However, as it was demonstrated in this work, we can observe that the excessive medicalization of childbirth goes beyond scientific reasons, also based on "ideologies" of a strong conservative nature and lined up with the current civil rights denial policy. This way, we can conclude that science is not neutral nor immune to sociopolitical contexts.

The activists from the humanized childbirth movement, in turn, argue that the C-section is a saving surgery in case of risk for the mother or baby. However, there are also scientific evidence suggesting that the pre-scheduled C-section, when not indicated by clinical reasons, causes three times more maternal deaths than the normal childbirth [39], besides increasing the risk of prematurity and neonatal death [40]. The fact that a great number of C-sections is accomplished in low-risk women and with a higher purchasing power strengthens the idea of the humanized childbirth activists that non-clinical factors influence this choice [41, 42]. These activists base themselves on clinical and epidemiological literature to claim that the relation of maternal deaths following C-sections in low- and middle-income counties like Brazil are 100 times higher than in high-income countries, with up to one third of all babies dying, according to data based on 12 million pregnancies [43]. That is, activists for the humanized childbirth consistently search for scientific arguments to legitimize their certainties. Therefore, even though the "ideology" is undisputed, in the fights for the humanized childbirth the activists use scientific arguments to accuse the doctors of ideological practices in relation to their "preferences" for the cesarean.

Here we observe that the "scientific evidence" becomes an argument of defense and that "ideology" is a category of accusation between the two poles.

The goal of this paper is not to advocate nor to accuse one or the other pole, but rather to evidence interpretations of the common sense both on the part of doctors and activists. Neither is the goal to question the scientific arguments defended by both poles, but rather to assume that one of the functions of social scientists is to diagnose the socially problematic consequences of the scientific development itself. In an exercise of relativization of both poles, one of the major conclusions that this study assumes is that, for the doctors, the preference for the cesarean does not have as a major factor the economic aspects and the comfort of the scheduled procedures, but rather the premise of the total control of the event of the childbirth, thus decreasing the uncertainties related to the unpredictability e of the events that surround it. This premise comes endorsed by the scientificity concerning the difficulty of modern women to give birth in a spontaneous way. The activists for the humanized childbirth, in turn, advocate for an absolute autonomy of the women on their childbirth, even being able, through a document called "childbirth plan", to decide all the procedures that will involve the event, including the accomplishment or not of episiotomy, anesthesia, position of the childbirth, and home childbirth. It can be inferred that some excesses in front of childbirth plans restraining any type of medicalization can make it difficult to make necessary decisions in the defense of the life of the mother and the baby in face of unexpected risks during the childbirth.

Thus, the great challenge is the need of a greater closeness between doctors and activists for the humanized childbirth, without prejudices and rejection from both parts, so that to guarantee the quality of the obstetric assistance. For the childbirth humanizing, an improvement of the relations between health professionals and users of the services is necessary. It is equally necessary significant transformations in the training of new obstetricians in relation to the appreciation of new knowledge and practices; acquisition of a more dialogic and horizontal position of the team with the patients; rediscussion of the excessively biological model of medicine; and adoption of bigger political accountability of the managers, aiming at the improvement of less invasive techniques.

Acknowledgements

I thank Marina Fagundes Gueiros and Ananyr Fajardo for the final version of the text in English.

Author details

Jaqueline Ferreira
Institute of Collective Health Studies at the Federal University of Rio de Janeiro, Brazil

*Address all correspondence to: jaquetf@gmail.com

References

[1] Good BJ. Medicine, Rationality and Experience. Cambridge: Cambridge University Press; 1994.

[2] Kleinman A. Patients and Healers in the context of culture. Berkeley: UC Press; 1980.

[3] Latour B, Woolgar S. A vida de Laboratório: a produção dos fatos científicos. Rio de Janeiro: Relume Dumará; 1997.

[4] Organização Mundial de Saúde. Declaração da OMS sobre Taxas de Cesáreas. Hum Reprod Program. 2015 Sep 10;1-8.

[5] ANS. O modelo de atenção obstétrica no setor de saúde suplementar no Brasil: cenários e perspectivas. Agência Nac Saúde Supl. 2008;158.

[6] Leal M do C, Pereira APE, Domingues RMSM, Filha MMT, Dias MAB, Nakamura-Pereira M, et al. Intervenções obstétricas durante o trabalho de parto e parto em mulheres brasileiras de risco habitual. Cad Saude Publica. 2014 Aug;30(suppl 1):S17–S32.

[7] Rattner D. Sobre a hipótese de estabilização das taxas de cesárea do Estado de São Paulo, Brasil. Rev Saude Publica. 1996;30(1):19-33.

[8] Castro A. Commentary: increase in cesarean sections may reflect medical control not women's choice. BMJ. 1999 Nov;319(7222):1401-1402.

[9] Declercq E. É a intervenção médica no parto inevitável no Brasil? Cad Saude Publica. 2014;30(suppl 1):S39–S40.

[10] Weidle WG, Medeiros CRG, Grave MTQ, Dal Bosco SM, Weidle WG, Medeiros CRG, et al. Escolha da via de parto pela mulher: autonomia ou indução? Cad Saude Colet. 2014;22(1):46-53.

[11] Tornquist CS. Armadilhas da Nova Era: natureza e maternidade no ideário da humanização do parto. Rev Estud Fem. 2002;10(2):483-492.

[12] Tornquist CS. Parto e poder: o movimento pela humanização do parto no Brasil [thesis]. Florianópolis: Universidade Federal de Santa Catarina; 2004.

[13] Carneiro RG. Cenas de parto e políticas do corpo: uma etnografia de práticas femininas de parto humanizado [thesis]. São Paulo: Universidade Estadual de Campinas; 2011.

[14] Faya-Robles A. Régulations en santé materno-infantile en milieu populaire à partir de la notion de risque. Anthropol Santé. 2014;(9).

[15] Leal M do C, Gama SGN da. Nascer no Brasil. Cad Saude Publica. 2014;30(suppl 1):S5–S5.

[16] CREMERJ. Conselho Regional de Medicina do Rio de Janeiro [Internet]. CREMERJ. 2020 [cited 2020 Aug 12]. Available from: https://www.cremerj.org.br/

[17] Eliot F. Profissão Médica. São Paulo: UNESP; Porto Alegre: Sindicato dos Médicos; 2009.

[18] Palharini LA, Figueirôa SF de M. Gênero, história e medicalização do parto: a exposição "Mulheres e práticas de saúde." Hist Cienc Saude-Manguinhos. 2018;25(4):1039-1061.

[19] Simpósio: Parto e Aborto. Discussão de Temas Polêmicos [Internet]. CREMERJ / Grupo de Trabalho Materno Infantil. 2019 [cited 2019 Mar 29]. Available from: https://www.cremerj.org.br/eventos/exibe/1036

[20] Souza MJ de. Discurso de ódio e dignidade humana: uma análise da

repercussão do resultado da eleição presencial de 2014. Trab Linguist Apl. 2018;57(2):922-953.

[21] Soares CM, Freitas MS de, Teixeira CF, Paim JS. Análise do posicionamento das Entidades Médicas - 2015-2016. Saúde em Debate. 2017;41(spe3):74-86.

[22] Alvim M. Como disputas ideológicas no país chegaram ao parto [Internet]. BBC NEWS - BRASIL. 2019 [cited 2020 Oct 9]. Available from: https://www.bbc.com/portuguese/brasil-46643198

[23] Jornal do Cremerj. Ministério da Saúde se posiciona contra o termo Violência Obstétrica [Internet]. Cremerj - Informes. 2019 [cited 2020 Sep 8]. Available from: https://www.cremerj.org.br/informes/exibe/4270

[24] Constantino R. É preciso fazer uma cesariana para extirpar o comunismo da Fiocruz [Internet]. Gazeta do Povo. 2014 [cited 2020 Jul 15]. Available from: https://www.gazetadopovo.com.br/rodrigo-constantino/artigos/e-preciso-fazer-uma-cesariana-para-extirpar-o-comunismo-da-fiocruz/

[25] Parente RCM, Bergqvist LP, Soares MB, Filho OBM. The history of vaginal birth. Arch Gynecol Obstet. 2011;284(1):1-11.

[26] Rosenberg KR. The evolution of modern human childbirth. Am J Phys Anthropol. 1992;35(S15):89-124.

[27] Rosenberg K, Trevathan W. Bipedalism and human birth: The obstetrical dilemma revisited. Evol Anthropol Issues, News, Rev. 1995 Jun 2;4(5):161-168.

[28] Wittman AB, Wall LL. The Evolutionary Origins of Obstructed Labor: Bipedalism, Encephalization, and the Human Obstetric Dilemma. Obstet Gynecol Surv. 2007 Nov;62(11):739-748.

[29] Robbie E. Davis-Floyd, Sargent CF. Childbirth and authoritative knowledge: cross-cultural perspectives. Berkeley: University of California Press; 1997.

[30] Diniz CSG. Humanização da assistência ao parto no Brasil: os muitos sentidos de um movimento. Cien Saude Colet. 2005;10(3):627-637.

[31] Rattner D. Humanização na atenção a nascimentos e partos: ponderações sobre políticas públicas. Interface - Comun Saúde, Educ. 2009;13(suppl 1): 759-768.

[32] Chacham AS, Maia MB, Camargo MB. Autonomia, gênero e gravidez na adolescência: uma análise comparativa da experiência de adolescentes e mulheres jovens provenientes de camadas médias e populares em Belo Horizonte. Rev Bras Estud Popul. 2012;29(2):389-407.

[33] El Dib RP. Como praticar a medicina baseada em evidências. J Vasc Bras. 2007 Mar;6(1):1-4.

[34] Uchôa SA da C, Camargo Jr KR de. Os protocolos e a decisão médica: medicina baseada em vivências e ou evidências? Cien Saude Colet. 2010;15(4):2241-2249.

[35] Fleck L. Gênese e desenvolvimento de um fato científico. 1st ed. Belo Horizonte: Fabrefactum; 1935. 2010

[36] Kuhn T. A estrutura das revoluções científicas. São Paulo: Perspectiva; 2006.

[37] Rezende J. Obstetrícia. Rio de Janeiro: Guanabara Koogan; 1998.

[38] Rothman B. The Encyclopedia of Chilbearing. New York: The Oryx Press; 1993.

[39] Mascarello KC, Horta BL, Silveira MF. Maternal complications and

cesarean section without indication: systematic review and meta-analysis. Rev Saude Publica. 2017;51:105.

[40] Chang HH, Larson J, Blencowe H, Spong CY, Howson CP, Cairns-Smith S, et al. Preventing preterm births: analysis of trends and potential reductions with interventions in 39 countries with very high human development index. Lancet. 2013 Jan;381(9862):223-234.

[41] Potter JE, Hopkins K, Faúndes A, Perpétuo I. Women's Autonomy and Scheduled Cesarean Sections in Brazil: A Cautionary Tale. Birth. 2008 Mar;35(1):33-40.

[42] Freitas PF, Sakae TM, Jacomino ; Maria Eduarda M. Lebarbechon Polli. Fatores médicos e não-médicos associados às taxas de cesariana em um hospital universitário no Sul do Brasil. Cad Saude Publica. 2008;24(5):1051-1061.

[43] Sobhy S, Arroyo-Manzano D, Murugesu N, Karthikeyan G, Kumar V, Kaur I, et al. Maternal and perinatal mortality and complications associated with caesarean section in low-income and middle-income countries: a systematic review and meta-analysis. Lancet. 2019;393(10184):1973-1982.